Notes on
Medical Bacteriology

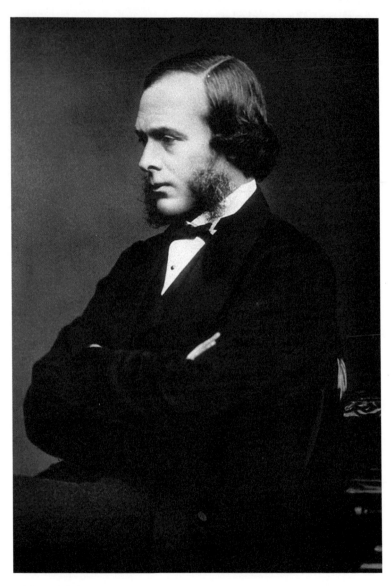

LORD LISTER
Professor of Surgery in Glasgow Royal Infirmary from 1861 to 1869

Notes on
Medical Bacteriology

J. Douglas Sleigh
Formerly Professor,
The Department of Bacteriology,
University of Glasgow,
Royal Infirmary,
Glasgow

Morag C. Timbury
Formerly Director,
Central Public Health Laboratory,
Public Health Laboratory Service,
Colindale,
London

FIFTH EDITION

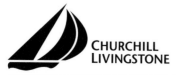
**CHURCHILL
LIVINGSTONE**

NEW YORK EDINBURGH LONDON MADRID MELBOURNE
SAN FRANCISCO AND TOKYO 1998

CHURCHILL LIVINGSTONE
A Division of Harcourt Brace and Company Limited

Robert Stevenson House, 1–3 Baxter's Place, Leith Walk, Edinburgh EH1 3AF, UK.

First published 1981
Fifth edition 1998

ISBN 0 443 05847 4

International edition ISBN 0 443 05848 2

British Library Cataloguing in Publication Data
A catalogue record for this book is available from the British Library.

Library of Congress Cataloging in Publication Data
A catalog record for this book is available from the Library of Congress.

Medical knowledge is constantly changing. As new
information becomes available, changes in treatment,
procedures, equipment and the use of drugs become
necessary. The authors and the publishers have, as far as it is
possible, taken care to ensure that the information given in
this text is accurate and up to date. However, readers are
strongly advised to confirm that the information, especially
with regard to drug usage, complies with current legislation
and standards of practice.

The
publisher's
policy is to use
paper manufactured
from sustainable forests

Printed in Singapore

Contents

Preface to the Fifth Edition

This book is intended for medical students studying for the Professional Examination in Microbiology, and is based on the course we gave to the Royal Infirmary students in the University of Glasgow. It aims to give a concise account of medical bacteriology but we have included notes on mycology and parasitology, which students also require for their microbiology course. Virology is mentioned only briefly because it is the subject of a companion book (Morag C. Timbury, *Notes on Medical Virology*, 11th edn, Churchill Livingstone, Edinburgh). Laboratory microbiology has been shortened for this edition to avoid overloading students with technical facts, and we have tried to emphasize those clinical aspects of the subject which seem to us of most importance in present-day medical practice. The main section of the book on bacterial disease is described from the point of view of the clinical presentations of infection, so that students may get an understanding of the ways in which various bacteria affect different parts of the body and how their properties can determine the nature and outcome of the infection.

For this edition, the book has had considerable revision to take account of the new or emerging pathogens and of the molecular technology which is revolutionizing microbiology. Students are advised to supplement this book by reading from larger or more specialized textbooks, and some suggestions for further reading are listed on page 463.

We are again grateful to colleagues who have helped us through discussion and advice. In Glasgow these are Ms E. Curran, Dr C.G. Gemmell, and Drs G.R. Jones and D.J. Platt and in London, Dr P. Chiodini, Dr Barry Evans, Mr P.N. Hoffman and Dr A. Christine McCartney. We also thank Dr D.M. Fleming for his help with the chapter on general practice. The cover of the book is based on an electromicrograph of a *Staphylococcus epidermidis* adhering to a heart valve, provided by Dr A. Christine McCartney. Colour photographs, except where otherwise attributed, are from the teaching collection in the Department of Bacteriology in the Royal Infirmary, Glasgow.

Both of us owe a particular debt to the late Sir James Howie, who was Professor of Bacteriology in the University of Glasgow (1951–1963) and later Director of the Public Health Laboratory Service (1963–1973). A whole generation of medical microbiologists was inspired by him, and he was responsible for our early years of training when we were members of his department in Glasgow. Sir James was a splendid teacher and writer, who could convey the maximum information in the fewest possible words – the prime objective of this book.

Glasgow   J. Douglas Sleigh
London   Morag C. Timbury

Bacterial biology

1. Introduction

Medical students need to learn bacteriology in order to diagnose and treat bacterial infections successfully.

Bacterial disease is still widespread and common, but its spectrum is changing because diseases which were once familiar are now rare and new infections are being recognized. Increasingly, the work of bacteriology laboratories is concerned with infection in patients in general hospitals – as distinct from hospitals for infectious diseases, the fever hospitals of former years – and in general practice.

The following are among the most important aspects of bacteriology which doctors must know in order to deal with infection:

- **Pathogenesis**: the ways in which bacteria produce disease in the human body – essential information for diagnosis and treatment.
- **Diagnosis**: laboratory investigation depends on taking correct specimens and being able to assess the results obtained from the laboratory.
- **Treatment**: bacterial disease was one of the first conditions in medicine for which specific and highly effective therapy became available.
- **Epidemiology**: the spread, distribution and prevalence of infection in the community.
- **Prevention**: many bacterial diseases have been virtually eradicated by immunization, public health measures and improved living standards.

HISTORY OF BACTERIOLOGY

Contagion. Since biblical times it has been known that some diseases spread from person to person.

The following are some of the pioneers responsible for the science of bacteriology as it is today.

Antony van Leeuwenhoek: a Dutch draper who made a microscope and in 1675 observed 'animalcules' in samples of water, soil and human material.

Louis Pasteur, the founder of modern microbiology: over a long period of brilliant and active research from 1860 to 1890, he developed methods of culture and showed that microorganisms cause disease. He also established the principles of immunization.

Joseph Lister was Professor of Surgery in Glasgow Royal Infirmary. He applied Pasteur's observations to the prevention of wound sepsis – then an almost inevitable and often fatal complication of surgery. In 1867 he developed an antiseptic technique to kill bacteria in wounds and in the air – with carbolic acid: this revolutionized surgery.

Robert Koch was a German general practitioner who discovered the bacterial causes of many diseases – including tuberculosis, in 1882. He introduced agar as a setting agent for bacteriological media, although the discovery is attributed to Frau Hesse from observations made in her kitchen. Koch defined the criteria for identifying an organism as the cause of a specific disease. These are the famous *Koch's postulates* and are as important today as when he propounded them:

1. The organism is found in all cases of the disease and its distribution in the body corresponds to that of the lesions observed.
2. The organism should be cultured outside the body in pure culture for several generations.
3. The organism should reproduce the disease in other susceptible animals.

Nowadays, a fourth postulate would be added:

4. Antibody to the organism usually develops during the course of the disease.

Note: Many infectious diseases of which the cause is clearly identified do not fulfil the third nor even occasionally the second of Koch's postulates.

Immunization

The first successful immunization was the demonstration by *Edward Jenner* in 1796 that a related but mild virus disease – cowpox – gave protection against subsequent attack by smallpox. Later,

Pasteur's observations led to the development of the vaccines now widely and successfully used in medicine against disease, e.g. diphtheria, tetanus, poliomyelitis.

Antibiotics

The discovery of penicillin in 1929 by **Alexander Fleming** – a Scot from Ayrshire – ushered in the antibiotic era. Generally derived from soil microorganisms, antibiotics kill or inhibit growth of a wide variety of pathogenic bacteria without harming their human host.

Public health

The development of a safe water supply, effective disposal of sewage, good housing and improved nutrition have also been major factors in the decline of epidemic infectious disease.

2. Structure and taxonomy of bacteria

Bacteria form a heterogeneous group of unicellular organisms. Their cellular organization is described as *prokaryotic* (i.e. having a primitive nucleus), and differs from that of *eukaryotic* cells, in which the chromosomes are in a nucleus surrounded by a nuclear membrane, as in plants and animals.

Genome. The most fundamental difference between bacteria and eukaryotes is that the bacterial chromosome, or *genome*, is a single circular molecule of double-stranded DNA: there is no nuclear membrane. Bacteria may from time to time harbour *plasmids* (smaller circular DNA molecules), some of which code for certain accessory functions.

STRUCTURE

Shape: Bacteria have a rigid wall, which determines their shape. They may be:

- spherical – cocci
- cylindrical – bacilli or rods
- helical – spirochaetes.

Arrangement: depends on the plane of successive cell divisions. Examples of different arrangements are chains, e.g. streptococci; clusters, e.g. staphylococci; diplococci, e.g. pneumococci; angled pairs or palisades, e.g. corynebacteria.

Gram's stain divides bacteria into Gram-positive or Gram-negative, an important step in classification and identification. The Gram-staining reaction reflects the structure of the cell wall.

Basic structure: a diagram of a typical but composite bacterium is shown in Figure 2.1. Bacteria have a rigid cell wall which surrounds the *protoplast*: this consists of a cytoplasmic membrane

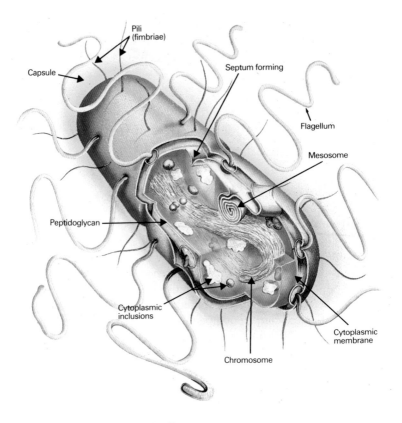

Fig 2.1   Diagram of bacterial cell.

enclosing internal components and structures, such as ribosomes and the bacterial chromosome.

External structures

External structures which protrude from the cell into the environment are present in many bacteria. These structures are:

1. **Flagella**: long filaments, which produce motility by rotation and have characteristic patterns of distribution on the bacterial cell (Fig. 2.2): composed of protein sub-units – *flagellin*.

2. **Fimbriae or pili**: finer, shorter filaments extruding from the cytoplasmic membrane; also protein (*pilin*). Common fimbriae are responsible for attachment and adhesion; sex fimbriae are associated with conjugation when genes are transferred from one bacterial cell to another.

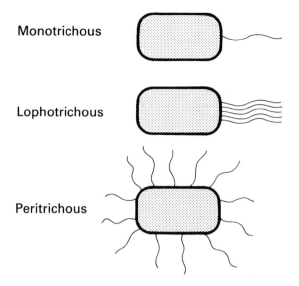

Monotrichous

Lophotrichous

Peritrichous

Fig. 2.2   Distribution of flagella on bacteria.

3. **Capsules**: amorphous material which surrounds many bacterial species as their outermost layer; usually polysaccharide, occasionally protein. Capsules often inhibit phagocytosis, and so their presence correlates with virulence in certain bacteria.

Cell wall

In addition to conferring rigidity upon bacteria, the cell wall protects against osmotic damage. It is porous and permeable to substances of low molecular weight.

Chemically, the rigid part of the cell wall is *peptidoglycan*: this is a mucopeptide composed of strands of alternating *N*-acetylglucosamine and *N*-acetylmuramic acid residues. Structural rigidity is conferred by interstrand peptide cross-links between *N*-acetylmuramic acid molecules.

Structure of the cell wall differs in Gram-positive and Gram-negative bacteria: this is illustrated in Figure 2.3.

Gram-negative cell wall

This differs from that of Gram-positive bacteria by the presence of an *outer membrane*, which contains lipopolysaccharide (LPS). It also contains specific proteins (outer membrane proteins), which

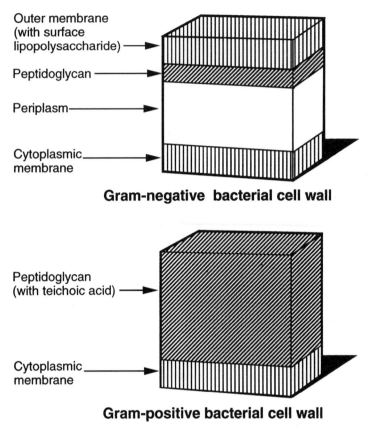

Outer membrane
(with surface
lipopolysaccharide) ➙

Peptidoglycan ➙

Periplasm ➙

Cytoplasmic
membrane ➙

Gram-negative bacterial cell wall

Peptidoglycan
(with teichoic acid) ➙

Cytoplasmic
membrane ➙

Gram-positive bacterial cell wall

Fig. 2.3 Diagram showing the structure of Gram-negative and Gram-positive bacterial cell walls.

include pore-forming proteins through which hydrophilic molecules are transported. Other proteins are receptor sites for phages and bacteriocins. The lipid is embedded in the outer membrane, whereas the polysaccharide which is anchored to the lipid projects from the cell surface. The *periplasm* or *periplasmic space* separates the peptidoglycan layer from the cytoplasmic membrane.

Gram-positive cell wall

The peptidoglycan layer of the cell wall of Gram-positive bacteria is much thicker than in Gram-negative bacteria. There is no periplasm and the peptidoglycan is closely associated with the cytoplasmic membrane.

Teichoic or *teichuronic acids* are part of the cell wall of Gram-positive bacteria: they maintain the level of divalent cations outside the cytoplasmic membrane.

Antigens: the cell wall may contain antigens, such as the polysaccharide (Lancefield) and protein (Griffith) antigens of streptococci.

Bacteria with deficient cell walls

Bacteria can survive with deficient cell walls: these can be induced in the laboratory by growth in the presence of some antibiotics and a hyperosmotic environment to prevent lysis.

Bacteria without cell walls are of four types:

1. **Mycoplasma**: a genus of naturally occurring bacteria which lack cell walls; stable and do not require hypertonic conditions for maintenance.

2. **L-forms**: cell-wall-deficient forms of bacteria, usually produced in the laboratory but sometimes spontaneously formed in the body of patients treated with penicillin; more stable than protoplasts or spheroplasts; they can replicate on ordinary media.

3. **Spheroplasts**: derived from Gram-negative bacteria; retain some residual but non-functional cell-wall material; osmotically fragile; produced artificially by lysozyme or by growth with penicillin or any other agent capable of breaking down the peptidoglycan layer: must be maintained in hypertonic medium.

4. **Protoplasts**: derived from Gram-positive bacteria and totally lacking cell walls; unstable and osmotically fragile; produced artificially by lysozyme and hypertonic medium; require hypertonic conditions for maintenance.

Cytoplasmic membrane

The cytoplasmic membrane is a trilaminar structure formed of proteins buried in a phospholipid bilayer. It acts as a semipermeable membrane through which there is uptake of nutrients by passive diffusion. It is also the site of numerous enzymes involved in the active transport of nutrients and in various other cell metabolic processes. Chemically, bacterial cytoplasmic membranes lack the sterols usually found in their eukaryotic cell equivalents.

Mesosomes

These are convoluted invaginations of cytoplasmic membrane, often at sites of septum formation, and are involved in DNA segregation during cell division. They are the site of respiratory enzyme activity, and may perform a function similar to that of mitochondria in eukaryotic cells.

Nuclear material

The single circular chromosome which is the bacterial genome or DNA undergoes semiconservative replication bidirectionally from a fixed point – the *origin*. Chromosomal DNA is condensed into about 50 supercoiled domains associated with an RNA core. DNA-binding proteins (histone-like) regulate supercoiling and influence expression.

Ribosomes

Ribosomes are distributed throughout the cytoplasm and are the sites of protein synthesis. Composed of RNA and proteins; organized in two sub-units: 30s and 50s.

Cytoplasmic inclusions

Sources of stored energy, e.g. polymetaphosphate (volutin), poly-β-hydroxybutyrate (lipid), polysaccharide (starch or glycogen).

Spores

Spores produced by bacteria in the genera *Bacillus* and *Clostridium* enable them to survive adverse environmental conditions. Spore production is triggered by a process analogous to differentiation in higher cells. It takes place within and at the expense of the vegetative cell. Spores are dense and dehydrated, contain a high concentration of calcium dipicolinate and are resistant to heat, desiccation and disinfectants. They often remain associated with the cell wall of the bacillus from which they develop, and are described as 'terminal', 'subterminal', etc. When growth conditions become favourable, they germinate to produce vegetative cells.

TAXONOMY

Taxonomy consists of:

1. **Classification**: the division of organisms into ordered groups
2. **Nomenclature**: the labelling of the groups and of individual members within groups.

Bacterial taxonomy is at present undergoing considerable change, organisms being increasingly grouped to reflect the genomic information in their cells, as determined by various molecular methods. Although species are generally now defined as levels of DNA–DNA relatedness for identification purposes, simple phenotypic characteristics are used, which usually correlate with the genotype.

These characteristics include:

- morphology
- staining
- cultural characteristics
- biochemical reactions
- antigenic structure.

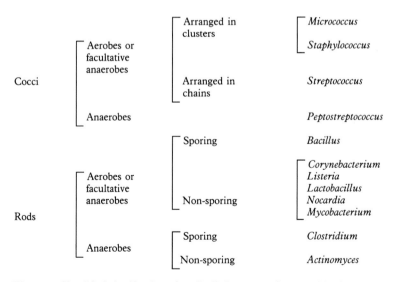

Fig. 2.4 Simplified classification of medically important Gram-positive bacteria.

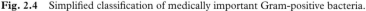

Antigenic differentiation:

- *serotype*: a single bacterial strain or type, defined by antigenic structure
- *serogroup*: a group of serologically related organisms
- *serovar*: term sometimes used interchangeably with, or instead of, 'serotype', on the basis of individual preference.

Figures 2.4 and 2.5 list most of the medically important bacterial genera classified on the basis of Gram's stain, morphology and aerobic or anaerobic growth: note that this classification has been simplified and retains nomenclature still widely used in medical bacteriology.

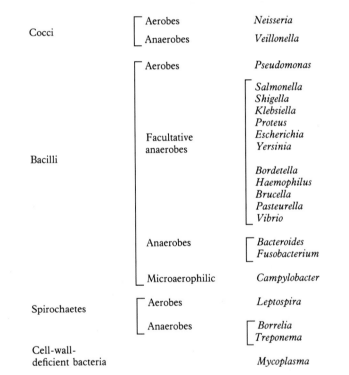

Cocci		
	Aerobes	*Neisseria*
	Anaerobes	*Veillonella*

Bacilli		
	Aerobes	*Pseudomonas*
	Facultative anaerobes	*Salmonella* *Shigella* *Klebsiella* *Proteus* *Escherichia* *Yersinia*
		Bordetella *Haemophilus* *Brucella* *Pasteurella* *Vibrio*
	Anaerobes	*Bacteroides* *Fusobacterium*
	Microaerophilic	*Campylobacter*

Spirochaetes		
	Aerobes	*Leptospira*
	Anaerobes	*Borrelia* *Treponema*

Cell-wall-deficient bacteria	*Mycoplasma*

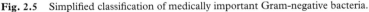

Fig. 2.5 Simplified classification of medically important Gram-negative bacteria.

3. Nutrition and growth of bacteria

Bacteria, like all cells, require nutrients for the maintenance of their metabolism and for cell division. Fast-growing bacteria divide approximately every 30 min.

Chemically, bacteria consist of:

- protein
- polysaccharide
- lipid
- nucleic acid
- peptidoglycan.

Bacterial growth requires:

- materials for the synthesis of structural components and for cell metabolism
- energy.

NUTRITIONAL REQUIREMENTS

Bacteria differ widely in their nutritional requirements. Some bacteria can synthesize all they require from the simplest elements. Others – including most pathogenic bacteria – are unable to do this: they need a ready-made supply of some of the organic compounds required for growth. Other necessary compounds can be synthesized from breakdown products of complex macromolecules (e.g. proteins, nucleic acids) which are taken into the cell and degraded by bacterial enzymes. These processes are illustrated diagrammatically in Figure 3.1.

Elements

Bacterial structural components and the macromolecules for cell metabolism are synthesized from the elements shown in Table

15

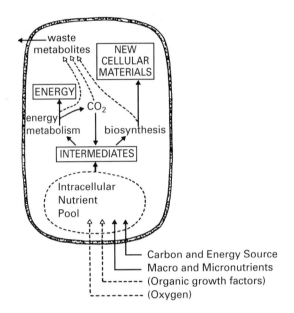

Fig. 3.1   Bacterial nutrition and metabolism.

3.1; all are therefore necessary for bacterial growth – whether available simply as elements or as part of complex molecules.

The four most important elements are:

1. hydrogen
2. oxygen
3. carbon
4. nitrogen.

Hydrogen and oxygen

These are obtained from water – essential for the growth and maintenance of any cell. Water must therefore be available in any situation of potential bacterial growth.

Carbon and nitrogen

Carbon and nitrogen are the principal elements for which an external source must be found.

The principal source of carbon is carbohydrate (usually sugars). Sugars are degraded by either oxidation or fermentation (i.e. without oxygen). This degradation provides energy in the form of

Table 3.1 Essential elements required for bacterial growth

Group	Element	Role
I Elements required for the synthesis of structural components	Carbon Hydrogen Oxygen Nitrogen Phosphorus Sulphur	Required for synthesis of carbohydrate, lipid, protein, nucleic acid
II Elements required for other cellular functions	Potassium	Major cation; activates various enzymes
	Calcium	Enzyme cofactor (e.g. proteinases): key role in spore formation
	Magnesium	Multi-enzyme cofactor: stabilizes ribosomes, membranes, nucleic acid; required for enzyme substrate binding
	Iron	Electron carrier in oxidation – reduction reactions; many other functions
III Trace elements	Copper Cobalt Manganese Molybdenum Zinc	Activators and stabilizers of a wide variety of enzymes

adenosine triphosphate (ATP), the universal energy storage compound.

The main source of nitrogen is ammonia, usually in the form of an ammonium salt: salts are either available in the environment or are produced by the bacterium as a result of the deamination of amino acids released from proteins.

Organic growth factors

These are organic compounds that cannot be synthesized by many bacteria; an exogenous supply is therefore required, although often only in small amounts. Some examples are listed below:

- **Amino acids**: required by many bacterial species which cannot synthesize them. Bacteria possess enzymes that degrade proteins to amino acids; these form an intracellular pool from which the appropriate amino acid is withdrawn to become incorporated into bacterial proteins.

- **Purines and pyrimidines**: the precursors of nucleic acids and coenzymes. In bacteria which require them, they are converted into nucleosides and nucleotides before incorporation into DNA and RNA.
- **Vitamins**: many pathogenic bacteria lack the ability to synthesize vitamins – most of which are required for the formation of coenzymes.

Classification based on nutritional requirements

Depending on their requirements, bacteria can be classified as *autotrophs* or *heterotrophs*.

Autotrophs are free-living, non-parasitic bacteria, most of which can use carbon dioxide as their carbon source. The energy needed for their metabolism can be obtained from:

- sunlight – photoautotrophs
- inorganic compounds, by oxidation – chemoautotrophs.

Heterotrophs are generally parasitic bacteria, requiring more complex *organic compounds* than carbon dioxide, e.g. sugars, as their source of carbon and energy.

Human pathogenic bacteria are heterotrophs: they are parasitic and have evolved to adapt to an environment – the human body – in which many of their nutrients are ready-made in complex form and are freely available. Such bacteria have lost the biosynthetic mechanisms necessary for a free-living existence in a harsher environment, e.g. soil or water.

Prototrophs and auxotrophs

Prototrophs are wild-type bacteria with 'normal' growth requirements. *Auxotrophs* are mutants which require an additional growth factor not needed by the parental or wild-type strain: the growth factor may be a different type of chemical compound, e.g. amino acid, purine or pyrimidine base, vitamin.

Nutrient uptake

Most nutrients are small molecules which diffuse freely across the bacterial cytoplasmic membrane to enter the cell. Some are at a higher concentration within the bacterial cell than in the external environment, so their uptake is an energy-dependent process.

Sugars are nutrients of relatively large size, and therefore diffuse slowly into the bacterial cell.

Enzymes which facilitate the rapid uptake of larger nutrient molecules are present in many bacteria. Usually associated with the cell membrane and energy-dependent, they may be:

- *inducible*, i.e. produced only in the presence of the substrate, or
- *constitutive*, i.e. produced constantly and independently of the substrate.

ENVIRONMENTAL CONDITIONS GOVERNING GROWTH

Water

Moisture is an absolute requirement for the growth of all bacteria: at least 80% of the bacterial cell consists of water. The availability of water, for example, largely determines the size of the population of bacteria that can be supported by the skin.

Oxygen

Bacteria differ in their need for molecular oxygen for growth or – in the case of anaerobic bacteria – in their need for its exclusion: this is illustrated in Table 3.2. The response to oxygen has considerable practical significance, because specimens from patients must be incubated in the proper atmosphere for the bacteria to grow.

Table 3.2   Effect of oxygen on bacterial growth

Bacteria	Growth	
	In free oxygen	In absence of oxygen
Aerobes		
Strict aerobes	+	–
Facultative anaerobes	+	+
Anaerobes		
Strict anaerobes	–	+
Microaerophiles	–	+ (can grow with trace of both oxygen and carbon dioxide)

Carbon dioxide

Required by all bacteria and usually available as a product of metabolism. Slow-growing or fastidious organisms may not generate enough carbon dioxide, so this must be supplied exogenously: this requirement may become increased by environmental change, e.g. the transfer of bacteria from growth in vivo to culture in vitro. Many pathogenic bacteria therefore require the addition of 5–10% carbon dioxide to the incubator atmosphere for *primary isolation* in vitro from clinical material.

Temperature

Bacteria also differ with regard to the optimal temperature range for their growth:

• Psychrophile – below 20°C
• Mesophile   – between 25°C and 40°C
• Thermophile   – between 55°C and 80°C.

Most medically important species are mesophiles, and grow best at temperatures around 37°C (i.e. body temperature).

Hydrogen ion concentration

Not surprisingly, the optimal pH for bacteria that have evolved in association with humans is similar to physiological pH, i.e. 7.2–7.4. A few species have evolved to become adapted to ecological niches where the pH is either higher or lower than normal.

BACTERIAL GROWTH AND DIVISION

Bacterial growth is the result of a balanced increase in the mass of cellular constituents and structures. The biosynthetic processes on which this increase depends are fuelled by energy, usually from ATP.

Cell division is initiated when the increase in cellular constituents and structures reaches a critical mass. Bacteria divide by *binary fission*.

Bacterial chromosome is a circular double-stranded DNA molecule. It replicates semiconservatively and bidirectionally: the replicated genome segregates between the daughter cells, and cross-walls then form as the parent cell divides into two daughter cells.

Bacterial growth cycle

The growth cycle of a bacterial population (on transfer into fresh medium) is shown in Figure 3.2.
Four main phases can be recognized:

1. **Lag phase**: bacteria do not divide immediately, but initially undergo a period of adaptation, with active macromolecular synthesis.
2. **Exponential (log) phase**: cell division then proceeds at a logarithmic rate determined by the nutrient content of the medium and conditions of culture (e.g. aeration). During the exponential phase, the population can double approximately every 30 min (with fast-growing bacteria): this is known as the *doubling time*, or *mean generation time*, and it can be calculated from the slope of the plot of the growth curve.
3. **Stationary phase**: is reached when one or more essential nutrients become depleted: cell division ceases and there is no further growth (represented by the plateau in Fig. 3.2): the bacteria have achieved their *maximal cell density* or yield. Cells grown in a special apparatus called a *chemostat*, into which fresh nutrients are added and from which waste products are removed continuously, can remain in the log phase and do not enter the stationary phase.
4. **Decline phase**: after a period in the stationary phase, the bacteria start to die although the total number of cells (viable and non-viable) remains constant.

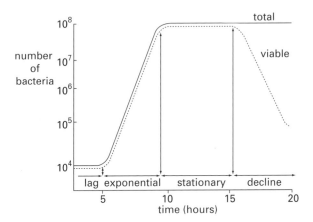

Fig. 3.2   The bacterial growth cycle.

Growth in vivo

Bacterial growth in the human body is very different from that in artificial culture in the laboratory. In general, the growth rate in vitro is much faster. Various factors influence bacterial growth in vivo:

- mean bacterial generation time
- nutritional status of patient
- redox (reduction-oxidation) potential (Eh)
- hydrogen ion concentration (pH)
- presence of metals, e.g. iron, calcium
- localization of nutrients
- cellular defences (reticuloendothelial system)
- humoral defences (immunoglobulin, complement)
- host enzymes (proteases, hyaluronidase).

4. Bacterial genetics

Genetics is the study of inheritance and variation. Except in the case of RNA viruses, all inherited characteristics are encoded in DNA. Bacteria have two types of DNA that contain their genes:

- chromosomal
- extrachromosomal, i.e. plasmid.

THE BACTERIAL CHROMOSOME

Bacteria are prokaryotes, i.e. their chromosome is not contained within a nuclear membrane (unlike those of eukaryotes). The chromosome is:

- circular, double-stranded DNA
- attached to the bacterial cell membrane (Fig. 4.1).

Genetic information is encoded in the sequence of purine and pyrimidine bases of the nucleotides which make up the DNA strand.

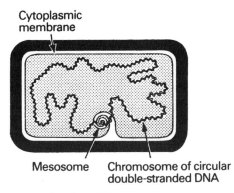

Fig. 4.1 Diagram to show bacterial genome.

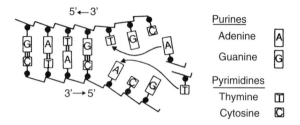

Fig. 4.2   Diagram to show bidirectional replication of bacterial DNA.

Three bases comprise one *codon* and each triplet codon codes for one amino acid or a regulatory sequence, e.g. 'start' and 'stop' codons. In this way, the sequence of bases in genes determines the amino acids which form the protein which is the gene product.

DNA replication is semiconservative, i.e. each strand of DNA is conserved intact during replication and becomes one of the two strands of the new daughter molecules (Fig. 4.2). The main replicase enzyme involved in DNA replication is *DNA-dependent DNA polymerase*, although many other enzymes take part in the process.

Repair mechanisms exist in bacteria: these excise incorrect nucleotide sequences with nucleases, replace them with the correct nucleotides and religate the sequence.

Restriction enzymes are endonucleases, and are a type of defence mechanism found in many bacteria against incoming foreign nucleic acids. They cleave double-stranded DNA at specific sequences (usually six nucleotides). The pattern of DNA fragments produced can be demonstrated by gel electrophoresis and is reproducible and constant.

PLASMIDS

Plasmids are extrachromosomal DNA molecules. Smaller than the chromosome, they consist of circular, double-stranded DNA, most often within the size range 1–200 MDa (megadaltons).

Replication is autonomous: plasmids multiply independently of the host cell (i.e. they are *replicons*), but also divide with the cell so that they are inherited by daughter cells. *Multiple or single copies* of the same plasmid may be present in each bacterial cell.

Different plasmids often coexist in the same cell – usually, one or two plasmids but occasionally as many as eight. In some genera, the majority of strains are plasmid-free.

Transmissibility. Some plasmids (but not all) can transfer to other bacteria of the same species and also of different species. Transfer takes place normally by conjugation, and the ability to transfer is mediated by the *tra* or transfer promotion genes. Some plasmids cannot transfer themselves but can nevertheless be mobilized by co-resident *tra*$^+$ plasmids ($^+$ signifies wild-type, i.e. expressing transfer genes).

Maintenance of the plasmid in the cell requires the expression of other plasmid genes.

Plasmid types

There are many types of plasmid. Below are some examples:

1. **R-plasmids**: plasmids which contain genes that code for antibiotic resistance (Fig. 4.3).

2. **Col factors**: found in many species of enterobacteria and produce extracellular toxins (colicines) that inhibit strains of the same or different species of bacteria.

3. **F or fertility factor**: this much-studied plasmid has been a useful tool for mapping genes on the bacterial chromosome. Genes are now mapped by molecular technology, in which the nucleotide sequences can be accurately determined.

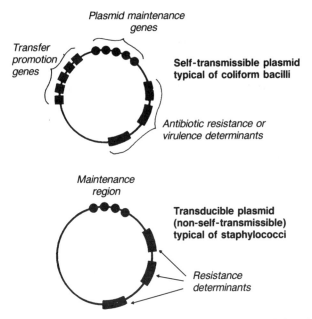

Fig. 4.3 The structure of two types of plasmid that code for antibiotic resistance in bacteria.

4. **Genetic engineering**: multi-copy plasmids with a high level of genetic expression are widely used as vectors in genetic engineering. Genes that code for certain proteins (such as interferon) are ligated into the DNA of the plasmid vector and introduced into cells such as *Escherichia coli*, yeasts or mammalian cells, where they are expressed, producing large amounts of the protein concerned.

GENETIC VARIATION IN BACTERIA

This can occur as a result of:

• mutation
• gene transfer.

Mutation

Mutation is due to a chemical alteration in DNA. Mutants are variants in which one or more bases in their DNA are changed: this change is heritable and irreversible (unless there is back-mutation to the original sequence). The gene defect may result in alteration in:

• the process of transcription
• the amino acid sequence of the protein which is the gene product.

Mutation can involve any of the numerous genes in bacterial DNA. Many mutations are never detected, because detection depends on the mutation affecting a recognizable function (e.g. causing antibiotic resistance); others are lethal and therefore also undetected.

Molecular basis of mutation

Mutation involves change in the sequence of bases in DNA. Change of a single base alters the genetic code, so that the triplet involved codes for a different amino acid: the new amino acid then becomes substituted for the correct amino acid in the protein product of the gene affected.

There are three types of mutation:

1. **Base substitution**: change of a single base to one of the three other bases, with consequent alteration in the triplet of the code.

DNA base sequence	–CAT–ACT–GAG–GTT–AGT–

↓		|	|	|	|
transcription/translation		|	|	|	|
↓		|	|	|	|
amino acid sequence	–his– thr– glu– val–

↓ (under glu)

Deletion mutation   –CAT–ATG–AGG–TTA–
delete **C** in **ACT**   –his– met– arg– leu–
↓ (under met)

Insertion mutation   –CAG–TAC–TGA–GGT–
insert **G** in **CAT**   –glut– tyr– cys– gly–

Fig. 4.4 Mutation. The effect of the deletion and insertion of a single base on the amino acid sequence of the gene product.

This may be:

- *transition*, in which purine/pyrimidine orientation is preserved, e.g. GC changes to AT
- *transversion*, with altered purine/pyrimidine orientation, e.g. GC changes to CG.

2. **Deletion**: loss of a base, to affect the reading of subsequent triplets – *frame-shift* mutation (Fig. 4.4). Deletion sometimes involves several bases rather than a single base.

3. **Insertion** of an additional base or a mobile DNA *insertion sequence* (see section on transposons below) also alters the reading frame of the DNA (Fig. 4.4).

Gene transfer

There are three types of gene transfer which alter the DNA gene content of bacteria:

1. Transformation
2. Transduction
3. Conjugation.

Transformation

Transformation is when fragments of exogenous bacterial DNA are taken up and 'absorbed' into recipient cells.

Recombination with the bacterial chromosome takes place (Fig. 4.5) to *transform* the cell, which then expresses the new genes. Transformation is detected by an alteration in the behaviour and

Bacterial
chromosome

Exogenous fragment
of bacterial DNA

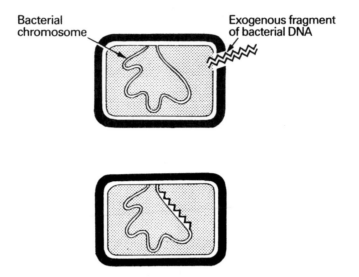

Fig. 4.5   Transformation. Gene transfer by the uptake and subsequent recombination of a fragment of exogenous bacterial DNA.

characteristics (i.e. the phenotype) of the recipient bacteria. As in other bacterial systems, recombination depends on extensive DNA homology and on the function of a gene known as the *recA* gene. The recipient bacteria must be competent – usually a transitory state in microbial cultures – and the frequency of transformation in nature is low.

Transduction

Fragments of chromosomal DNA are transferred into a second bacterium by phage (bacterial virus): this is known as *transduction*. During phage replication, a piece of bacterial DNA becomes, by accident, enclosed within a phage particle in place of the normal phage DNA (Fig. 4.6). When this particle infects a second bacterial host cell, the DNA from the first bacterium is released and becomes recombined with the chromosome of the second bacterium. The bacterial genes transferred in this way are therefore expressed.

Plasmid DNA can also be transferred to the second bacterium by transduction. The donated plasmid can then function (and replicate) independently, i.e. without recombining with the chromosome of the bacterial cell.

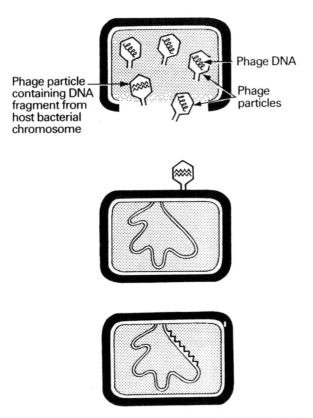

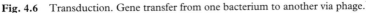

Fig. 4.6 Transduction. Gene transfer from one bacterium to another via phage.

β-lactamase production in *Staphylococcus aureus* is plasmid-mediated, and the responsible plasmids transfer between staphylococcal strains by transduction.

Transduction otherwise seems to be a relatively uncommon event in nature.

Phage conversion: phage DNA (as distinct from plasmid DNA) becomes integrated into the bacterial chromosome. The phage genes cause changes in the phenotype of the host bacterium, for example toxin production in *Corynebacterium diphtheriae* and the production of certain O antigens in salmonellae. Integration of phage DNA into the bacterial genome acts as a switch, to cause the DNA expression of otherwise unexpressed bacterial genes. However, when the phage is lost from the bacterium so, of course, are the new characteristics. The continuing presence of the phage DNA is therefore necessary for the maintenance of the altered phenotype.

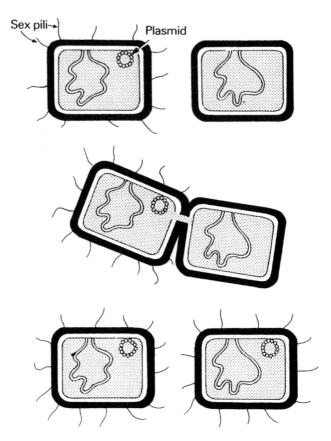

Fig. 4.7   Plasmid gene transfer by conjugation.

Conjugation

Conjugation is the major way in which bacteria – particularly enterobacteria – acquire additional genes. In conjugation, plasmid DNA
is transferred from donor to recipient bacterium by direct contact,
probably via a hollow-cored tube formed by a sex pilus (Fig. 4.7).
The formation of the pilus is coded by plasmid *tra* genes.

TRANSPOSONS

Sometimes called 'jumping genes', *transposons* are segments of DNA
that can transpose or move from plasmid to plasmid or from plasmid
to chromosome (and vice versa). In this way, plasmid genes can
become part of the chromosomal complement of genes. When

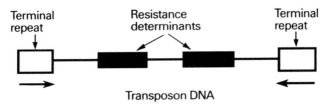

Fig. 4.8 Transposon. Diagram to show structure of transposon DNA, with inverted terminal repeat regions.

transposons transfer to a new site, it is usually a copy of the transposon that moves, the original transposon remaining in situ. Transposons belong to a family of transposable elements that includes insertion sequences. Insertion sequences are flanked by terminal DNA sequences that comprise inverted or direct repeats. The repeat sequences are responsible for the ability to translocate and insert into DNA. Transposons also have terminal repeat sequences in their DNA (Fig. 4.8).

For their insertion, transposons do not require extensive homology between the terminal repeat sequences of the transposon (which are responsible for integration) and the site of insertion in the recipient DNA, although certain sites are preferred. Unlike classical recombination in bacteria, transposition is independent of the function of the *recA* gene. However, transposons do not exist in the free state, but only in integrated form within plasmid or chromosome.

Transposons code for toxin production and for resistance to antibiotics, e.g. ampicillin, trimethoprim, as well as for other functions. Some examples of transposons which mediate antibiotic resistance are:

Transposon (Tn)	*Antibiotic resistance*
Tn1	Ampicillin
Tn4	Ampicillin, streptomycin, sulphonamide
Tn5	Kanamycin
Tn7	Trimethoprim, low-level streptomycin
Tn9	Chloramphenicol
Tn10	Tetracycline

Transposition is, therefore, a mechanism which enables genetic flexibility among plasmids and bacterial chromosomes.

5. Laboratory methods: specimens for investigation

Bacterial disease is diagnosed principally by the culture and subsequent identification of the organisms responsible. The main techniques involved in the laboratory diagnosis of bacterial disease are:

- microscopy
- culture
- bacterial identification
- tests of antimicrobial drugs
- serology
- molecular methods.

MICROSCOPY

Light (bright-field) microscopy

Preparations are made either directly from clinical samples (e.g. sputum, urine) or from bacterial cultures. These are usually examined after staining with dyes, but are sometimes unstained ('wet'). Standard light microscopy of stained films with the oil-immersion objective gives a magnification of about × 1000.

Fluorescence microscopy

This uses ultraviolet light. Bacteria or cells stained with auramine or other suitable fluorescent dyes alter the wavelength and become visible as bright objects against a dark ground.

Staining

Gram's stain

The most widely used stain in medical bacteriology: it not only reveals the shape and size of the bacteria but enables them to be classified immediately into two categories – Gram-positive and

Gram-negative.

Method: crystal violet, then iodine solution; decolorize with acetone or alcohol; counterstain (e.g. with dilute carbol fuchsin).

Observe:

- *Gram-positive* bacteria, which resist decolorization and stain blue-black
- *Gram-negative* bacteria, which are decolorized and so stain pink with the counterstain
- *Tissue cells* are Gram-negative: Gram's stain allows polymorphs to be distinguished from other cells, but does not reveal much cytological detail.

Staining for acid- and alcohol-fast bacilli

This is usually used to demonstrate tubercle bacilli.

1. **Ziehl-Neelsen method**: concentrated carbol fuchsin (heated); decolorize with acid *and* alcohol; counterstain with methylene blue or malachite green.

Observe: for red bacilli against a blue ground (see Fig. 14.1).

2. **Auramine method**: auramine-phenol; decolorize with acid *and* alcohol; apply potassium permanganate.

Observe: for fluorescent yellow bacilli in a dark field under ultraviolet light.

The auramine method is now preferred by many laboratories.

Other stains

Medical bacteriologists use various special stains in addition to those listed above, e.g. for demonstration of volutin granules (Albert's or Neisser's stain), capsules, spores, spirochaetes, flagella.

Immunofluorescence

This combines serology with fluorescence microscopy by using antibody labelled with a fluorescent dye (e.g. fluorescein isothiocyanate, lissamine rhodamine) to detect specific antigens and so identify bacteria.

CULTURE

Bacteria grow well in vitro on artificial media. They differ in their growth requirements, so many different kinds of media must be used, but the majority of pathogenic bacteria grow on blood agar – the mainstay of diagnostic bacteriology. Most pathogenic bacteria are heterotrophs, (see p. 18) and require organic materials for growth.

Media

The constituents of culture media include:

- water
- sodium chloride and other electrolytes
- peptone (a protein digest)
- meat or yeast extract
- blood (usually defibrinated horse blood).

Most media are prepared from commercially supplied dehydrated ingredients.

Solid media

Dispensed in plastic Petri dishes: solid media are solidified fluid media.

Agar: the setting agent is derived from seaweed. It melts at 90°C but does not solidify until cooled to 40°C. Added to a concentration of 1.5%, it gives the medium the consistency of a firm jelly.

Method of inoculation: specimens or cultures of bacteria are plated or stroked out on the medium with a wire loop, in such a way as to ensure a reducing concentration of inoculum. This ensures that, after incubation, separated colonies will develop, where individual bacteria have been deposited (Fig. 5.1). *Colonial morphology* enables many bacterial species to be identified presumptively.

Selective media are solid media containing ingredients which inhibit unwanted contaminants (e.g. from the normal flora) but allow certain pathogens to grow.

The most widely used media are listed in Table 5.1.

Liquid media

Dispensed in tubes or screw-capped bottles.

Growth is recognized by turbidity in the fluid.

Simple media include peptone water and nutrient broth. *Robertson's meat medium* (nutrient broth with minced meat) can support the growth of both aerobic and anaerobic bacteria.

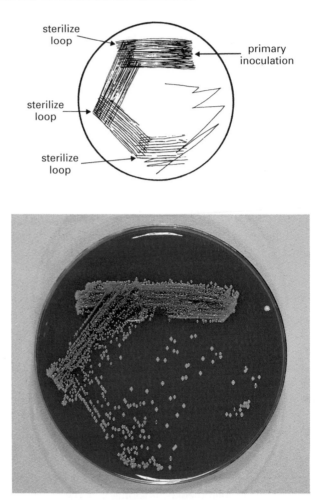

Fig. 5.1   Plating. Diagram illustrating the method of inoculating a plate of solid medium with bacteria to achieve separated colonies, and a blood agar plate inoculated in this way after overnight incubation.

Enrichment media (e.g. tetrathionate and selenite F broths) are fluids which encourage the preferential growth of a particular bacterium: they contain inhibitors for contaminants which might otherwise overgrow the pathogen.

Media for blood cultures: two bottles, each with a rubber seal and a perforated metal cap, are inoculated by the injection of aseptically collected blood through the hole in the cap, using a syringe.

Table 5.1   Solid media

Medium	Main constituents	Use
Nutrient agar	Nutrient broth, agar	General culture
Blood agar	Nutrient agar, 5–10% horse blood	General culture; the most widely used medium in medical bacteriology
Chocolate agar	Heated blood agar	Isolation of *Haemophilus influenzae*, *Neisseria gonorrhoeae*
MacConkey agar	Peptone-water agar, bile salt, lactose, neutral red	Culture of enterobacteria: lactose-fermenting colonies are coloured pink
CLED agar (cystine–lactose electrolyte-deficient medium)	Peptone, L-cystine, lactose, bromothymol blue	Culture of enterobacteria: lactose-fermenting colonies are coloured yellow
Desoxycholate citrate agar	Nutrient agar, sodium desoxycholate, sodium citrate, lactose, neutral red	Selective medium for salmonellae, shigellae
Xylose–lysine–desoxycholate (XLD) agar	Nutrient agar, xylose, lactose, sucrose, lysine, sodium desoxycholate, ferric ammonium citrate, phenol red	Selective medium for salmonellae, shigellae
Löwenstein-Jensen*	A mineral salt solution, glycerol, malachite green, whole egg	Culture of *Mycobacterium tuberculosis*
Antibiotic sensitivity ('Isosensitest')	Peptone in a semi-synthetic medium designed to avoid antibiotic inhibitors	Antibiotic sensitivity tests

* *Note*: This is rendered solid by heating, which 'sets' the egg: it does not contain agar.

One bottle contains a broth suitable for the growth of aerobes, the other a medium designed to cultivate anaerobes.

Transport medium

For the preservation of delicate pathogens during transit to the laboratory. For example, *Stuart's transport medium*, a semi-solid, non-nutrient agar with thioglycollic acid (as reducing agent), electrolytes and sometimes pieces of charcoal. Originally devised for *Neisseria gonorrhoeae*, but now used as a general transport medium.

Incubation

Atmosphere

Most human pathogens grow in air, but the addition of 10% carbon dioxide is essential for the isolation of some species and enhances the growth of many others.

Anaerobic bacteria require incubation without oxygen: plates of media are inoculated and are placed in a sealed jar from which the air is removed. Hydrogen and carbon dioxide are liberated inside the jar by means of a commercial gas-generating system: the remaining oxygen combines with the hydrogen in the presence of a catalyst to form water.

Many laboratories use a cabinet capable of handling a large number of plates. Anaerobic conditions are maintained within the cabinet by the use of a system similar in principle to that described above: the gases, however, are delivered from cylinders.

Temperature

The optimal temperature for the growth of most pathogens is body heat, 37°C: a few bacteria require a higher and some a lower temperature.

BACTERIAL IDENTIFICATION

Bacteria isolated by culture are identified as follows:

1. **Colonial and microscopic morphology**
2. **The conditions required for growth**
3. **Biochemical tests**: these determine the ability of the bacterium to metabolize particular substrates. Often performed on a number of substrates, presented in a commercially prepared kit. This allows a wide range of tests to be carried out rapidly and accurately. API (Analytical Profile Index) systems (Fig. 5.2) are widely used.

   Method: after inoculation and incubation, the results are scored to give a numerical profile. This is compared to a profile compiled statistically from type cultures, and correspondence

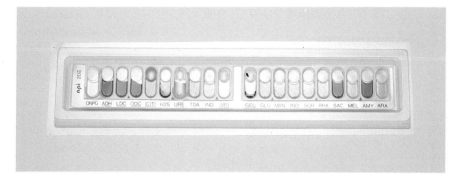

Fig. 5.2   API (Analytical Profile Index) strip. A commercial kit of 20 biochemical tests used to identify enterobacteria. Also available for various other bacteria.

enables identification to be made with a known degree of certainty.

4. **Recognition of enzymes**: although enzyme production is the basis of most of the reactions included in the biochemical tests, some bacteria can be identified primarily by production of a characteristic enzyme. For example, coagulase clots plasma and is characteristic of *Staphylococcus aureus* (Fig. 7.2); lecithinase produces opacity in egg or serum medium, and if inhibited by *Clostridium perfringens* antitoxin, identifies this organism – the Nagler reaction (Fig. 18.1).

5. **Antigenic structure**: serology depends mainly on the recognition of antigens in flagella, cell wall, or capsule, or liberated from the bacteria as toxins. Particularly useful for the large numbers of biochemically similar enterobacteria (e.g. salmonella).

6. **Typing of bacterial strain**: to trace epidemic spread of an organism, it is often necessary to identify individual strains or types within a bacterial species. This can be done by:
   - *Antigenic typing*: uses differences in antigenic structure.
   - *Bacteriophage typing*: uses differences in the susceptibility of the bacterium to a series of bacterial viruses (bacteriophages).
   - *Bacteriocin typing*: uses differences in the production of bacteriocins – proteins released by bacteria which inhibit the growth of other members of the same species.
   - *Plasmid typing*: uses differences in the plasmids contained by the bacterium. Any plasmid DNA is extracted, then separated into its constituent bands by gel electrophoresis so that these can be compared.

TESTS OF ANTIMICROBIAL DRUGS

Sensitivity tests

One of the most important functions of a diagnostic bacteriology laboratory, and a large part of the day-to-day workload.

There are two principal methods: disc diffusion and tube dilution

Disc diffusion

By far the most widely used method.

Method: paper discs impregnated with antibiotic solutions (at a concentration related to blood or urine levels attained by the drug) are placed on the surface of a plate inoculated all over with either the specimen or the bacterial culture under test (Fig. 5.3).

Stokes' method: the outside of the plate can be inoculated with a standard organism (e.g. the Oxford strain of *Staphylococcus aureus*). The zones round the discs can then be compared to those produced against the test organism in the middle of the plate (Fig. 5.4).

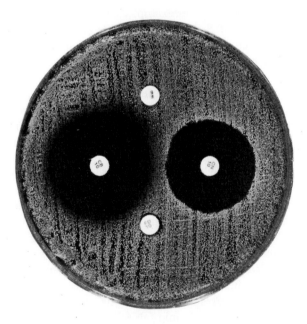

Fig. 5.3   Antibiotic sensitivity test, showing zones of inhibition of the growth of the test organism round discs containing antibiotics to which it is sensitive. Resistance is shown by the growth of the organism right up to the disc.

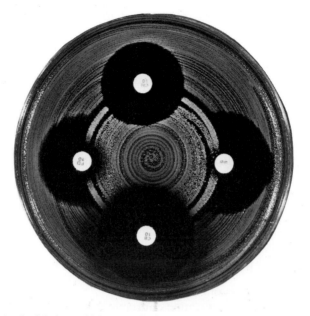

Fig. 5.4   Antibiotic sensitivity test – Stokes' method. The fully sensitive standard organism is on the outside. Reduced zones around two of the discs indicate resistance in the test organism.

Observe: zones of inhibition round the discs after inoculation.

Primary **sensitivity testing**: the specimen is inoculated directly onto a sensitivity plate. Often successful with infected urines, it may fail to give a readable result with other specimens.

Secondary **sensitivity testing**: the inoculum is the bacterium isolated from the specimen: often preferred, and is essential when the growth is mixed. Unfortunately, it involves a day's delay in reporting.

Tube dilution

Laborious: only done in special circumstances, e.g. in tests on bacteria from cases of infective endocarditis, for which treatment is difficult.

Method: a series of tubes with doubling dilutions of the antibiotic in broth are inoculated with the bacterium under test.

Observe: tubes in which bacterial growth is inhibited after incubation. The lowest concentration in which there is no growth represents the MIC or *minimum* (bacteriostatic) *inhibitory concentration*.

MBC or *minimum bactericidal concentration* is estimated by sub-culture from the tubes of an MIC test onto solid media; growth on subculture indicates the presence of surviving bacteria and that the concentration has not been bactericidal. MBC is estimated as the lowest concentration of antibiotic in which the bacteria have been killed (i.e. no growth on subculture from the appropriate tube).

Tests of combined antibacterial action are carried out by the tube dilution method, but using combinations of two antibiotics. This is only done when indicated clinically, e.g. in infective endocarditis due to a resistant organism. When the dilutions are cross-titrated, so that each dilution of one is combined with each dilution of the other in a 'chessboard' format, it may be possible to demonstrate synergy or antagonism.

Estimation of level of antimicrobial agents in blood

This is carried out in order to:
- check that the concentration of drug in the blood is below that associated with toxicity
- confirm that the blood contains an adequate therapeutic level of the drug.

Method: specimens of serum are taken before and after a dose of drug to estimate 'trough' and 'peak' levels respectively. They can be tested in one of two ways:

1. *Immunological assays*: fast, accurate and now widely used. Tests are run on computerized assay equipment with commercially prepared kits. Available for relatively few antibiotics – principally aminoglycosides and vancomycin, but these are the drugs most frequently in need of assay.

2. *Bioassay*: measuring zones of inhibition produced by serum in wells in an agar plate inoculated with a suitable bacterial culture. These are compared to zones produced by standard concentrations of the drug, and the level in the serum calculated.

SEROLOGY

Some diseases – fewer now than formerly – are diagnosed by demonstration of antibody to the causal organism in the patient's blood.

Titre is the term for the highest dilution of serum at which antibody activity is demonstrable, usually expressed as the reciprocal of the serum dilution, e.g. 64 if antibody was detected at a final serum dilution of 1 in 64.

Methods

The main immunological techniques for antibody detection are:

- agglutination
- precipitation
- complement fixation
- immunofluorescence
- enzyme-linked immunosorbent assay (ELISA).

Agglutination

Antibody in the patient's serum is detected by its ability to cause visible aggregation of suspensions of bacteria.

Indirect (Coombs) agglutination: sometimes the antibody in a patient's serum is incomplete, and although it combines with bacteria it does not cause them to agglutinate – later addition of rabbit anti-human globulin causes the antibody-coated bacteria to agglutinate.

Precipitation

The antigen is in soluble form, and antibody is detected usually by the formation of a visible line of precipitate as a result of diffusion in an agar gel.

Complement fixation

Combination of antigen with antibody 'fixes' or uses up complement. When an indicator system (sheep erythrocytes coated with rabbit antibody) is then added, haemolysis takes place if there is free or unfixed complement.

Observe:

- *Absence of haemolysis*: indicating complement fixation due to initial reaction of antibody in the patient's serum with the original antigen – a positive result.

- *Presence of haemolysis*: due to persistence of complement – a negative result.

Immunofluorescence

Usually indirect immunofluorescence, in which smears containing the organism (antigen) are exposed to patient's serum, followed by anti-human globulin labelled with a fluorescent dye. Serum antibody that has reacted with antigen attaches to the labelled anti-human globulin: when viewed by ultraviolet microscopy, the antigen fluoresces.

Enzyme-linked immunosorbent assay (ELISA)

Like immunofluorescence, depends on demonstrating antibody with anti-human globulin, in this case tagged with an enzyme. Antibody in patient's serum, having attached to antigen, is detected by a colour change produced by the bound enzyme on the addition of a suitable substrate.

MOLECULAR METHODS

These are being introduced slowly but steadily into diagnostic bacteriology.

Nucleic acid hybridization methods may be used for the direct detection of specific nucleotide sequences, in either a clinical sample or an extract of it. The sensitivity of these procedures is often enhanced by increasing the amount of nucleic acid present by bacterial culture or, if the organism cannot be grown, by a nucleic acid amplification technique, notably the polymerase chain reaction.

Recognized problems include:

- destruction of bacterial nucleic acids in the sample by nucleases in the inflammatory exudate
- relative insensitivity of direct methods
- false positive results due to nucleic acid fragments from previous amplifications contaminating equipment and being amplified again when a subsequent sample is processed.

SPECIMENS FOR INVESTIGATION

Laboratory diagnosis in bacteriology depends on:

- careful collection of the appropriate specimens. These must be accurately labelled, and if there is a risk of serious infection

being transmitted by the specimen, this must be indicated.
- transport to the laboratory without delay.

Specimen collection

1. **Urine**: a mid-stream specimen, with precautions to avoid contamination.
2. **Faeces**: collect in a plastic container; if not available, take a rectal swab.
3. **Sputum**: a morning specimen in a wide-mouthed container. *Tuberculosis*: if suspected, collect specimens on three consecutive mornings.
4. **Serous fluids** (e.g. pleural, synovial, ascitic fluids): collect in a sterile container, with citrate to prevent clotting.
5. **Cerebrospinal fluid**: collect by lumbar puncture into a sterile container.
6. **Blood culture**: blood, aseptically collected, is injected into each of two screw-capped bottles (see p. 36).
7. **Clotted blood** (for serological tests, antibiotic assays): 5–10 ml in a clean, dry container.

Swabs are widely used to collect samples from infected sites. They consist of a shaft (wooden, plastic or metal) with a cotton-wool tip which is rubbed over or inserted into the lesions and re-placed in a stoppered tube for transport to the laboratory. Essential for sampling some areas, e.g. throat, cervix, but where *pus* is available it is always better to collect this in a sterile container for examination.

Labelling

All specimens must be labelled with the patient's name and ward (or home address) and accompanied by a *request form* giving other details. These should include the nature of the specimen, clinical history, antibiotic therapy, date and time of collection, etc., and are essential for the interpretation of results.

Risk of serious infection

Specimens which may present a hazard to laboratory staff (e.g. blood samples positive for hepatitis B virus, sputum from a known case of open pulmonary tuberculosis) must be labelled '*Dangerous specimen*'.

Doctors must remember that they may infect themselves when taking a specimen, and gloves should always be worn.

Transport

Most specimens need to be sent to the laboratory without delay: some bacteria die off quickly outside the body; others may overgrow and give a false impression of their original numbers.

If delay cannot be avoided, specimens should be kept cool, except blood cultures and CSF, which should be incubated at 37°C.

Stuart's transport medium: swabs should be placed in this medium: delicate organisms are preserved.

LABORATORY INVESTIGATION

Diagnosis of an infection can be achieved by:

1. **Direct demonstration**: presumptive diagnosis of certain infections can be made by detecting the causal organism morphologically in a stained smear from the specimen.

Immunofluorescence: demonstration of the causal organism by immunofluorescence not only detects its presence in the material under examination but also identifies it serologically.

2. **Isolation** on culture of the infecting organism: the most widely used and best method of diagnosis. It also enables the antibiotic sensitivity of the causal bacterium to be determined.

3. **Serology**: the demonstration of antibody to the causal organism: in general, less satisfactory for the diagnosis of bacterial infections than isolation. However, of great value in a few infections (e.g. Legionnaires' disease, leptospirosis, syphilis), in which the organism responsible is difficult to culture.

6. Sterilization and disinfection

Doctors must know how to render articles safe from the risk of transmitting infection. This does not always require *sterility*, which means the complete destruction of all organisms, including spores. The degree of bacterial inactivation which is necessary depends on the circumstances. For example, pasteurized milk is far from sterile but is safe, because any human pathogens of bovine origin that it might have contained have been killed.

STERILIZATION

Involves rendering an article sterile.

Bacteria in the vegetative – or non-sporing – state are readily killed by heat, e.g. at 56°C for 30 min or at 100°C for a few seconds.

Spores are survival mechanisms possessed by members of the genera *Bacillus* and *Clostridium*: spores are very resistant to heat and other inactivating agents, and are destroyed only by longer and more intensive application of the various methods used to kill bacteria.

Sterilization – as distinct from disinfection – requires the destruction of spores and is therefore difficult and often costly.

The various methods of sterilization are shown in Table 6.1.

Autoclaves

Steam is a very efficient sterilizing agent because when it condenses to form water it:

- liberates latent heat, which participates in bacterial killing;
- contracts in volume, enhancing penetration.

An *autoclave* consists of a double-walled or jacketed chamber: steam circulates within the jacket and is supplied under pressure

Table 6.1   Methods of sterilization

Method	Equipment	Use
Moist heat (steam under pressure), e.g. at 121°C for 15 min or 134°C for 3 min	Autoclave	Surgical dressings; instruments; almost any article or fluid which is not heat-sensitive
Dry heat at 160°C for 1 h	Hot-air oven	Glassware; powders; ointments
Ethylene oxide (gaseous)	Special chamber	Plastic and rubber goods; certain sophisticated instruments; poor penetration, therefore articles must be clean
Gamma irradiation	Carefully shielded cobalt-60 source or electron accelerator – expensive; special plant required; used commercially	Plastic goods; orthopaedic prostheses
Subatmospheric steam at 80°C with formaldehyde vapour*	Special chamber	Heat-sensitive equipment, e.g. plastic cannulas
Filtration through cellulose membranes	Filtration apparatus	Heat-sensitive fluids (will not remove viruses)

*Subatmospheric steam without formaldehyde is often used to render equipment safe (but not sterile) by killing vegetative bacteria.

(and therefore at higher than normal temperature) to the closed inner chamber in which the goods for sterilization are placed (Fig. 6.1).

Porous-load autoclaves

Modern, fast and reliable equipment. Before the sterilization phase, air is removed from porous loads (e.g. theatre packs) by establishing a partial vacuum in the chamber, admitting steam, and repeating this a number of times. Thus air in fabrics and packs is diluted out and replaced with steam. The cycle is short; all loads are penetrated efficiently.

Centralized sterilization facilities using porous-load autoclaves are available in most hospitals today:

- *Hospital Sterilization and Disinfection Unit (HSDU)*, in which packs of sterilized dressings, equipment, etc. are prepared and

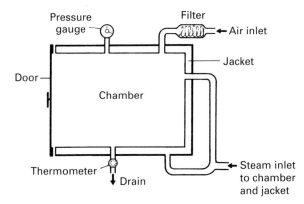

Fig. 6.1   Diagram of an autoclave (simplified).

then transported to the various wards, clinics and theatres. Disinfection of heat-labile equipment is also carried out. Most of the sterilization needs of the hospital are undertaken in the HSDU, by specially trained and supervised staff.

● *Theatre Sterile Supply Unit (TSSU)*: usually a subdepartment of HSDU specializing in theatre equipment, e.g. pre-set trays of surgical instruments.

Other sterilization methods

The following are used:

● *Dry heat*: by microbiology laboratories for glassware
● *Ethylene oxide gas; gamma irradiation*: largely by commercial suppliers, for plastic goods
● *Filtration*: by pharmaceutical firms, for the sterilization of drugs for injection.

Sterile single-use plastic articles

Syringes, catheters, tubing, infusion bags, etc. are now supplied as pre-sterilized single-use (i.e. disposable) articles. The ready availability and comparative cheapness of these has revolutionized medical practice.

DISINFECTION

Disinfectants are chemicals which inactivate vegetative bacteria but are rarely capable of killing spores. Disinfection renders equip-

Table 6.2   Hospital disinfection procedures

Disinfection purpose	Disinfection procedure	Antimicrobiological activity
Skin		
Hands – ward staff	Soap and water Alcohol rub with/without additional bactericides (e.g. chlorhexidine, hexachlorophane)	Wide, mainly Gram-positive but including viruses
Hands – surgeons	Aqueous surgical scrubs with chlorhexidine Povidone-iodine Chlorhexidine in alcohol	Wide, mainly Gram-positive Wide, including viruses Wide, mainly Gram-positive but including viruses
Patients at operation	Alcoholic chlorhexidine	Wide, mainly Gram-positive but including viruses
	Povidone-iodine	Wide, including viruses
Cleansing wounds, burns, pressure sores, ulcers	Aqueous chlorhexidine } Cetrimide Sterile saline	Wide, mainly Gram-positive
Environment		
Floors, walls	Phenolics Hypochlorite	Wide Wide, including viruses
Spills of blood, body fluids	Hypochlorite	Wide, including viruses
Instruments		
Endoscopes Thermometers	Gluteraldehyde Single-use 70% alcohol Single-use sheath	Wide, including viruses Wide, including viruses

ment *safe*, as distinct from sterile. However, the activity of disinfectants is reduced or even abolished by the presence of blood, faeces or other organic matter.

Table 6.2 lists the most common disinfection procedures used in hospitals today.

Decontamination of instruments in general practice

Table 6.3 shows methods of decontaminating the types of instruments and equipment in common use in general practice. Note that pre-sterilized, single-use equipment is increasingly being used in general practice (and in hospitals).

Bedpans

Safe disposal of faeces is a major problem in hospitals. Two main methods are now used:

Table 6.3   Recommended methods for decontamination of instruments used in general practice

Instrument	Recommended methods	Acceptable alternatives
High-risk items Surgical scissors and forceps Intrauterine device sets Uterine sounds Tenaculums Neurological examination pins	Sterilize or single-use (pre-sterile)	None
Medium-risk items Vaginal specula* Fitting rings/diaphragms Ring pessaries Proctoscopes/sigmoidoscopes Auriscope 'nozzles' Laryngeal mirrors Nasal speculums Tongue depressors Peak flowmeter mouthpieces	Sterilize or single-use	Boil
Thermometers – oral or rectal	70% alcohol for 10 min or single-use	None
Low-risk items Ear syringe nozzles	Sterilize or boil	Chemical disinfection or wash
Skin thermometers	70% alcohol for 10 min or single-use	Wash

Reproduced with permission from P N Hoffman et al 1988 BMJ 297: 34.
*Note: must be sterile for high-risk procedures (e.g. IUCD insertion).

- disposable papier-mâché bedpans: placed in a special apparatus which macerates the pan and flushes away the contents;
- stainless steel or plastic bedpans: locked into a disposal washer-disinfecter unit which empties them and flushes them out with hot water, so that the surface of the bedpan reaches 80°C for at least 1 min.

PUBLIC HEALTH ASPECTS – SAFE MILK AND WATER SUPPLIES

Pasteurization of milk

One of the most successful applications of bacteriology: milk is raised to a temperature of either 63–66°C for 30 min or – in the flash method – to 72°C for 15 s. Milk so treated is not sterile, as anyone who keeps it for a few days at room temperature will discover; but it is safe from contamination with viable *Mycobacterium tuberculosis*, brucellae, campylobacter, *Coxiella burneti* and other pathogenic vegetative bacteria. Long-life or UHT (ultra heat treatment) milk is treated at 132°C for at least 1 s.

Treatment of water

The natural habitat of some saprophytic bacteria (e.g. legionellae) is water, and many soil bacteria gain access to water during heavy rain. In addition, microorganisms of faecal origin from the human and animal intestine may find their way into water supplies and cause outbreaks of water-borne infection, causing diseases such as enteric fever, dysentery, cholera, hepatitis A and gastroenteritis.

Before entering the piped supply, reservoir or drinking water is treated by:

- *filtration* through sand supported on gravel and clinker;
- *chlorination*.

Medically important bacteria

7. Staphylococcus

Gram-positive cocci are arranged in grape-like clusters:

- *Staphylococci*: pathogenic or commensal parasites
- *Micrococci*: free-living saprophytes, with little pathogenic potential – but are the occasional cause of opportunistic infections.

STAPHYLOCOCCI

Species

1. *S. aureus* – the main pathogen – responsible for pyogenic infections: identified by a positive coagulase test.

2. *S. epidermidis* (*S. albus*) – a universal skin commensal.

3. *S. saprophyticus* – similar to *S. epidermidis*, but resistant to novobiocin.

Habitat: the body surfaces and, by dissemination, air and dust.

S. aureus: the nose – around 50–75% of healthy people carry it: less often, the skin (especially axilla and perineum), throat or gut.

S. epidermidis: normally present in the resident skin flora. Also the gut or upper respiratory tract.

Laboratory characteristics

Morphology and staining: Gram-positive cocci (diameter about 1 μm), arranged in clusters (Fig. 7.1).

Culture: grow well on ordinary media aerobically and, although less well, anaerobically; optimal temperature 37°C.

Colonial appearance:

S. aureus: typically golden, but pigmentation varies from orange to white.

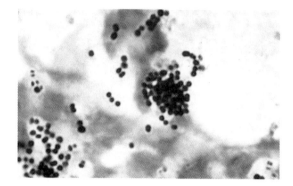

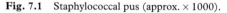

Fig. 7.1 Staphylococcal pus (approx. × 1000).

S. epidermidis: white colonies.

Selective media: staphylococci tolerate sodium chloride in concentrations of 5–10%. Salt-containing media are useful in isolating staphylococci from samples containing large numbers of other bacteria.

Identification of S. aureus: by the detection of *Protein A* – commercial kits for detecting this surface protein have replaced traditional coagulase tests; confirm identity by test for DNAase (or coagulase – see Fig. 7.2).

Typing: strains of *S. aureus* can be distinguished by the pattern of their susceptibility to an internationally recognized set of over 20 bacteriophages (phages).

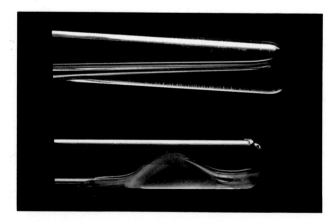

Fig. 7.2 Photograph of a positive tube coagulase test (bottom).

Table 7.1 Toxins and toxic components produced by *Staphylococcus aureus*

Toxin	Activity
Haemolysins α, β, γ and δ	Cytolytic; lyse erythrocytes of various animal species
Coagulase	Clots plasma
Fibrinolysin	Digests fibrin
Leucocidin	Kills leucocytes
Hyaluronidase	Breaks down hyaluronic acid
DNAase	Hydrolyses DNA
Lipase	Lipolytic (produces opacity in egg-yolk medium)
Protein A	Antiphagocytic
Epidermolytic toxins A and B	Epidermal splitting and exfoliation
Enterotoxin(s)	Causes vomiting and diarrhoea
Toxic shock syndrome toxin-1	Shock, rash, desquamation

Toxins:
S. aureus forms a large number of extracellular toxins and enzymes. Not all strains produce the whole range listed in Table 7.1; most of the products probably play a role in pathogenicity.

S. epidermidis produces few toxins.

Pathogenicity

S. aureus is an important pyogenic organism, causing:

- Superficial infections: pustules, boils, carbuncles, abscesses, impetigo, sycosis barbae, conjunctivitis, wound infections (including postoperative sepsis)
- Deep infections: septicaemia, endocarditis, pyaemia, osteomyelitis, pneumonia
- Toxic food poisoning
- Toxic shock syndrome
- Skin exfoliation: toxic epidermal necrolysis (Ritter–Lyell's disease).

S. epidermidis: of lower pathogenicity but an important pathogen of implanted metal and plastic devices and prostheses.

S. saprophyticus: a cause of urinary tract infection in sexually active women.

Antibiotic sensitivity

S. aureus readily appears in multiply resistant form – especially in hospitals.

Antibiotics active against *S. aureus* are:

- Penicillin (50% of domiciliary and 80% or more of hospital strains are now resistant)
- Flucloxacillin (stable to β-lactamase produced by penicillin-resistant strains)
- Macrolides
- Fusidic acid
- Vancomycin
- Cephalosporins.

Antibiotic resistance

Penicillin resistance is due to production of *β-lactamase*, which breaks down the β-lactam ring of penicillin. The β-lactamase is plasmid-coded and transferred by transduction via bacteriophage.

MRSA (methicillin-resistant *Staphylococcus aureus*): strains of *S. aureus* resistant to methicillin (and related penicillins) have now spread to many hospitals in Britain and elsewhere. Often, they are also resistant to a variety of other antibiotics, e.g. tetracycline, erythromycin and sometimes also gentamicin. Although the infections caused by MRSA are not necessarily more severe than those due to other staphylococci, some strains possess the capacity to spread with ease and they have caused hospital epidemics which have been difficult to control. Serious MRSA infections require treatment with vancomycin.

S. epidermidis is often resistant to penicillin; most strains are sensitive to at least some of the other anti-staphylococcal antibiotics. Vancomycin is particularly useful.

MICROCOCCI

Micrococci have little pathogenic potential: occasional cause of opportunistic infections.

ANAEROBIC GRAM-POSITIVE COCCI

These are considered with the other anaerobic cocci (see Ch. 19).

8. Streptococcus, enterococcus and pneumococcus

CLASSIFICATION

This is extremely complex, and still incomplete. An important basis for classification is the type of haemolysis produced around colonies growing on blood agar (Table 8.1).

The main classes are:

1. **Pyogenic streptococci**: this class includes the most pathogenic human species: the main pathogen is *Streptococcus pyogenes*. Pyogenic streptococci have polysaccharide Lancefield group antigens in their cell wall: *S. pyogenes* is in Lancefield group A; other pyogenic streptococci belong to Lancefield groups B, C, G, R and S.

2. **Enterococci**: all enterococci have the same glycerol-teichoic acid group antigen of Lancefield group D. Their normal habitat is the gut. Formerly, they were classified as streptococci.

3. **Viridans streptococci**: a heterogeneous group, sometimes called indifferent or other streptococci: strains may possess one of

Table 8.1 Classification of streptococci, enterococci and pneumococci, based on haemolysis

Haemolysis	Appearance	Designation	Streptococcal class
Complete	Colourless, clear, sharply-defined zone	β	Pyogenic streptococci
Partial	Greenish discoloration	α	Viridans streptococci
Partial	Greenish discoloration	α	Pneumococci
None	No change	γ or non-haemolytic	Enterococci

Note: Some strains produce variable haemolysis.

a variety of Lancefield group antigens (A, C, E, F, G, H, K, M, O or Q) or none at all.

4. **Pneumococci**: important invasive pathogens. Bacteria are arranged in pairs or short chains and are surrounded by a capsule; colonies, like those of viridans streptococci, are α-haemolytic.

Laboratory characteristics of streptococci

Morphology and staining: Gram-positive spherical or oval cocci, in pairs or chains (Fig. 8.1); 0.7–0.9 μm diameter.

Culture: grow well on blood agar; enrichment of media with blood, serum or glucose may be necessary.

Selective media containing an aminoglycoside antibiotic or 1:500 000 crystal violet inhibit other bacteria in a mixed culture, but permit growth of streptococci.

Aerobic but grow well, sometimes better, *anaerobically*; growth enhanced by 10% carbon dioxide. The major fermentative product is lactic acid: it accumulates in cultures and rapidly terminates growth. Culture in buffered glucose medium (e.g. Todd–Hewitt broth) increases the yield of organisms.

Colonial morphology: usually small, compared to enterococci.

Haemolysis: see Table 8.1.

Biochemical reactions: all give a negative catalase reaction. Streptococci can be characterized by their biochemical activities, and a commercial API system which combines 20 tests is useful in identification, particularly of species belonging to the viridans group.

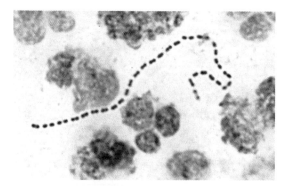

Fig. 8.1   Streptococcal pus (approx. × 1000).

Serology: identifies *Lancefield groups*: 20 are recognized, designated A-H and K-V. The antigens that define the groups are either polysaccharide or teichoic acid.

Method: classically a precipitin reaction with antigen extracted by acid treatment; now carried out by slide agglutination using commercially-prepared kits.

Bacitracin: *S. pyogenes* is generally more sensitive to bacitracin than are other haemolytic streptococci. This property is the basis of a disc-diffusion sensitivity test for the *presumptive* identification of Lancefield group A streptococci. However, some streptococci of groups B, C and G are also bacitracin-sensitive by this test, and this gives rise to confusion.

The main medically important Lancefield groups with the species usually responsible for human disease are as follows:

Group A: *S. pyogenes*
Group B: *S. agalactiae*
Group C: *S. equisimilis*
Group D: *Enterococci*
Group G: no species recognized
Groups R and S: *S. suis*.

PYOGENIC STREPTOCOCCI

STREPTOCOCCUS PYOGENES (LANCEFIELD GROUP A STREPTOCOCCI)

The most pathogenic member of the genus: produces a large number of powerful enzymes and toxins.

Habitat: present as a commensal in the nasopharynx of a variable proportion of healthy adults and, more commonly, children. The carriage rate in children is about 10%.

Laboratory characteristics

Culture: blood agar with small, typically matt or dry colonies surrounded by β-haemolysis.

Capsule: some strains produce a hyaluronic acid capsule during the logarithmic phase of growth, and develop mucoid colonies on blood agar.

Toxins: the following extracellular products have been characterized:

1. *Streptokinase*: a protease which lyses fibrin.
2. *Hyaluronidase*: attacks hyaluronic acid – the cement of connective tissue – causing increased permeability. Antibodies to this enzyme are produced after infection.
3. *DNAases (deoxyribonucleases)*: four immunologically distinct types – A, B, C and D; B enzyme is the most common. Antibodies to DNAase – especially B enzyme – are demonstrable in most patients after recent infection with *S. pyogenes*.
4. *NADase (nicotinamide adenine dinucleotidase)*: kills leucocytes. Antibody formed after infection.
5. *Haemolysins*: two *streptolysins* (toxins which lyse erythrocytes) are produced; their characteristics are shown in Table 8.2.
6. *Erythrogenic toxin*: produced as a result of the presence of a lysogenic phage in the streptococci. Responsible for the characteristic erythematous rash in scarlet fever. Injection of erythrogenic toxin intradermally produces a localized area of erythema within 8–16 h in non-immune people; presence of antibody to the toxin results in neutralization of the toxin, and no reaction is produced; the *Dick test*.
7. Other enzymes are produced and include:
   - *leucocidin*
   - *protease*
   - *amylase*.

Note: All these enzymes and toxins probably contribute to the invasiveness and pathogenicity of *S. pyogenes*.

Serotypes: *S. pyogenes* (Lancefield group A) can be subdivided into *Griffith types*, depending on three surface protein antigens:

- *M*: type-specific, i.e. there is a distinct M antigen for each type or strain: only found in virulent or pathogenic strains. M antigens impede phagocytosis and antibody to them enhances phagocytosis. 65 distinct M serotypes have been identified.

Table 8.2 Streptolysins of *Streptococcus pyogenes*

Haemolysin	Stability to oxygen	Active aerobically	Active anaerobically	Antigenic
Streptolysin O	–	–	+	+
Streptolysin S	+	+	+	–

- *R*: fewer R antigens than there are M antigens, and the same R antigen can be found on several different M types.
- *T*: each T antigen may be found on several different M types; used in conjunction with M typing for identifying different types of *S. pyogenes*.

Immunity to infection with *S. pyogenes* is specific for each individual M type.

Pathogenicity

S. pyogenes causes:

- Tonsillitis and pharyngitis
- Peritonsillar abscess (quinsy)
- Scarlet fever
- Otitis media
- Mastoiditis and sinusitis
- Wound infections; may lead to cellulitis and lymphangitis
- Impetigo
- Erysipelas (an acute lymphangitis of the skin)
- Puerperal sepsis.

Post-streptococcal complications:

- Rheumatic fever
- Glomerulonephritis.

Antibiotic sensitivity

The drug of choice is penicillin. In patients hypersensitive to penicillin, use erythromycin.

Antibiotic resistance: all strains are sensitive to penicillin but there is often resistance to tetracycline. Resistance to erythromycin, although uncommon, is increasing.

LANCEFIELD GROUP B STREPTOCOCCI

Group B contains only one species: *S. agalactiae* – increasingly recognized as an important human pathogen. Three main types, with subdivisions, are recognized: human strains (mainly type I) are distinct from animal strains.

Habitat: commensal of female genital tract; this may be secondary to anorectal carriage. Common in animals – especially cattle – in which it causes bovine mastitis.

Laboratory characteristics

Culture: grows on ordinary and bile-containing media (e.g. MacConkey agar).

Colonies: usually β- but may be α- or non-haemolytic; typically produces red or orange pigment when incubated anaerobically on serum- and starch-containing media (e.g. Islam's medium).

Identification: Lancefield grouping.

Pathogenicity

An important pathogen in neonates, causing meningitis and septicaemia: also associated with septic abortion and puerperal or gynaecological sepsis.

Antibiotic sensitivity

Penicillin, erythromycin.

LANCEFIELD GROUP C STREPTOCOCCI

Rarely cause human disease: primarily veterinary pathogens.

Laboratory characteristics

Culture: blood agar; colonies often large and mucoid due to hyaluronic acid capsules. Usually β-haemolytic.

Toxins: elaborate a number of extracellular substances antigenically similar to those of *S. pyogenes*.

Identification: Lancefield grouping.

Biotypes: four species can be distinguished by biochemical and other tests. *S. equisimilis* is the most common species isolated from humans.

Note: Some strains of *S. milleri* (see under viridans streptococci) have group C antigen.

Pathogenicity

Low pathogenicity for humans. Occasionally cause tonsillitis (especially in closed institutional communities), and rarely, endocarditis, septicaemia, meningitis or skin infections.

Antibiotic sensitivity

Pencillin.

LANCEFIELD GROUP G STREPTOCOCCI

A heterogeneous group: no species have so far been recognized. Share a number of characteristics with Lancefield groups A and C streptococci.

Habitat: human throat, gut and vagina.

Laboratory characteristics

Colonies: there are two colonial forms – large and small; both produce β-haemolysis. The large-colony strains are related to streptococci of groups A and C. Small-colony strains are closely related, and perhaps identical, to the strains of *S. milleri* that possess the group G antigen.

Pathogenicity

As for group C streptococci.

LANCEFIELD GROUPS R AND S STREPTOCOCCI

One species, *S. suis*, is recognized.
Habitat: pigs.

Laboratory characteristics

Culture: on blood agar colonies are usually β- but occasionally α-haemolytic.

Identification: Lancefield grouping differentiates two types: *S. suis* (Serotype 1) – S antigen; *S. suis* (Serotype 2) – R antigen.

Pathogenicity

Both types cause serious infections in pigs. Serotype 2 strains cause zoonotic infection, notably meningitis and septicaemia, in farmers, abattoir workers and butchers.

ENTEROCOCCI

Formerly classified as faecal streptococci, these organisms have now been placed in a separate genus, *Enterococcus*. The two medically important species are *E. faecalis* and *E. faecium*. Most infections are caused by *E. faecalis*.
Habitat: human and animal gut.

Laboratory characteristics

Morphology: oval cocci, usually in pairs; do not readily chain.

Culture: grow on ordinary and bile-containing media: heat-resistant and able to grow at 45°C; also able to grow in the presence of 6.5% sodium chloride.

Colonies: large, whitish; haemolysis variable but generally non-haemolytic; lactose-fermenting colonies on MacConkey agar (pink) and on CLED agar (yellow).

Identification: colonial and cultural characteristics; antibiotic sensitivity pattern; demonstration of Lancefield group D antigen.

Pathogenicity

Urinary and biliary tract infections, abdominal wound infection, endocarditis.

Antibiotic sensitivity

Enterococci are usually sensitive to ampicillin, moderately resistant to penicillin, and resistant to the cephalosporins. Vancomycin-resistant strains, usually of *E. faecium*, are an increasing problem in hospitals.

VIRIDANS OR INDIFFERENT STREPTOCOCCI

An ill-defined group of streptococci which typically show α-haemolysis on blood agar, but haemolysis is variable and some strains are non-haemolytic. Most human strains are commensals of the upper respiratory tract, and are of low pathogenicity.

Clinical laboratories do not usually differentiate species, but simply report *S. viridans*. Species identification within the viridans group depends on the results of a range of biochemical tests. Species do not possess a characterizing Lancefield group antigen.

The principal species are listed in Table 8.3.

STREPTOCOCCUS PNEUMONIAE (PNEUMOCOCCUS)

Probably the most common, and nowadays the most important, pathogen amongst the streptococci: also known as pneumococcus.

Habitat: normal commensal of the upper respiratory tract.

Table 8.3   Viridans (indifferent) streptococci

Species	Haemolysis on blood agar	Lancefield group antigens	Habitat	Disease
S. mitior (*S. mitis*)	α (β or none)	O,K,M,Q or none		Endocarditis
S. sanguis	α (β or none)	H,K or none	Human oropharynx	Endocarditis
S. mutans	None	E or none		Endocarditis; dental caries
S. salivarius	None	K or none		Rarely, endocarditis
S. milleri	None (α or β)	A,C,F,G or none	Human oropharynx, gut, vagina	Abscesses (deep abdominal, liver, lung, brain)
S. bovis	α (or none)	D	Animal, sometimes human, gut	Endocarditis

Note: *S. milleri* is now recognized as an important cause of sepsis, and is sometimes classified with the pyogenic streptococci.
( ) = less common reactions.

Laboratory characteristics

Morphology: lanceolate diplococci (Fig. 8.2) arranged longitudinally in pairs, with the pointed ends outwards: sometimes form short chains. Normally capsulated with carbohydrate antigenic capsule, which is correlated with virulence.

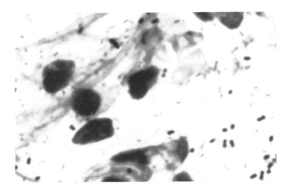

Fig. 8.2   Sputum: pneumococcus and haemophilus (approx. × 1000).

Culture: blood agar, sometimes broth enriched with serum or glucose.

Colonies: α-haemolytic, typically 'draughtsmen', i.e. with sunken centre due to spontaneous autolysis of older organisms. Young colonies may resemble dew-drops, due to large capsules before autolysis.

Differentiation from viridans streptococci by:
• optochin sensitivity: viridans streptococci are resistant
• bile solubility: addition of bile to broth cultures lyses pneumococci but not viridans streptococci
• inulin fermentation: viridans streptococci do not ferment inulin.

Antigenic structure:

Capsule: contains the polysaccharide carbohydrate antigen: type-specific. 84 capsular types are recognized.

Identification: by a variety of serological tests directed against the antigen. The standard reference method is capsule swelling – the *quellung reaction* – observed microscopically when pneumococci are mixed with specific antisera.

C substance: a cell-wall-associated antigen common to all pneumococci: consists of choline teichoic acid.

Protein M antigen: resembles but is unrelated to M antigens of *S. pyogenes*. Not associated with virulence.

Virulence correlates with the presence of a capsule, probably because this prevents or inhibits phagocytosis.

Transformation: the transfer of DNA – and some of the genetic markers for which it codes – from one bacterial strain to another was first demonstrated in pneumococci by Griffiths in 1928.

Pneumococcal types: not all types are equally common. The majority of human infections are associated with the lower-numbered serotypes.

Common infecting types are included in the polyvalent vaccine used in prophylactic immunization. Some of the infecting types are particularly invasive and liable to cause serious infections such as pneumonia and septicaemia (types 1 and 3) and meningitis (types 7 and 12). Types 6 and 18 are important in children.

Pathogenicity

Pneumococci are important pathogens and cause a considerable amount of both morbidity and mortality today, despite their sensitivity to penicillin. They may cause:

- Lobar pneumonia
- Acute exacerbation of chronic bronchitis (often with *Haemophilus influenzae*)
- Meningitis
- Otitis media
- Sinusitis
- Conjunctivitis
- Septicaemia (especially in splenectomized patients).

Antibiotic sensitivity

In the UK almost all strains remain sensitive to penicillin but penicillin resistance is a significant problem in some countries, including Spain, South Africa and Hungary. Resistance to erythromycin, tetracycline and trimethoprim is more commonly encountered in the UK.

9. Enterobacteria

Gram-negative bacilli which belong to the tribe *Enterobacteriaceae*. Often called *coliforms*, they are intestinal parasites of humans and animals: many are human pathogens.

Table 9.1 lists the main medically important species.

Laboratory characteristics

Morphology and staining: Gram-negative bacilli, 2–3×0.6 μm. Non-motile, or motile by peritrichous flagella (Fig. 9.1). Non-sporing.

Culture: grow well on ordinary media, e.g. blood agar, MacConkey agar, CLED agar; aerobic and facultatively anaerobic; grow in a wide range of temperatures.

Identification:
- *Lactose fermentation* on indicator media assists in initial identification: e.g. MacConkey agar contains lactose and a pH

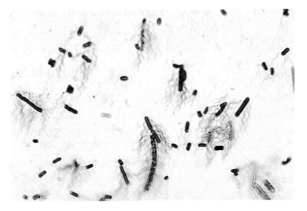

Fig. 9.1   Flagella. Peritrichous flagella demonstrated by a silver-impregnation staining method (magnified × 2000).

Table 9.1 Medically important enterobacteria

Genus	Species	Principal diseases
Escherichia	*E. coli*	Wound and urinary infection, gastroenteritis
Shigella	*S. dysenteriae* *S. flexneri* *S. boydii* *S. sonnei*	Dysentery
Salmonella	*S. typhi* *S. paratyphi A, B, C*	Enteric fever
	S. typhimurium Many other serotypes	Food poisoning
Klebsiella	*K. pneumoniae* *K. oxytoca*	
Morganella	*M. morgani*	
Proteus	*P. mirabilis* *P. vulgaris*	Urinary infections, other forms of sepsis
Providencia	*P. stuartii* *P. rettgeri* *P. alcalifaciens*	
Yersinia	*Y. pestis* *Y. pseudotuberculosis* *Y. enterocolitica*	Plague, septicaemia, enteritis, mesenteric adenitis
Enterobacter	*E. cloacae* *E. aerogenes*	
Serratia	*S. marcescens*	Generally of lower pathogenicity
Citrobacter	*C. freundii*	

indicator, so that lactose-fermenting colonies are pink. On CLED medium, the colour of lactose fermentation is yellow.

- *Biochemical tests* are used to identify species of enterobacteria, usually by means of test kits based on 10 (API 10E) or 20 (API 20E) biochemical tests (see Fig. 5.2).
- *Serological tests* for somatic and flagellar antigens are used mainly for the final identification of *Salmonella* and *Shigella* species. A diagram of the sites of the main antigens in enterobacteria is shown in Fig. 9.2.

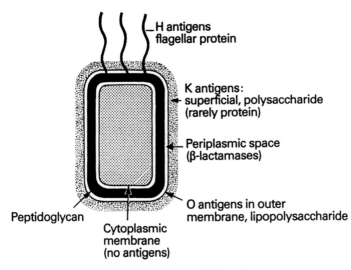

H antigens
flagellar protein

K antigens:
superficial, polysaccharide
(rarely protein)

Periplasmic space
(β-lactamases)

O antigens in outer
membrane, lipopolysaccharide

Peptidoglycan

Cytoplasmic
membrane
(no antigens)

Fig. 9.2   Antigenic structure of Gram-negative bacteria.

Strain identification within a species can also be done by bacterio-phage typing or by analysis by restriction fragment length polymorphism of bacterial DNA.

Toxins:

Endotoxins are O antigens and are lipopolysaccharides consisting of sugars and lipid A. Present in the cell wall of Gram-negative bacilli (see Ch. 2), they are liberated when the bacterial cells lyse and are responsible for many pathological effects of enterobacterial infection.

Exotoxins are *proteins* liberated extracellularly from the intact bacterium by some species of enterobacteria.

Antibiotic sensitivity

Antibiotic sensitivity is unpredictable, because enterobacteria readily acquire resistance-coding plasmids, which can spread to other strains. *The main antibiotics* used against enterobacteria are:

- Ampicillin/amoxycillin
- Aminoglycosides
- Trimethoprim
- Chloramphenicol
- Ciprofloxacin

- Cephalosporins
- Nitrofurantion*
- Nalidixic acid.*

Note: drugs marked * are used only for urinary tract infections.

ESCHERICHIA COLI

Habitat: a normal inhabitant of the human and animal intestine.

Laboratory characteristics

Isolation: grows well as large colonies after overnight incubation.

Identification: ferments lactose (hence pink colonies on Mac-Conkey agar, yellow on CLED agar). Produces yellow colonies on XLD medium. Further biochemical tests are required for accurate identification.

Typing is rarely required, but phage typing is available for certain serogroups, e.g. 0157.

Pathogenesis: although a normal gut commensal, many strains of *E. coli* have *enteropathogenetic mechanisms* which can be responsible for diarrhoea and other symptoms:

1. *Enterotoxins*: these are of two types, both plasmid-coded: LT – heat-labile, and ST – heat-stable.
2. *Adhesive factors*: now known as colonization factor antigens mediated by plasmid-coded pili.
3. *Entero-invasiveness*: confers the ability to penetrate intestinal epithelial cells.
4. *Vero cytotoxin* (VT) produces a cytopathic effect on Vero cells. There are two (VT1 and VT2), which are serologically distinct. Strains that produce VT (known as VTEC), notably *E. coli* 0157, cause diarrhoea with haemorrhagic symptoms.
5. *Attaching – effacing mechanism*: some strains adhere to intestinal epithelium to cause erosion (effacement) of the microvilli, resulting in formation of characteristic structures known as *pedestals*.

O antigens

Diarrhoea-producing strains of *E. coli* were originally detected by their O (or somatic) antigens. Although the picture is not

clear-cut (i.e. there is overlapping), serogroups possessing certain
O antigens tend to be found in each of the four main categories of
diarrhoea-producing strains:

- Enteropathogenic (EPEC): 055, 0111
- Enterotoxigenic (ETEC): 06, 078
- Entero-invasive (EIEC): 0124, 0164
- Enterohaemorrhagic (EHEC): 0157.

Pathogenicity

Sepsis: *E. coli* causes:

- Urinary tract infection
- Wound infection, especially after surgery of the lower
  intestinal tract (*E. coli* is often mixed with anaerobes in
  such cases)
- Peritonitis
- Biliary tract infection
- Septicaemia
- Neonatal meningitis.

  Diarrhoea: *E. coli* is a common cause of diarrhoea:

- Infantile gastroenteritis
- Tourist diarrhoea
- Haemorrhagic diarrhoea:
  – Haemorrhagic colitis
  – Haemolytic uraemic syndrome.

SHIGELLA

There are four species, most with several serotypes:

- *S. dysenteriae*
- *S. boydii*
- *S. flexneri*
- *S. sonnei* (one serotype).

  Habitat: human intestine.

Laboratory characteristics

Isolation: grow well on routine media: do not ferment lactose, and so colonies on MacConkey agar and lactose-containing media are colourless. *S. sonnei* is an important exception, which ferments lactose slowly with the production of pale pink colonies.

Enrichment culture of faeces in selenite F broth, with subsequent subculture on to MacConkey agar, improves isolation.

Identification:

- non-motile
- *biochemical tests*: produce acid, but not gas, from carbohydrates
- *determination of O antigens*.

Pathogenicity

The cause of dysentery: *S. dysenteriae* type 1, which produces protein exotoxins, causes the severe illness *shiga dysentery*. Dysentery due to other shigellae tends to be milder. *S. sonnei* is the cause of most dysentery in Britain. Shigellae have entero-invasive properties similar to those described above for *E. coli*.

SALMONELLA

Habitat: the gut of domestic animals (especially cattle) and poultry. Foodstuffs from animals are therefore important sources of infection. *S. typhi* and *S. paratyphi* differ from the other species in that humans are the only natural hosts.

Laboratory characteristics

Isolation: from faeces, culture on MacConkey agar (for pale, non-lactose-fermenting colonies) and on other indicator and selective media.

Identification:

Biochemical tests: salmonellae generally produce acid and gas from carbohydrates, except for *S. typhi* which does not produce gas.

Serology: by identification of antigens (see Fig. 9.2):

- O: somatic
- H: flagellar
- Vi: a surface antigen possessed by a few species, notably *S. typhi*.

More than 1500 serotypes ('species') are recognized: sharing of O and H antigens is common, and identification is complex, depending

Table 9.2 Selected salmonellae showing antigenic profiles (Kauffman–White scheme)

Serotype ('species')	Group	O antigens	H antigens Phase 1	Phase 2
S. paratyphi A	A	1.2.12.	a	–
S. paratyphi B	B	1.4.5.12.	b	1.2
S. agona	B	4.12.	f.g.s.	–
S. typhimurium	B	1.4.5.12.	i	1.2
S. paratyphi C★	C	6.7.	c	1.5
S. typhi★	D	9.12.	d	–
S. enteritidis	D	1.9.12.	g.m.	–

★Also possess Vi antigen.

on detection of several antigens (Table 9.2). A single strain can possess two different sets of H antigens at different times (*phase variation*), and so both sets must be analyzed for identification.

Typing: bacteriophage typing of particular serotypes can be carried out to trace outbreaks, e.g. *S. typhi, S. enteritidis, S. typhimurium*.

Pathogenicity

Enteric fever is due to *S. typhi* or *S. paratyphi A, B, C*.

Most other salmonella serotypes cause gastroenteritis or food poisoning (*S. typhimurium* was for many years the most common, now it is *S. enteritidis*, especially phage type 4). Some types (e.g. *S. dublin, S. virchow, S. cholerae-suis*) have a particular tendency to cause septicaemia.

Rarely, salmonellae cause osteomyelitis, septic arthritis and other purulent lesions.

KLEBSIELLA

Habitat: human and animal intestine. Some strains are saprophytes in soil, water and vegetation.

Laboratory characteristics

Isolation: grow well on ordinary media, with colonies which are often, but not always, large and mucoid.

Identification: biochemical tests.

Typing: sometimes useful in hospital outbreaks: antigenic analysis of the capsular polysaccharides which comprise the large capsules typical of this genus. More than 80 serotypes recognized.

Pathogenicity

- Urinary tract infection
- Septicaemia
- Meningitis (especially in neonates)
- Pneumonia (rare).

PROTEUS

There are two important species:
- *P. mirabilis*
- *P. vulgaris*.

Habitat: human and animal intestine.

Laboratory characteristics

Isolation: grow well on routine media, produce a swarming type of growth on ordinary media.

Identification: swarming growth allows presumptive identification. API tests permit formal identification. Proteus species produce a potent urease.

Pathogenicity

P. mirabilis is the most frequently isolated species, causing:

- Urinary tract infection: urinary urea is 'split' by the bacterial urease to produce ammonium salts: this results in alkaline urinary pH.
- Often isolated from the mixed flora of wounds, burns, pressure sores, chronic discharging ears – generally a low-grade pathogen in such circumstances.
- Septicaemia (rare).

YERSINIA

Habitat: yersinia are found in animals and sometimes – although rarely – cause disease in humans.

Laboratory characteristics

Isolation: on ordinary media. Colonies are often small and prolonged incubation of cultures is necessary.

Identification: small (1.5 × 0.5 μm) bacilli, which may show *bipolar* staining (i.e. darker at both ends of the bacilli). Biochemical (API) tests permit formal identification, the reactions being more reproducible at 22–27°C than at the 37°C temperature used for other enterobacteria. Identification of *Y. pestis* is by fluorescent antibody staining and by testing for susceptibility to specific bacteriophages.

Pathogenicity

- Plague: *Y. pestis* (formerly called *Pasteurella pestis*) causes bubonic and pneumonic plague ('The Black Death').

Y. pseudotuberculosis and *Y. enterocolitica* cause:
- Enteritis
- Mesenteric adenitis, sometimes associated with terminal ileitis – clinically, can closely mimic appendicitis
- A septicaemic illness similar to typhoid fever.

ENTEROBACTER; SERRATIA; PROVIDENCIA; MORGANELLA; CITROBACTER

These members of the enterobacteria can conveniently be considered together. The most frequently isolated species are: *Enterobacter cloacae, E. aerogenes; Serratia marcescens; Providencia rettgeri, P. stuartii; Citrobacter freundii; Morganella morgani.*

Habitat: human and animal intestine, but some strains are saprophytes. Moist environments in hospitals may be important reservoirs.

Laboratory characteristics

Isolation: grow well on routine media.
    Identification: biochemical (API) tests.

Pathogenicity

- Urinary tract infections (particularly chronic infection in complicated postoperative urological surgery)

- Wounds, skin lesions and respiratory infections in hospitalized patients
- Septicaemia.

Some species have been responsible for outbreaks of infection in intensive care areas, burns units and other special units.

Antibiotic resistance

Hospital strains are often multiply antibiotic-resistant.

10. Pseudomonas and other aerobic Gram-negative bacilli

These Gram-negative motile aerobic bacilli have very simple growth requirements and limited fermentation activity. They are widely distributed in water, soil and sewage.

Several of the human pathogens formerly classified in the genus *Pseudomonas* have been reclassified (see Table 10.1).

PSEUDOMONAS AERUGINOSA

Habitat: human and animal gastrointestinal tract, water, soil. Moist environments are important reservoirs in hospitals; able to survive and multiply in some aqueous antiseptics, saline and 'sterile' water in hospitals.

Laboratory characteristics

Morphology and staining: Gram-negative bacilli (1.5–3.0 × 0.5 μm); motile (polar flagella); non-sporing; non-capsulate.

Culture: a strict aerobe; grows readily on routine media over a wide temperature range (5–42°C).

Table 10.1 Reclassification of pathogenic aerobic Gram-negative bacilli

Genus	Species
Pseudomonas	*P. aeruginosa* *P. fluorescens* *P. putida*
Stenotrophomonas	*S. maltophilia*
Burkholderia	*B. cepacia* *B. mallei* *B. pseudomallei*

Colonies: are often but not always large and irregular, with a fluorescent, greenish appearance due to the production of *pyocyanin* (blue-green) and *fluorescein* (yellow) pigments and with a characteristic 'fruity' odour. Strains isolated from the sputum of patients with cystic fibrosis often give rise to large mucoid colonies, due to the formation of extracellular polysaccharide slime: such colonies may fail to produce pyocyanin.

Selective media: cetrimide agar inhibits many other organisms, but allows the growth of *P. aeruginosa*, which resists the action of quaternary ammonium compounds.

Identification: colonial morphology and pigment production. Biochemical tests are generally not helpful: *P. aeruginosa* tends to be inert in API tests.

Serotyping: a typing scheme exists based on heat-resistant O (somatic) antigens and heat-labile H (flagellar) antigens. Strain identification can also be done by restriction fragment length polymorphism of chromosomal DNA.

Pathogenicity

An important cause of hospital-acquired infections in debilitated patients, such as those with burns or malignancy, or as a result of therapeutic procedures (e.g. indwelling urinary tract catheters, mechanical ventilatory support).

- Urinary tract infection: often difficult to eradicate and particularly associated with breaches in the urinary tract mucosa: also common with indwelling catheters
- Wound infections, including pressure sores and varicose ulcers
- Chronic otitis media and otitis externa
- Lower respiratory tract infections:
  - in cystic fibrosis
  - in patients on ventilators
- Eye infections, secondary to trauma or surgery.

Antibiotic sensitivity

Resistant to many antibiotics. The major antipseudomonal drugs are:

- Aminoglycosides
- Certain β-lactams: penicillins (carbenicillin, ticarcillin, azlocillin, piperacillin); cephalosporins (ceftazidime); aztreonam
- Polymyxin (colistin).

OTHER PATHOGENIC SPECIES

PSEUDOMONAS FLUORESCENS AND *PSEUDOMONAS PUTIDA*

These fluorescent pseudomonads are similar to *P. aeruginosa* but of lower pathogenicity. Their ability to grow at 4°C has occasionally caused the contamination of blood and other stored fluids.

STENOTROPHOMONAS MALTOPHILIA

This sometimes causes human infections, mainly opportunistic infection in immunocompromised patients.

BURKHOLDERIA PSEUDOMALLEI AND *BURKHOLDERIA MALLEI*

B. pseudomallei (Whitmore's bacillus) causes melioidosis, a disease of animals and humans, endemic in South East Asia. Most human cases are asymptomatic, but there may be pulmonary consolidation, skin lesions and fatal septicaemia. The organism is a saprophyte of certain soils and waters, often with a large animal reservoir locally.

B. mallei causes glanders in horses. Rarely, human infections are acquired from animals or from laboratory work with the organism.

Other aerobic gram-negative bacilli

ACINETOBACTER CALCOACETICUS

Gram-negative coccobacilli (microscopic morphology may be confused with neisseria).

Habitat: widely distributed in nature.

Laboratory characteristics

Isolation: grows well on routine media.

Pathogenicity

Generally a low-grade opportunistic pathogen seen in hospitalized patients, particularly those in intensive care units. Readily colonizes wards and specialist units, often requiring closure for disinfection.

Antibiotic resistance

Usually resistant to many antibiotics, including those used to treat other forms of serious hospital sepsis.

11. Vibrio, aeromonas, campylobacter and helicobacter

VIBRIO

Widespread in nature, mainly in water: one species, *V. cholerae*, is the cause of cholera.

VIBRIO CHOLERAE

Habitat: water contaminated with faeces of patients or carriers.

Laboratory characteristics

Morphology and staining: Gram-negative slender bacilli (2 × 0.5 µm), sometimes comma-shaped with a pointed end. Often arranged in pairs or short chains, giving a spiral appearance. Actively motile by one long polar flagellum; non-capsulate; non-sporing.

Culture: aerobe; grows readily on ordinary media as glistening colonies over a wide temperature range (optimum 37°C). Growth is inhibited at acid pH (optimal pH for growth is alkaline, pH 8.0–8.2).

Enrichment medium: alkaline peptone water (pH 8.6) promotes the rapid growth of *V. cholerae* from mixtures of other bacteria, e.g. faecal samples.

Selective medium: TCBS medium – thiosulphate citrate bile sucrose agar, pH 8.6.

Observe: for large yellow sucrose-fermenting colonies after incubation for 18–24 h. Enterobacteria may grow, but growth is inhibited and the colonies are small.

Identification: by slide agglutination of suspect colonies with specific antisera.

Biochemical reactions: oxidase-positive; fermentation of sucrose and mannose, but not arabinose, is typical of *V. cholerae*, and a distinguishing feature from other vibrios. Use of the API 20E system (Fig. 5.2) gives a characteristic biochemical profile.

Antigenic structure:

O antigens: 139 O serogroups are recognized. Epidemic cholera is caused by *V. cholerae* serogroup O1, which is divided into three sero-types, *Ogawa*, *Inaba* and *Hikojima*. However, antigenic structure (and therefore serotype) may change within the human gut.

Biotypes: two biotypes of *V. cholerae* O1, classical and El Tor, can be differentiated (biotyping is the distinguishing of different bacterial strains within a species by various biological and bio-chemical reactions). Any serotype can be of either classical or El Tor biotype.

Non-O1 vibrios, deficient in the O1 antigen, were classified as non-cholera vibrios – but a cholera epidemic has been reported, due to serogroup 0139 – a non-O1 vibrio.

Phage typing: is of limited value in epidemiological studies.

Toxins: endotoxins (cell-wall lipopolysaccharide) and exotoxins are recognized. The enterotoxin is an exotoxin which stimulates persistent and excessive secretion of isotonic fluid by the intestinal mucosa.

Pathogenicity

V. cholerae O1 is the cause of cholera in humans, a febrile diarrhoeal illness which is often severe. In the acute disease, vibrios are present in enormous numbers – about 10^8/ml of faeces. In 1992 a serious outbreak of cholera-like diarrhoeal disease in Bangladesh was caused by *V. cholerae* 0139. Strains in serogroups 02–0138 – non-cholera vibrios – may be associated with milder diarrhoeal illness.

Viability: readily killed by heat and drying; dies in polluted waters but may survive in clean stagnant water (especially if alkaline) or sea water for 1-2 weeks.

Antibiotic sensitivity

Sensitive to macrolides (e.g. erythromycin), ciprofloxacin and aminoglycoside antibiotics.

Strains resistant to tetracyclines, ampicillin and co-trimoxazole have emerged in cholera-endemic areas.

VIBRIO PARAHAEMOLYTICUS

V. parahaemolyticus is a halophilic (i.e. salt-tolerant) marine vibrio isolated from shellfish, particularly in countries with warm coastal water, e.g. South East Asia.

It causes an acute gastroenteritis in which vibrios are excreted in large numbers in the stools. Faecal samples plated on TCBS agar yield large blue-green colonies typical of *V. parahaemolyticus*, which fails to ferment sucrose.

AEROMONAS AND PLESIOMONAS

Gram-negative bacilli; aerobes, facultative anaerobes; motile; oxidase-positive.

Aeromonas hydrophila and *Plesiomonas shigelloides* are the medically important species, but infections are rare and are usually in patients with some other serious disease: occasionally isolated from blood, CSF and exudates. Both organisms may be isolated from human faeces, but the significance of this finding is uncertain. They are *not* accepted as an established cause of diarrhoeal disease.

CAMPYLOBACTER

Strictly microaerophilic vibrios. Species that cause human or animal diarrhoeal illness are thermophilic, growing best at 43°C. The main human pathogenic species is *C. jejuni*. Other species occasionally found in human gastrointestinal disease include *C. coli* and *C. lari*.

Habitat: various animal species, including chickens, domestic animals and seagulls (*C. lari*).

Laboratory characteristics

Morphology and staining: small, Gram-negative, curved or spiral rods (Fig. 11.1). Highly motile, by a single flagellum at one or both poles.

Culture: microaerophilic; grow best in an atmosphere containing a mixture of 7% oxygen and 10–15% carbon dioxide, with the remainder an inert gas, usually nitrogen or hydrogen. Growth takes place at 37°C, but the optimal temperature for *C. jejuni* is 43°C. Grow readily on simple media.

Selective medium (necessary for isolation from faeces and other samples containing numerous other bacteria): lysed blood agar with vancomycin, polymyxin and trimethoprim.

Incubate: for 24–48 h at 43°C under microaerophilic conditions.

Observe: effuse colonies that look like spreading fluid droplets.

Identification: by Gram-film appearance, motility, growth temperature requirements (25°C: no growth; 37°C: growth; 43°C:

Fig. 11.1   Campylobacter (approx. × 1000).

enhanced growth) and oxidase test (campylobacters are oxidase-positive).

Antibiotic sensitivity

Most strains are sensitive to macrolides (e.g. erythromycin): resistant strains usually sensitive to ciprofloxacin and chloramphenicol.

HELICOBACTER

Helicobacter pylori (formerly known as *C. pylori* or *C. pyloridis*) is found closely associated with gastric mucosa and causes chronic active gastritis: it plays a role in gastric and duodenal ulceration and probably also in gastric cancer.

Laboratory characteristics

Morphology and staining: small, Gram-negative, spiral rods; motile by polar flagella.

Culture: on blood or chocolate agar in a moist microaerophilic atmosphere. For isolation from clinical specimens, use campylobacter selective medium (see above). Small colonies grow after 3–7 days at 37°C.

Biochemical reactions: catalase-positive; oxidase-positive; strongly urease-positive.

Typing: a variety of nucleic acid methods have been developed, but there is no agreed typing scheme.

Antibiotic sensitivity

Sensitive to amoxycillin, tetracycline, metronidazole, macrolides (especially clarithromycin) and to bismuth salts.

12. Parvobacteria

Parvobacteria (parvus = small) is a convenient but old-fashioned name for a number of quite different, small, Gram-negative bacilli which generally require enriched media for isolation and culture. This heterogeneous group contains several important human pathogens, which cause a wide variety of diseases. They are un-related and classified in separate genera: consequently the term 'parvobacteria' lacks taxonomic respectability.

The following genera are considered here as parvobacteria:

- *Haemophilus*
- *Brucella*
- *Bordetella*
- *Pasteurella*
- *Francisella*
- *Actinobacillus*
- *Gardnerella*
- *Streptobacillus.*

HAEMOPHILUS

Habitat: mainly the respiratory tract: often part of the normal flora, but may also cause respiratory disease, usually as a secondary invader. Some species are associated with other mucosal surfaces, e.g. conjunctiva, genital tract.

Laboratory characteristics

Morphology and staining: small, Gram-negative coccobacilli (see Fig. 8.2); non-sporing, non-motile.

Culture: require enriched media, such as blood or chocolate agar; optimum temperature around 37°C. Most species grow poorly in the absence of oxygen, and growth is enhanced in an

Table 12.1   Growth factors for *Haemophilus species*

Factor required	Species
X and V	*H. influenzae, H. aegyptius,*
	H. haemolyticus
X	*H. ducreyi*
V	*H. parainfluenzae, H. parahaemolyticus*

atmosphere with added CO_2. Enriched media are necessary because *Haemophilus species* need one or both of two growth factors:
- Heat-stable X factor – haemin or some other iron-containing porphyrin
- Heat-labile V factor – di- or tri-phosphopyridine nucleotide.

Requirement for growth factors can help to differentiate between species (Table 12.1).

Pathogenicity

The diseases caused by *Haemophilus species* are listed in Table 12.2.

HAEMOPHILUS INFLUENZAE

The main pathogenic species.

Habitat: the upper respiratory tract; most strains found in the normal flora are non-capsulated.

Laboratory characteristics

Morphology: small, Gram-negative coccobacillus; a minority of strains are capsulated.

Table 12.2   Pathogenicity of *Haemophilus species*

Species	Disease
H. influenzae	Exacerbations of chronic bronchitis
	Sinusitis, otitis media
	Meningitis
	Epiglottitis
H. aegyptius	Conjunctivitis
H. ducreyi	Chancroid
H. parainfluenzae *H. haemolyticus* *H. parahaemolyticus*	Commensals of the upper respiratory tract; rarely cause disease

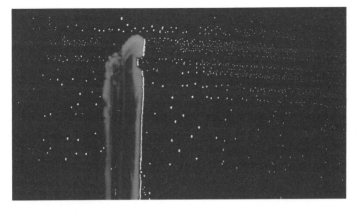

Fig. 12.1 Satellitism. A blood agar plate showing enhancement of the growth of colonies of *Haemophilus influenzae* next to the streak of *Staphylococcus aureus* which supplies V factor.

Culture: on chocolate or blood agar: a streak of *Staphylococcus aureus* across the plate produces V factor and enlarges the size of adjacent colonies of *H. influenzae* – satellitism (Fig. 12.1).

Colonial morphology: small, translucent, non-haemolytic colonies: capsulated strains form larger iridescent colonies.

Selective medium: the addition of bacitracin to chocolate agar inhibits the growth of many Gram-positive bacteria found in the upper respiratory tract (e.g. viridans streptococci), and use of this medium facilitates the isolation of *H. influenzae* from sputum specimens.

Identification: by testing:
- on nutrient agar for growth requirements, using discs impregnated with X and V factors
- in a special substrate for the ability to synthesize porphyrin: strains able to do this do not require X factor.

Serotypes of capsulated strains: six are recognized, on the basis of capsular polysaccharide antigens – Pittman types a, b, c, d, e, f. Type b is the main pathogen.

Pathogenicity

Non-capsulated strains are mainly responsible for exacerbations of chronic bronchitis and bronchiectasis.

Capsulated strains (predominantly type b) can cause various invasive infections, mainly in children from 2 months to 3 years old:

- Meningitis
- Acute epiglottitis
- Osteomyelitis } these infections are often accompanied by septicaemia
- Arthritis
- Cellulitis (orbital).

Vaccine: a vaccine (Hib), which protects against invasive *H. Influenzae* type b infections, was introduced into the UK schedule for childhood immunization in 1992 (see p. 413).

Antibiotic sensitivity

Sensitive to:

- Ampicillin
- Co-trimoxazole
- Tetracycline
- Erythromycin
- Trimethoprim
- Ciprofloxacin
- Chloramphenicol (reserve for meningitis and epiglottitis)
- Second and third generation cephalosporins

Antibiotic resistance

Resistance to ampicillin due to β-lactamase production is now present in 5–10% of UK strains.

HAEMOPHILUS AEGYPTIUS

Similar to, in fact sometimes regarded as a variety of, *H. influenzae*. Formerly called the Koch-Weeks bacillus.

Pathogenicity

Acute conjunctivitis.

HAEMOPHILUS DUCREYI

The cause of the sexually transmitted disease *chancroid*, or soft sore.

Laboratory characteristics

Morphology: slender, Gram-negative, ovoid bacilli; slightly larger than *H. influenzae*; bacteria en masse from clinical specimens have the configuration of 'shoals of fish'.

Table 12.3   Animal hosts and geographical distribution of *Brucella species*

Strain	Usual animal host	Geographical distribution
B. melitensis	Goats, sheep	Mediterranean countries
B. abortus	Cattle	World-wide
B. suis	Pigs	Denmark and USA

Culture: on 20–30% rabbit blood agar or other special enriched medium: incubate at 35–37°C for 3–5 days, with added moisture and CO_2. *Growth factors*: only X factor is required.

Antibiotic sensitivity

Erythromycin, co-trimoxazole, tetracycline. Other effective agents are new cephalosporins and ciprofloxacin.

BRUCELLA

Predominantly infect domestic animals, from which infection may be transmitted to humans.

There are three main species *Brucella melitensis*; *B. abortus* and *B. suis*, each with a number of biotypes. Some of the subtypes are associated with a particular geographical location.

Habitat: chronically infected domestic animals (Table 12.3).

Laboratory characteristics

Morphology and staining: short, slender, pleomorphic, Gram-negative bacilli; non-motile, non-sporing, non-capsulate.

Culture: in enriched medium, such as glucose serum, broth or agar; small transparent colonies develop after several days' incubation at 37°C in aerobic conditions. CO_2 is required for the growth of *B. abortus*.

Identification of the different species is done by a variety of biochemical and serological tests, and the ability of certain dyes to inhibit growth. Biotypes are recognized within species, and some biotypes do not give the typical reactions.

Antigenic structure: the three species share two antigens, A and M, but these are present in different proportions. Typical melitensis strains contain an excess of M antigen, whereas typical abortus and suis strains contain an excess of A antigen. Mono-specific antisera can be prepared, and these are of use in identification.

Pathogenicity

The cause of undulant fever or brucellosis – a chronic, debilitating febrile illness, usually without any localizing signs: the bacteria persist intracellularly and are therefore difficult to eradicate by antibiotic therapy.

Antibiotic sensitivity

Sensitive to many antibiotics: tetracycline combined with strepto-mycin is the usual treatment.

BORDETELLA

The important member of the genus is *Bordetella pertussis*, the cause of whooping cough. *B. parapertussis* causes a milder form of whooping cough, which is uncommon in Britain. *B. bronchiseptica* is an animal pathogen.

BORDETELLA PERTUSSIS

Habitat: the human respiratory tract, usually associated with acute disease.

Laboratory characteristics

Morphology and staining: short, sometimes oval, Gram-negative bacilli: freshly isolated strains may be capsulated.

Culture: special enriched medium is required for primary isolation: the most widely used medium is charcoal blood agar. This has largely replaced the traditional Bordet–Gengou medium, which contains 30% blood, potato extract, glycerol and agar. The media are usually made selective by the addition of penicillin or cephalexin.

Colonial morphology: colonies like 'split pearls' or 'mercury drops' appear after 3 or more days of incubation in a moist aerobic atmosphere at 35°C.

Identification is confirmed serologically by slide agglutination with a polyvalent antiserum reacting with all three main antigens.

Antigenic structure: surface antigens (agglutinogens) designated 1–6 are recognized: all freshly isolated strains possess agglutinogen 1.

Serotypes: there are three main serotypes, based on the presence of the six surface antigens: type 1,2; type 1,3; type 1,2,3.

Pathogenicity

The cause of whooping cough, a disease seen mainly in pre-school children and especially severe in those under 1 year of age. Affects the lower respiratory tract, causing bronchospasm and the characteristic *paroxysmal cough*.

Antibiotic sensitivity

Erythromycin.

PASTEURELLA

PASTEURELLA MULTOCIDA

The main pathogenic member of the genus, also known as *Pasteurella septica*.
   Habitat: respiratory tract of many animals, notably dogs.

Laboratory characteristics

Morphology: small, sometimes capsulated, ovoid Gram-negative bacilli, often showing bipolar staining.
   Culture: on nutrient agar or blood agar, aerobically at 37°C. Does not grow on MacConkey agar – a differentiating feature from enterobacteria.

Pathogenicity

An important animal pathogen. In humans, it may cause septic wounds after dog or cat bites.

Antibiotic sensitivity

Penicillin, tetracyclines, erythromycin, aminoglycosides.

FRANCISELLA

FRANCISELLA TULARENSIS

The cause of tularaemia.
   Habitat: rodents and other small mammals.

Laboratory characteristics

Morphology: pleomorphic, capsulated, small Gram-negative cocco-bacilli, often showing bipolar staining.
   Culture: on blood agar enriched with cystine and glucose.

Pathogenicity

Tularaemia, a plague-like disease of rodents, is contracted by contact with animal hosts or their products. It is widespread in the USA, and is occasionally seen in parts of Europe, but not yet in the UK.

Antibiotic sensitivity

Streptomycin or gentamicin are the drugs of choice. Tetracyclines are also generally effective.

ACTINOBACILLUS

Facultatively anaerobic, non-branching Gram-negative coccobacilli that can grow on nutrient agar. The type species *Actinobacillus lignieresi* is responsible for actinobacillosis in cattle and sheep, a disease which resembles actinomycosis in humans. *A. actinomycetemcomitans*, present in the normal oral flora of humans, is sometimes found along with *Actinomyces species* in human actinomycosis.

GARDNERELLA

GARDNERELLA VAGINALIS

Previously known as *Haemophilus vaginalis* and *Corynebacterium vaginale*.
   Habitat: vagina; male urethra. Found in small numbers in the vaginal secretions of up to 50% of normal women, and in the discharge of patients with bacterial vaginosis.

Laboratory characteristics

Morphology and staining: small, Gram-negative, sometimes Gram-variable, bacilli: non-motile, non-sporing.

Culture: requires enriched media such as blood agar or dextrose-starch agar. Facultative anaerobe – growth enhanced by 5% CO_2 and moisture; optimum temperature around 37°C; optimum pH 6.8. After incubation for 48 h, small domed colonies develop. These are surrounded by a zone of β-haemolysis on human or rabbit (but not horse or sheep) blood agar, and by a zone of clearing on dextrose–starch agar, due to starch hydrolysis.

Identification: by Gram-film appearance; negative catalase reaction (corynebacteria are catalase-positive); ability to grow aerobically and anaerobically; sensitivity to metronidazole, using a high potency disc.

Pathogenicity

In association with anaerobes, believed to be the cause of bacterial vaginosis – but asymptomatic vaginal carriage is common.

Antibiotic sensitivity

Sensitive to high concentrations of metronidazole – the drug of choice for the treatment of bacterial vaginosis.

STREPTOBACILLUS

STREPTOBACILLUS MONILIFORMIS

Habitat: *Streptobacillus moniliformis* is a normal inhabitant of the nasopharynx of rats.

Laboratory characteristics

Morphology and staining: *S. moniliformis* is a slender, filamentous bacterium with club-shaped ('moniliform') terminal swellings. Gram-negative, but may be Gram-positive in young cultures.

Culture: requires enriched media for growth.

Pathogenicity

Causes one form of rat-bite fever in humans.

13. Corynebacterium and related bacteria

CORYNEBACTERIUM

Gram-positive bacilli with a characteristic morphology; non-sporing; non-capsulate; non-motile.

Widely distributed in nature: several human and animal species are important pathogens.

CORYNEBACTERIUM DIPHTHERIAE

Habitat: the throat and nose of humans.

Laboratory characteristics

Morphology and staining: pleomorphic Gram-positive rods (3 × 0.3 μm) or clubs. These divide by 'snapping fission', so that adjacent cells lie at different angles to each other forming V-, L- and W-shapes – a so-called *Chinese-character* arrangement. Adjacent cells may also be parallel to one another, in *palisades*.

Some strains stain irregularly due to the intracellular deposition of polymerized phosphate – forming the metachromatic or volutin granules characteristic of, but not exclusive to, *C. diphtheriae*. The granules, usually two or three per cell, show up with special stains – bluish-black by Albert's method, deep blue with Neisser's methylene blue.

Culture: an aerobe and facultative anaerobe; optimum temperature 37°C. Does not grow well on ordinary agar – media containing blood or serum are required. Selective media are necessary for isolation from clinical specimens.

Selective media:
- *Loeffler's serum medium*: *C. diphtheriae* grows rapidly – faster than other upper respiratory tract bacteria present in clinical

material. The morphology develops particularly well, and smears made as soon as 8 h after inoculation may show a typical appearance.

- *Blood tellurite agar* (e.g. Hoyle's or McLeod's medium): after 48 h incubation, corynebacteria produce characteristic grey-black colonies due to their ability to reduce potassium tellurite to tellurium.

Colonial appearance: three colonial types are recognized: *gravis, intermedius* and *mitis,* so named from the type of clinical disease they were most likely to cause. Other corynebacteria also grow on tellurite media, to form colonies that can be confused with those of *C. diphtheriae.*

Identification: by biochemical tests and demonstration of toxin production. Other corynebacteria may mimic *C. diphtheriae* in films and on culture. Some isolates of *C. diphtheriae,* especially mitis strains, are not toxigenic and are therefore non-virulent.

Biochemical reactions: acid production from a range of carbohydrates and other biochemical tests are used to differentiate *C. diphtheriae* from other corynebacteria. Gravis (but not intermedius or mitis) strains ferment starch and glycogen.

Typing: serotyping, phage typing and bacteriocin typing have all been used to subdivide strains of *C. diphtheriae* for epidemiological studies.

Toxin: responsible for virulence; can be demonstrated by guinea pig inoculation or by a gel precipitation test.

1. *Guinea pig inoculation*: inject subcutaneously a suspension of the isolated strain of *C. diphtheriae* into two guinea pigs, one protected with diphtheria antitoxin. If the strain is toxigenic, the unprotected animal dies in 2–3 days but the protected animal survives.

2. *Gel-precipitation (Elek) test*: a filter-paper strip previously immersed in diphtheria antitoxin is incorporated into serum agar before it has set. The strain of *C. diphtheriae* under investigation is then streaked onto the agar at right angles to the filter-paper strip. Incubate at 37°C. *Observe* after 24 h and 48 h for lines of precipitation, indicating toxin-antitoxin interaction (Fig. 13.1).

Diphtheria toxin: the exotoxin of *C. diphtheriae* is produced only by strains carrying a bacteriophage: its formation in vitro is stimulated in culture media with low iron content. The toxin interferes with protein synthesis in mammalian cells by splitting the molecule of

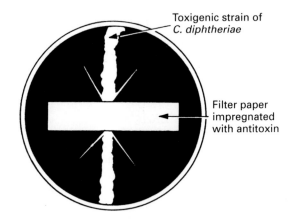

Fig. 13.1   Elek test for demonstration of toxin production by *Corynebacterium diphtheriae*. The toxin combines with antitoxin to produce antigen-antibody complexes, which form visible lines of precipitation in the agar.

NAD (nicotinamide adenine dinucleotide) – an essential cofactor for the transferase involved in peptide bond formation by ribosomes. The toxin acts locally on the mucous membranes of the respiratory tract to produce a grey, adherent pseudomembrane consisting of fibrin, bacteria, and epithelial and phagocytic cells. After absorption into the bloodstream, it acts systemically on the cells of the myocardium, the nervous system (only motor nerves are affected) and the adrenal glands. The toxin can be rendered non-toxic but still antigenic by treatment with formaldehyde: the *toxoid* so formed is used in prophylactic immunization.

Schick test: a skin test formerly used to demonstrate immunity, i.e. circulating diphtheria antitoxin. Toxin was injected into the skin of the forearm, and this caused an erythematous reaction in those who were susceptible. Immunity checks in individuals at special risk are now carried out by the measurement of antitoxin levels in serum.

Pathogenicity

C. diphtheriae is the cause of diphtheria. Usually the mucous membranes of the upper respiratory tract are affected but sometimes, especially in tropical countries, skin lesions are produced. The serious systemic manifestations follow absorption of the exotoxin.

Antibiotic sensitivity

C. diphtheriae is sensitive to penicillin, erythromycin and other antibiotics.

OTHER CORYNEBACTERIA

CORYNEBACTERIUM ULCERANS

May be responsible in humans for diphtheria-like throat lesions, but usually with little evidence of toxaemia.

Laboratory characteristics

Biochemical reactions distinguish it from *C. diphtheriae*.
   Toxins: two are produced – one immunologically identical to the toxin of *C. diphtheriae*, the other identical to the toxin of *C. pseudotuberculosis*, an important animal pathogen.

HUMAN COMMENSALS

There are many so-called *diphtheroid bacilli*, e.g. *C. hofmannii* in the throat and *C. xerosis* in the conjunctiva.
   Habitat: normally present in the skin (especially within sebaceous ducts) and mucous membranes.

Laboratory characteristics

Morphology and staining: less pleomorphic and more strongly Gram-positive than *C. diphtheriae*; metachromatic granules are few or absent. Tend to be arranged in palisades, with less pronounced Chinese lettering, than *C. diphtheriae*.
   Culture: grow well on ordinary agar.

Pathogenicity

Occasional opportunistic pathogens, causing e.g. endocarditis on prosthetic valves, infection in implanted artificial joints, peritonitis in patients receiving chronic ambulatory peritoneal dialysis (CAPD).

CORYNEBACTERIUM JEIKEIUM

A skin commensal diphtheroid with a particular ability to cause opportunistic infections. Notable because of its resistance to many antimicrobial agents: vancomycin is the only drug to which all strains are sensitive.

PROPIONIBACTERIUM

Gram-positive, non-sporing, anaerobic bacilli, formerly classified as anaerobic corynebacteria. A differential feature from other similar bacteria is that they produce propionic acid as the major end-product from glucose fermentation: this can be detected by gas-liquid chromatography.

There are two main species. *P. acnes* and *P. granulosum*.

Habitat: the human skin.

Pathogenicity

Association with the skin disease acne vulgaris.

ERYSIPELOTHRIX

ERYSIPELOTHRIX RHUSIOPATHIAE

A slender, Gram-positive, non-motile bacillus of uncertain classification. Aerobe and facultative anaerobe.

Habitat: healthy pigs, but widely distributed in other animals and birds; found on the skin and scales of fish; causes swine erysipelas.

Pathogenicity

Responsible in humans for erysipeloid, a rare skin infection.

LISTERIA

Six species are recognized, but almost all human infections are due to *Listeria monocytogenes*.

LISTERIA MONOCYTOGENES

Morphologically similar to erysipelothrix and diphtheroids, but flagellated below 33°C. Non-motile at 37°C, but exhibits active tumbling motility at 25°C in young broth cultures.

Habitat: wild and domestic animals: ubiquitous in the environment, and found throughout the food chain.

Laboratory characteristics

Culture: aerobic and facultatively anaerobic; optimal temperature 37°C, but will survive and grow at 6°C.

Colonies on horse-blood agar are non-pigmented and surrounded by a narrow zone of complete (β) haemolysis with an indistinct margin.

Typing: on the basis of O and H antigenic structure, 13 serotypes are recognized – but almost all infections are caused by three of these serotypes, type 4b being the commonest.

Pathogenicity

Causes listeriosis in humans and animals.

Antibiotic sensitivity

Sensitive in vitro to a number of antibiotics. Ampicillin is usually used in treatment, often in combination with gentamicin.

14. Mycobacterium

Mycobacteria are referred to as *acid-fast*, because after mordanting in stain they resist decolorization with strong acids. Their cell wall has a high lipid content: acid fastness is the result of the formation of complexes between the dye and mycolic acid, one of the cell-wall lipids.

The main medically important mycobacteria are listed in Table 14.1, together with some of their properties.

Table 14.1 Medically important mycobacteria

Species	Habitat and source	Disease	Cultural characteristics on Löwenstein–Jensen medium
M. tuberculosis	Infected humans	Tuberculosis	Rough, dry, yellow colonies: slow grower
M. bovis	Infected cattle	Tuberculosis	White, smooth colonies (inhibited by glycerol): slow grower
M. africanus	Infected humans	Tuberculosis	Colonies like those of *M. bovis*
M. leprae	Infected humans	Leprosy	No growth
Mycobacteria other than tuberculosis bacilli (MOTT)	Mainly soil, water; sometimes birds, animals	Pulmonary infection, cervical adenitis, skin ulcers	Colonies often pigmented: some grow slowly, others rapidly; may exhibit unusual temperature requirements

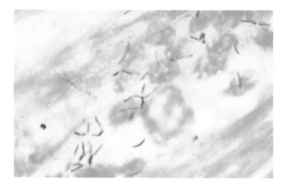

Fig. 14.1   *Mycobacterium tuberculosis* (approx. × 1000).

MYCOBACTERIUM TUBERCULOSIS

Laboratory characteristics

Morphology: slender, beaded bacilli; non-sporing.

Staining: Ziehl–Neelsen stain: bacilli are stained with con-centrated carbol fuchsin, heated, and then decolorized with 20% sulphuric acid and alcohol: the bacilli retain a bright red colour (Fig. 14.1). Nowadays, tubercle bacilli are usually detected under fluorescent microscopy, with a uramine stain.

Culture: does not grow on ordinary media. Grows well, but slowly on Löwenstein–Jensen medium (contains egg, asparagine, glycerol and, to inhibit contaminants, malachite green) – usually after 2–3 weeks' incubation at 37°C. Cultures should be kept for 6–8 weeks before being discarded (Fig. 14.2).

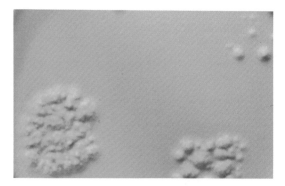

Fig. 14.2   *Mycobacterium tuberculosis*: culture, showing 'rough, tough and buff' colonies.

Pathogenicity

The cause of tuberculosis – a slowly progressive, chronic infection – usually of the lungs, but many other organs and tissues can become affected. Tuberculosis is increasing in incidence, especially in Africa, due to its emergence in AIDS cases.

MYCOBACTERIUM BOVIS

The main cause of infection in tubercular cattle: humans become infected by the ingestion of milk containing *M. bovis*.

Laboratory characteristics

Culture: grows, but relatively poorly, on Löwenstein–Jensen medium.

Pathogenicity

Similar to human tubercle bacilli, but particularly liable to infect children – causing enlarged, caseous cervical lymph nodes ('scrofula') and tuberculosis of the bones, joints and kidneys. Rare nowadays in the UK, due to the eradication of the disease in cattle.

Antibiotic sensitivity

Both *M. tuberculosis* and *M. bovis* are sensitive to a wide range of drugs (listed below). Because resistant variants arise readily, therapy should always comprise a combination of drugs.

First-line drugs	*Second-line drugs*
Isoniazid	Streptomycin
Rifampicin	Capreomycin
Pyrazinamide	Cycloserine
Ethambutol	Thiacetazone
	Ethionamide

MYCOBACTERIUM LEPRAE

The cause of leprosy – still a scourge in many parts of the world today.
Habitat: found only in cases of human infection.

Laboratory characteristics

Cultivation: in vivo by inoculation of the foot-pads of mice or of armadillos: the animals develop slow-growing granulomas at the site of injection. Does not grow in vitro.

Antibiotic sensitivity

Sensitive to dapsone (a sulphone), rifampicin, clofazimine.

MOTT (MYCOBACTERIA OTHER THAN TUBERCULOSIS BACILLI)

A group of miscellaneous mycobacteria, of low pathogenicity for humans.

Classification is still controversial. The principal species, together with the diseases they cause, are listed in Table 14.2.

Laboratory characteristics

Culture: on Löwenstein–Jensen medium, sometimes at lower (25°C) or higher (45°C) temperatures than normal. Several species produce pigmented growth in the dark (scotochromogens) and some only after exposure to light (photochromogens), whereas others are non-pigmented.

Table 14.2   MOTT (mycobacteria other than tuberculosis bacilli)

Species	Disease
M. avium complex:	
M. avium	Pulmonary;
M. intracellulare	lymphadenopathy;
M. scrofulaceum	disseminated infection in AIDS patients
M. fortuitum	Pulmonary
M. marinum	Granulomatous ulcers of skin
M. kansasii	
M. malmoense	Pulmonary
M. xenopi	

Pathogenicity

Pulmonary infection: MOTT are sometimes simply 'passengers' which accompany tuberculosis. However, they are a major problem in AIDS cases – especially the *M. avium* complex.

Antibiotic sensitivity

Variable, often resistant to several of the standard antituberculous drugs.

15. Actinomyces and nocardia

Actinomyces and nocardia are morphologically similar Gram-positive branching rods and filaments. Actinomyces are micro-aerophilic or anaerobic on primary isolation, although some species grow in air after a few subcultures. Nocardia are aerobic organisms.

ACTINOMYCES

Most actinomyces are soil organisms but some – and these are the potentially pathogenic species – are commensals of the mouth of humans and animals (Table 15.1).

Species are identified by colonial appearances, ability to grow aerobically and biochemical tests.

ACTINOMYCES ISRAELII

Laboratory characteristics

Morphology and staining: Gram-positive bacteria, which grow in filaments that readily break up into rods and may show branching. Non-motile, non-sporing, not acid-fast. In tissue, colonies develop to form diagnostic yellowish 'sulphur granules', which are visible

Table 15.1 Some *Actinomyces species*

Species	Host/habitat	Disease association
A. israelii	Oropharynx and gut of humans	Human actinomycosis
A. naeslundii *A. viscosus* *A. odontolyticus*	Oropharynx of humans	Dental plaque and caries; human actinomycosis
A. bovis	Oropharynx of cattle	Lumpy jaw in cattle

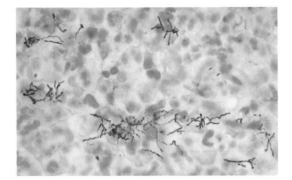

Fig. 15.1 Actinomycotic pus (approx. × 1000).

to the naked eye and which are found in pus discharged through draining sinuses (Fig. 15.1).

Culture:

Solid media: on blood or serum glucose agar incubated anaerobically at 37°C for 7 days or more; growth is enhanced by 5% carbon dioxide. *Observe:* small, white to cream, adherent, nodular colonies.

'Shake' cultures: in semi-solid glucose agar kept at 37°C for 5–10 days. *Observe*: maximal growth in a turbid band 10–15 mm below the surface, where conditions are microaerophilic.

Isolation of this exacting microorganism from clinical material is difficult, especially as the pus usually contains other, faster-growing, bacteria. Presumptive diagnosis is made by the demonstration of typical Gram-positive branching filaments in a sulphur granule. Whenever possible, a washed, crushed sulphur granule should be cultured in preference to pus.

Pathogenicity

Actinomycosis is a mixed infection: *A. israelii* is the most important actinomycete involved. The infection is endogenous in origin, and results in a chronic granuloma with abscess formation: profuse pus discharges by draining through sinuses. Infection probably starts after local trauma, e.g. the extraction of carious teeth, appendicectomy. The typical sites of the disease are: cervicofacial – 65% of cases; abdominal (usually ileocaecal) – 20% of cases; and, rarely, thoracic, affecting the lung.

Intrauterine contraceptive devices, especially those made of plastic, may be colonized with *A. israelii*. The significance of this is uncertain but, perhaps in association with other organisms, a low-grade intrauterine infection may result.

Antibiotic sensitivity

Sensitive to penicillin, clindamycin, tetracycline, erythromycin.

NOCARDIA

Habitat: majority of species are soil saprophytes; a few are pathogenic to humans.

Laboratory characteristics

Morphology and staining: similar to actinomyces, but some species are partially acid-fast.

Culture: slow-growing, aerobic organisms which require 5–14 days' incubation on nutrient agar.

Colonies: wrinkled, rosette- or star-shaped colonies, initially white, then yellow and finally pink or red.

Pathogenicity

Generally cause chronic granulomatous suppurative infections.

NOCARDIA ASTEROIDES

Affects lungs, sometimes with secondary spread to other organs, e.g. brain. Pulmonary nocardiosis usually develops as an opportunistic infection in immunocompromised patients.

NOCARDIA MADURAE AND NOCARDIA BRASILIENSIS

Madura foot or *mycetoma* is a tropical form of nocardiosis which affects the skin, subcutaneous tissue and bones of the foot to produce a destructive infection with multiple discharging sinuses. The bacteria are implanted by contaminated thorns or splinters.

Antibiotic sensitivity

Sensitive to sulphonamides and to co-trimoxazole. Treatment may have to be continued for many months.

16. Neisseria and moraxella

NEISSERIA

The neisseriae are Gram-negative diplococci: the two pathogenic species, *N. gonorrhoeae* (the gonococcus) and *N. meningitidis* (the meningococcus) have exacting growth requirements.

NEISSERIA GONORRHOEAE

Habitat: the human urogenital tract.

Laboratory characteristics

Morphology and staining: Gram-negative cocci, 0.6–1.0 μm, characteristically (when intracellular) in pairs. In purulent clinical material, many of the diplococci are intracellular within polymorphs; the remainder are extracellular, in the exudate (Fig. 16.1).

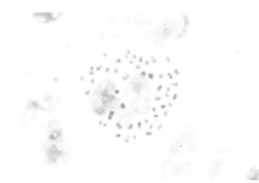

Fig. 16.1   Gonococcal pus (approx. × 1000).

118   NOTES ON MEDICAL BACTERIOLOGY

Culture: requires an enriched medium (usually a lysed-blood or chocolate agar) and incubation in a moist aerobic atmosphere containing 5–10% CO_2.

Selective media: are necessary to inhibit other bacteria – e.g. Thayer–Martin medium or MNYC medium: both contain mixtures of antibiotics to which *N. gonorrhoeae* is resistant.

Colonies: oxidase-positive, grey, glistening colonies after 24 h incubation, becoming larger, opaque and somewhat irregular at 48 h: test suspect colonies with tetramethyl-*p*-phenylenediamine (the 'oxidase reagent'). Oxidase-positive colonies rapidly turn dark purple.

Identification: Biochemical test or serological by using a 'Phadebact' monoclonal 'GC' test kit.

Typing: for epidemiology, by auxotyping (analysis of nutritional requirements) or serotyping.

Pathogenicity

The cause of the sexually transmitted disease gonorrhoea, a purulent infection of the urethra and, in females, also of the uterine cervix. Dies rapidly outside the human host, but may remain viable in pus for some time.

Antibiotic sensitivity

Sensitive to penicillin, ampicillin, tetracycline, macrolides, spectinomycin, cefuroxime, ceftriaxone, ciprofloxacin and other drugs.

Low-level, chromosomally mediated, penicillin resistance was first recognized in the 1950s and is now present in some strains. Highly resistant β-lactamase-producing strains are now common (up to 50% of isolates) in some developing countries, although rarer (less than 5% of isolates) in the UK. This type of resistance is plasmid-mediated.

NEISSERIA MENINGITIDIS

Habitat: the human nasopharynx: present in 10–25% of normal people.

Laboratory characteristics

Morphology and staining: as for *N. gonorrhoeae*. Films of the CSF in meningococcal meningitis have a similar appearance to that of genital tract exudate in gonorrhoea, but organisms are scantier.

Culture: requirements similar to those of *N. gonorrhoeae*, although somewhat less exacting.

Selective media: in meningitis, the organism is present in CSF in pure culture and selective media are not required for isolation.

Identification: by biochemical test.

Antigenic structure: there are three main groups (A, B, C) and five subsidiary groups (X, Y, Z, Z^1 (29E) and W135). Not all isolates are groupable. Groups B and C are the most common in the UK. Group B strains are poorly immunogenic.

Pathogenicity

Cause of meningococcal meningitis: in those susceptible, spread from the nasopharynx results in septicaemia, which is usually

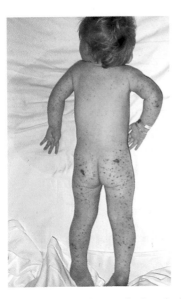

Fig. 16.2 Meningococcal septicaemia: haemorrhagic rash. (Photograph by Dr D. H. M. Kennedy.)

followed by rapid involvement of the meninges. The septicaemia may be accompanied by a haemorrhagic rash (Fig. 16.2), with death due to adrenal haemorrhage (Waterhouse-Friderichsen syndrome) before the development of clinical meningitis.

Viability: dies quickly at room temperature outside the human host.

Antibiotic sensitivity

Sensitive to penicillin, cefotaxime, chloramphenicol, rifampicin. Sulphonamide sensitivity was formerly the rule, but resistance is now common.

COMMENSAL NEISSERIAE (*NEISSERIA PHARYNGIS*)

Habitat: regularly present in the mucous membranes of the mouth, nose and pharynx; less frequently in the genital tract.

MORAXELLA

Gram-negative cocci or short bacilli arranged in pairs: strictly aerobic, non-motile, oxidase-positive. *M. lacunata* causes a purulent conjunctivitis.

MORAXELLA CATARRHALIS

Formerly classified as *Neisseria catarrhalis* and (more recently) as *Branhamella catarrhalis*, this bacterium shares many characteristics with the commensal neisseriae and grows well on ordinary media.

Laboratory characteristics

Identification: by biochemical tests.

Pathogenicity

This nasopharyngeal organism is now recognized as a cause of lower respiratory tract infection – especially in adults with pre-existing respiratory disease, such as chronic obstructive airways disease.

Antibiotic sensitivity

The majority of clinically significant strains are β-lactamase producers, and are resistant to penicillin and ampicillin but sensitive to tetracycline and erythromycin.

17. Bacillus

Members of the genus *Bacillus* are aerobic, sporing, Gram-positive, chaining bacilli. *Bacillus species* are ubiquitous soil saprophytes but one, *B. anthracis*, is an important pathogen responsible for anthrax in animals and humans. Anthrax is now rare in developed countries.

BACILLUS ANTHRACIS

Habitat: infected animals, but spores are found in soil and pasture contaminated with vegetative cells from dead and dying animals.

Laboratory characteristics

Morphology: large (4–8 × 1.5 μm), non-motile, rectangular bacilli usually arranged in chains. Spores – oval and central – are not formed in tissue, but develop after the organism is shed or if it is grown on artificial media. The bacilli are capsulated in the animal body and on laboratory culture under certain conditions: the capsule consists of a polypeptide of D-glutamic acid.

Staining: Gram-positive; spores can be stained by modified Ziehl–Neelsen method.

McFadyean's reaction is used to demonstrate *B. anthracis* in the blood of animals, in a heat-fixed film stained with polychrome methylene blue. *Observe*: blue bacilli surrounded by purplish-pink amorphous material, due to disintegrated capsules and indicating a positive reaction: diagnostic of *B. anthracis* (Fig. 17.1).

Culture: aerobe and facultative anaerobe; grows readily on ordinary media over a wide temperature range (optimum 35°C): best temperature for sporulation is lower, 25–30°C.

Colonies: are large, dense, grey-white, matt and irregular: they are composed of parallel chains of cells, and this gives the margin

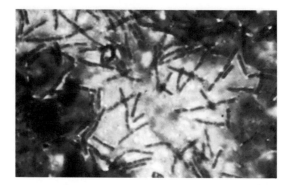

Fig. 17.1   *Bacillus anthracis*: McFadyean's reaction (approx. × 1000).

of the colony the so-called 'medusa head' or 'curled hair lock' appearance.

Blood agar: there is only slight haemolysis round the colony – a differential feature, because other *Bacillus species* are markedly haemolytic.

Broth cultures: develop a thick pellicle.

Gelatin stab cultures: show growth along the track of the wire, with lateral spikes longest near the surface – the 'inverted fir tree'; liquefaction is late, starting at the surface.

Antigenic structure: the antigenic components described include a complex group of toxins and the capsular polypeptide.

Pathogenicity

The cause of anthrax. A wide range of animal hosts is susceptible. Infection is characteristically septicaemic, with splenic enlargement. Humans are infected from animals or animal products.

Viability: vegetative cells are readily destroyed by heat, but spores demonstrate a variable, often high, level of heat resistance – in the dry state, up to 150°C for 1 h. Spores can remain viable for many years in contaminated soil.

Antibiotic sensitivity

B. anthracis is susceptible to many antibiotics: penicillin is the drug of choice.

OTHER BACILLUS SPECIES

Habitat: saprophytes in soil, water, dust and air and on vegetation.

Many species are recognized: some (e.g. *B. megaterium, B. cereus*) are large-celled like *B. anthracis*; others (e.g. *B. subtilis*) are small-celled and shorter and thinner with rounded ends. Saprophytic species differ from *B. anthracis* in being motile, non-capsulated and in producing a distinct zone of haemolysis around colonies on blood agar; furthermore, they fail to produce a fatal septicaemia in laboratory animals.

The spores of certain bacilli, e.g. *B. stearothermophilus, B. megaterium,* are used as a test of the efficiency of sterilization by steam under pressure (i.e. in autoclaves), by ethylene oxide or by ionizing radiation.

B. cereus is a cause of food poisoning (e.g. when contaminating rice). A number of species may cause opportunistic infections.

18. Clostridium

Clostridia are anaerobic, sporing, Gram-positive bacilli. Most species are soil saprophytes, but a few are pathogens. The most important are listed, with some of their principal properties, in Table 18.1.

Habitat: human and animal intestine; soil; water; decaying animal and plant matter.

Laboratory characteristics

Morphology and staining: large (3–8 × 0.5 μm) rods, sometimes pleomorphic; filamentous forms are common. Gram-positive, but may stain irregularly or be Gram-negative in older cultures.

Spores: all species form endospores, which may be 'bulging', i.e. wider than the bacterial body; sometimes useful in identification, e.g. *C. tetani*. Note that *C. perfringens* (the most common human pathogen) forms spores with difficulty.

Motile, with peritrichous flagella (*C. perfringens* is non-motile).

Table 18.1 Pathogenic properties of the main medically important species of clostridia

Species	Disease
C. perfringens	Gas gangrene, food poisoning
C. novyi	Gas gangrene
C. septicum	Gas gangrene, neutropenic enterocolitis
C. histolyticum	Secondary role in gas gangrene
C. sordellii	Secondary role in gas gangrene
C. difficile	Antibiotic-associated colitis
C. sporogenes	Doubtful pathogenicity in gas gangrene
C. tetani *	Tetanus
C. botulinum	Botulism

*Forms round, terminal spores; the other species have oval, central, subterminal or terminal spores.

127

Capsule: *C. perfringens* has a capsule, but most are non-capsulated.

Culture:

Blood agar anaerobically: in mixed culture, addition of an amino-glycoside makes an excellent selective medium for clostridia.

Robertson's meat medium.

Anaerobic requirement: variable. *C. tetani* and *C. novyi* are exacting anaerobes; *C. perfringens* and *C. histolyticum* can grow in the presence of limited amounts of oxygen.

Colonial morphology: the main human pathogenic species show three types of colonial morphology:

1. *C. perfringens*: round, opaque colonies; usually surrounded by a zone of β-haemolysis on blood agar.

2. *C. tetani, C. septicum*: irregular, translucent colonies with thin spreading edges on the surface of moist agar; marked tendency to swarm, especially *C. tetani*.

3. *C. novyi, C. sporogenes, C. botulinum*: matt to glossy colonies, the centre of which may be raised; margins irregular with filamentous rhizoid outgrowths; limited swarming may take place.

Biochemical activity:

Saccharolytic: many species ferment sugars; this produces reddening of the meat particles in Robertson's meat medium, with a rancid smell.

Proteolytic: production of enzymes that digest proteins is a common property of many clostridia: this causes blackening and digestion of the meat particles in Robertson's meat medium, with a foul smell. Although most clostridia liquefy gelatin, only those with considerable proteolytic activity are able to liquefy coagulated serum and egg.

Toxins: medically important clostridial species produce several toxins: the exotoxins of *C. tetani* and *C. botulinum* are amongst the most toxic substances known. Clostridial toxins are often lethal for laboratory animals.

Classification: the range of saccharolytic and proteolytic activity; tests for lecithinase and lipase activity; and detection of the fatty acid end-products of glucose metabolism (by gas chromatography) are used in classification.

Identification: often difficult; the characteristics and identification of four important pathogenic clostridia – *C. perfringens, C. tetani, C. botulinum and C. difficile* – are described below.

Antibiotic sensitivity

Sensitive to penicillin, metronidazole, clindamycin, tetracycline, erythromycin.

Resistant to aminoglycosides.

CLOSTRIDIUM PERFRINGENS (CLOSTRIDIUM WELCHII)

Laboratory characteristics

Morphology: a stubby bacillus, in which spores are hardly ever seen.

Culture: most strains grow well on blood agar anaerobically, producing β-haemolytic colonies, but some strains are non-haemolytic.

Biochemical activity: mainly saccharolytic: in tube cultures of litmus milk, a characteristic 'stormy clot' is formed due to the production of acid and large amounts of gas.

Typing: C. perfringens can be divided into five types – A, B, C, D and E – on the basis of the 12 toxins formed; all five types produce α toxin. Type A is the human pathogen; the other types are important pathogens of domestic animals.

Toxins:

1. *Alpha (α) toxin*: an enzyme, phospholipase C, which causes cell lysis due to lecithinase action on the lecithin in mammalian cell membranes.

2. *Other toxins*: include collagenase, proteinase, hyaluronidase, deoxyribonuclease. Several have haemolytic activity: some are described as 'necrotizing' or 'lethal', from their effects on laboratory animals.

Identification: the *Nagler reaction* identifies *C. perfringens* by neutralization of α toxin with specific antitoxin. Colonies are streaked on an agar plate containing egg yolk (which contains lecithin), half of the plate having been spread with antitoxin. A dense opacity is produced by growth of *C. perfringens* on the untreated half of the plate, but there is no opacity on the area with antitoxin (Fig. 18.1).

Pathogenicity

- *Gas gangrene*: wounds associated with the necrosis of muscle may become infected with *C. perfringens* and other clostridia,

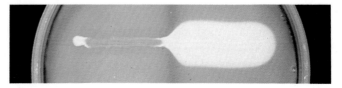

Fig. 18.1 Nagler reaction. The alpha toxin (a lecithinase) of *Clostridium perfringens* has produced opacity due to degradation of lecithin in the medium on the right. This action has been neutralized by the antitoxin on the left of the plate.

causing a severe and life-threatening spreading infection of the muscles.
- *Food poisoning*: when ingested in large numbers, some strains of *C. perfringens* produce an enterotoxin in the gut, causing diarrhoea and other symptoms of food poisoning.

CLOSTRIDIUM TETANI

Laboratory characteristics

Morphology: a longer, thinner bacillus than *C. perfringens*, with round terminal spores giving a characteristic 'drumstick' appearance (Fig. 18.2).

Toxin: a protein, and exceedingly potent. There are two components:
- *Tetanospasmin*: neurotoxic – the true tetanus toxin.
- *Tetanolysin*: haemolytic.

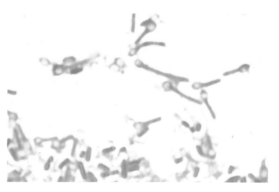

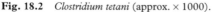

Fig. 18.2 *Clostridium tetani* (approx. × 1000).

Identification: by toxin neutralization tests:

In vitro: culture on a blood agar plate half-spread with tetanus antitoxin. Observation of haemolysis inhibited by the antiserum makes a presumptive identification: confirm, if necessary, by mouse inoculation.

In vivo: a fluid culture is injected into mice, some of which have been protected by previous inoculation of tetanus antitoxin. In a positive result, the unprotected animals die with typical tetanic spasms; protected animals survive.

Pathogenicity

The cause of tetanus – a classical toxin-mediated disease in which *C.tetani* in a wound elaborates the powerful neurotoxin, which spreads and acts on the central nervous system, causing severe muscle spasms.

CLOSTRIDIUM BOTULINUM

Laboratory characteristics

Toxin: protein, and even more potent than that of *C. tetani*, the toxin of *C. botulinum* is the most active known poison. It acts by preventing the release of acetylcholine at motor nerve endings in the parasympathetic system. Destroyed in 2 min at 60–90°C, dependent on type. There are seven *toxin types* – A, B, C, D, E, F and G – with serologically distinct but pharmacologically similar toxins.

Human botulism is usually due to toxin types A, B and E.

Identification: by testing for the toxin in a culture, patient's serum or food sample. Mice, some of which are protected with antitoxin to A, B and E toxins, are injected with the suspect material: if toxin is present, mice inoculated with the appropriate antitoxin survive; the others become paralyzed and die.

Pathogenicity

Produces a rare form of 'food poisoning' known as *botulism*, in which the symptoms are neurological rather than intestinal. It is caused by the ingestion of preformed toxin in food contaminated with the organism.

CLOSTRIDIUM DIFFICILE

Habitat: found in the faeces of 3–5% of healthy adults, and regularly present in the faeces of healthy infants. Found with its toxin in the faeces of patients suffering from antibiotic-associated colitis: in its severe form, this becomes pseudomembranous colitis.

Laboratory characteristics

Identification:
- *Isolation*: from faeces using selective media, e.g. cefoxitin-cycloserine-fructose agar; anaerobic incubation. Cultures produce a characteristic 'dung-like' aroma, and the irregular rough colonies fluoresce under ultraviolet light. Gas-liquid chromatography of pure broth subcultures demonstrates a characteristic pattern of volatile fatty acids.
- *Demonstration of toxin* by inoculation of cell cultures (e.g. human embryo fibroblasts) with broth culture of *C. difficile*: cell cultures containing antitoxin are also inoculated. *Observe*: cytotoxicity which is neutralized in the cultures containing *C. difficile* antitoxin. All enteropathogenic isolates of *C. difficile* are toxigenic.

Note: This test can be carried out on faeces, to demonstrate directly the presence of toxin.

Typing: a molecular typing scheme, using a PCR (polymerase chain reaction) method, is available: of value in investigating hospital outbreaks.

19. Bacteroides and other non-sporing anaerobes

The genera of non-sporing anaerobes are:

	Gram-positive	Gram-negative
Bacilli	Bifidobacterium Propionibacterium (see Ch. 13) Eubacterium	Bacteroides Prevotella Porphyromonas Fusobacterium Leptotrichia
Cocci	Peptostreptococcus	Veillonella

ANAEROBIC GRAM-NEGATIVE BACILLI

The classification of these organisms is complex, and there have been many revisions. Until recently, the genus *Bacteroides* included organisms now placed in the genera *Prevotella* and *Porphyromonas*. For the sake of simplicity and to conform with current terminology in clinical practice, the term 'bacteroides' is used elsewhere in this book as an all-embracing term for non-sporing Gram-negative anaerobic bacilli.

Habitat:

Colon: Gram-negative anaerobic bacilli are present in enormous numbers in the faeces (10^{10}/g or more). The majority belong to the genus *Bacteroides*, mostly *B. vulgatus*, *B. distasonis* and *B. fragilis*.

Female genital tract: Gram-negative anaerobic bacilli are common in the cervix and vaginal fornices: prevotella, mostly *P. melaninogenica*, predominate; porphyromonas is also common.

Mouth: always found in large numbers in the normal mouth. Most are prevotella, the commonest species being *P. oralis*; fusobacteria and leptotrichia are also present.

Laboratory characteristics

Morphology and staining: small, ovoid or short, Gram-negative, non-motile, non-sporing bacilli. Fusobacteria and leptotrichia tend to be long and spindle-shaped, but pleomorphism is common.

Culture: strict anaerobes: require media enriched with blood or haemin; the growth of many strains is improved by the addition of menadione (vitamin K3).

Fluid media: Robertson's cooked meat broth, preferably enriched: the medium should be boiled and promptly cooled before use, to remove dissolved oxygen and so improve anaerobiasis.

Selective media: incorporation of antibiotics to which 'bacteroides' are resistant aids isolation from mixed cultures, e.g. blood agar containing an aminoglycoside (neomycin, kanamycin, gentamicin) or an aminoglycoside and vancomycin.

Incubate: anaerobically with 10% carbon dioxide (which enhances growth) for a minimum of 48 h.

Observe:

- *Bacteroides*: light grey, opaque or translucent colonies, usually 1–2 mm in diameter after 48 h incubation.
- *Prevotella* slower growing than *Bacteroides*: *P. melaningogenica* characteristically produces black or brown pigmented colonies on blood agar, which fluoresce brick-red when exposed to long-wave ultraviolet light; *P. oralis* and some other species in this group are non-pigmented.
- *Porphyromonas*: slower growing than *Bacteroides*. *P. asaccharolytica* produces black or brown colonies on blood agar, similar to the pigmented colonies of *Prevotella*.
- *Fusobacteria*: some species produce dull granular colonies, which may be rhizoid or irregular.
- *Leptotrichia*: colonies are convoluted and often striate.

Identification: most anaerobes can be identified to generic level by the examination of Gram-stained smear, colonial morphology, growth inhibition by bile salts, antibiotic resistance, and gas chromatographical analysis of the fatty acid end-products of glucose metabolism. Species differentiation is time-consuming and costly, requiring biochemical tests, and is rarely attempted by routine diagnostic laboratories.

Pathogenicity

The most common isolate from clinical specimens is *B. fragilis*, and thus this species seems to have a special pathogenic potential.

Gram-negative anaerobic bacilli are important in abdominal and gynaecological (including puerperal) sepsis: they are usually found along with other organisms, notably coliform organisms. It appears that these combinations of anaerobic and aerobic bacteria potentiate the ability of each other to cause infection – *pathogenic synergy*.

Gram-negative anaerobic bacilli are also responsible for dental, periodontal and oropharyngeal disease.

Vincent's infection (Fig. 22.3) is caused by *Borrelia vincenti* in association with a variety of Gram-negative anaerobic bacilli, including one or more of *Prevotella intermedia*, *Fusobacterium nucleatum* and *Leptotrichia buccalis*.

Antibiotic sensitivity

Like other anaerobes, these organisms are sensitive to metronidazole. Many are also sensitive to clindamycin, chloramphenicol and cefoxitin.

Bacteroides are penicillin-resistant due to β-lactamase production, but many strains of the other genera are penicillin-sensitive. There is uniform resistance to the aminoglycosides.

BIFIDOBACTERIUM

Bifidobacterium is a genus of diverse, non-pathogenic bacteria. *B. bifidum* is the type species.

Habitat: dominant members of the colonic flora of infants (classically the breast-fed) and common also in the adult gut; normally present in the human vagina.

Laboratory characteristics

Morphology and staining: pleomorphic Gram-positive bacilli, characterized by club-shaped rods and by branching forms which are often Y-shaped; non-sporing, non-motile.

Culture: strict anaerobes.

ANAEROBIC COCCI

The classification of this heterogeneous group is confused. They must be clearly separated from microaerophilic and carbon dioxide-requiring cocci, which in the past have often been incorrectly considered anaerobic. One simple differential test is sensitivity to metronidazole: truly obligate anaerobic cocci are metronidazole-sensitive; the others are resistant.

Gram-positive anaerobic cocci are vancomycin-sensitive and are classified in the genus *Peptostreptococcus*. Gram-negative anaerobic cocci are vancomycin-resistant and are placed in the genus *Veillonella*.

Habitat: commensals in the skin, oropharynx, colon and female genital tract.

Pathogenicity

Local sepsis, in mixed infections with anaerobic Gram-negative bacilli and aerobes.

20. Lactobacillus

Members of this genus are widely distributed as saprophytes in vegetable and animal material (e.g. milk, cheese); others are common human and animal commensals.

Classification is complex. Lactobacilli attack carbohydrates to form abundant acid, and are tolerant of an acid environment (pH 3.0–4.0). The best-recognized species is *L. acidophilus*.

LACTOBACILLUS ACIDOPHILUS

Habitat: present in the mouth, gastrointestinal tract and female genital tract – most vaginal lactobacilli (Döderlein's bacilli) seem to be *L. acidophilus*.

Laboratory characteristics

Morphology and staining: large, often thick $(1–5 \times 1 \, \mu m)$ Gram-positive bacilli; non-branching, non-motile, non-sporing.

Culture: grows best, but slowly, under microaerophilic conditions in the presence of 5% CO_2 and at pH 6.0.

Selective media: acid media, e.g. tomato juice agar (pH 5.0), support the growth of lactobacilli but inhibit many other bacteria.

Pathogenicity

Lactobacilli are associated with dental caries.

21. Legionella and related genera

Legionella is a genus of which the base composition of the DNA is distinct from that of other bacteria.

There are 39 recognized species of legionellae but *L. pneumophila* is by far the most important human pathogen.

LEGIONELLA PNEUMOPHILA

The most common infecting strain is Serogroup 1.

Habitat: an environmental organism found in soil and water (including domestic water supplies and air-conditioning units).

Laboratory characteristics

Morphology and staining: slender rods. Gram-negative, but legionellae sometimes do not stain well.

Culture: requires media with iron and cysteine for isolation: use buffered charcoal yeast extract agar supplemented with L-cysteine and ferric pyrophosphate. *Incubate* for 21 days at 35–37°C in 5% carbon dioxide; colonies usually appear in 3–5 days.

Identification: by direct immunofluorescence.

Diagnosis is most often serological: however, better culture media are now increasing the rate of isolation from clinical material.

Table 21.1 Some species of legionella associated with human infection

*L. pneumophilia**	*L. dumoffii*
L. micadadei	*L. feeleii*
L. bozemanii	*L. longbeachae*

*Serogroup 1 is the most common infecting strain.
Note: Several other species have been reported as the cause of isolated cases of infection of occasional small outbreaks.

139

Pathogenicity

L. pneumophila serogroup 1 is the major cause of Legionnaires' disease – a severe form of pneumonia – and of the less serious respiratory disease, Pontiac fever. Other species also cause pneumonia – most often in immunocompromised patients.

Antibiotic sensitivity

Sensitive to erythromycin and rifampicin.

22. Spirochaetes

Spirochaetes are a group of helical organisms which share many properties with Gram-negative bacteria. Three genera contain species pathogenic to humans: *Treponema*, *Borrelia* and *Leptospira*.

Habitat: most are free-living and non-pathogenic, but a few are causes of important human disease.

Laboratory characteristics

Morphology and staining: unique helical structure, with a central protoplasmic cylinder bounded by a cytoplasmic membrane and cell wall of similar structure to that of Gram-negative bacteria (see Fig. 2.3). Between a thin peptidoglycan layer and the outer membrane run the *axial filaments*, now regarded as internal flagella. These are fixed at the extremities of the organism and meet to overlap in the middle of the cell. They constrict and distort the bacterial cell body to give rise to the typical helical structure (Fig. 22.1).

The larger spirochaetes (e.g. *Borrelia* species) are Gram-negative. Others stain poorly or not at all by the usual methods. Spirochaetes

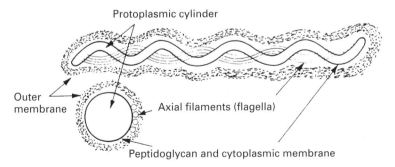

Fig. 22.1 The structure of a spirochaete.

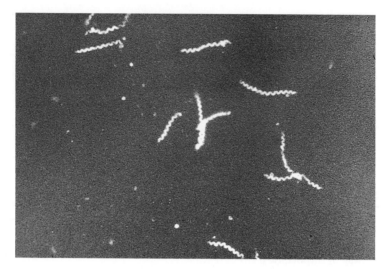

Fig. 22.2   Dark-ground photomicrograph of *Treponema pallidum*. (Reproduced with permission from Abbott Laboratories *Slide Atlas of Infectious Diseases*, 1982, Gower Medical Publishing, London. Photograph by Dr R.D. Caterall.)

are too slender and weakly refractile to be seen with the ordinary light microscope, but can be rendered visible by dark-ground microscopy (Fig. 22.2), by staining with heavy metals (e.g. silver), or by immunofluorescence.

Motile by:

● rotation about the long axis
● flexion
● true movement, i.e. from one site to another.

Antibiotic sensitivity

Sensitive to penicillin and a number of other antibiotics. Anaerobic spirochaetes are also sensitive to metronidazole.

GENERA

Three genera contain human pathogenic species:

1. Treponema
2. Borrelia
3. Leptospira.

TREPONEMA

The main treponemes are:
  T. pallidum
  T. pertenue
  T. carateum.
Morphologically indistinguishable from, and antigenically similar to, each other: cannot be cultivated in vitro.

Other treponemes are found as commensals in the mouth, genital secretions and intestine.

TREPONEMA PALLIDUM

Habitat: the lesions of primary and secondary syphilis.

Laboratory characteristics

Morphology: long, slender filamentous helices, with 6–12 evenly-spaced coils.

  Culture: cannot be cultivated in vitro, but can be propagated by inoculation of rabbit testes.

  Identification: in material from primary and secondary clinical lesions, by dark-ground or phase-contrast microscopy.

Pathogenicity

Cause of the sexually transmitted disease, syphilis.

  Viability: a strict parasite that dies rapidly outside the body; it is very sensitive to drying and to heat.

TREPONEMA PALLIDUM, SUBSPECIES *PERTENUE*

The cause of yaws, a chronic relapsing non-venereal treponematosis widespread in the tropics: characterized by ulcerative and granulomatous lesions in skin, mucous membranes and bone.

TREPONEMA CARATEUM

The cause of pinta, a non-venereal treponematosis with lesions confined to the skin. It affects dark-skinned people in Central and

South America, causing hyperkeratosis and depigmentation of skin.

OTHER TREPONEMES

A number of species are found as commensals in the mouth, genital secretions and intestine.

Some can be grown in vitro anaerobically.

BORRELIA

BORRELIA VINCENTI

Habitat: the oropharynx, as a commensal and potential pathogen.

Laboratory characteristics

Morphology and staining: large spirochaetes with three to eight irregular open coils; Gram-negative.

Culture: can be grown, with difficulty, in serum-enriched media; a strict anaerobe.

Identification: in exudates from clinical lesions by morphology, in Gram-stained film (Fig. 22.3).

Pathogenicity

In association with anaerobic fusiform bacilli (e.g. *Leptotrichia buccalis*), responsible for gingivostomatitis and Vincent's angina.

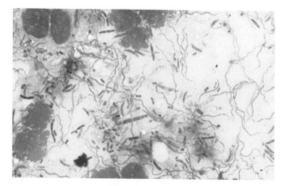

Fig. 22.3   Vincent's angina: film (approx. × 1000).

Antibiotic sensitivity

Pencillin.

BORRELIA BURGDORFERI

Habitat: ticks, small mammals, deer.
   Spread: by ticks of the genus *Ixodes*.

Laboratory characteristics

Morphology: flexible helical spirochaete; Gram-negative.
   Culture: microaerophilic, grows at 34°C in special medium.
   Serology: diagnose by detection of antibody by immuno-
fluorescence or ELISA.

Pathogenicity

The cause of Lyme disease – a generalized infection with arthritis,
neurological and cardiac complications; there is a characteristic
rash which spreads from the initial tick bite – *erythema chronicum
migrans*.

Antibiotic sensitivity

Amoxycillin, tetracycline.

BORRELIA RECURRENTIS: the cause of louse-borne relapsing
fever.

BORRELIA DUTTONI AND OTHER SPECIES: the causes of
tick-borne relapsing fever.
   Both diseases are encountered in parts of Asia, Africa and
South America.
   Relapsing fever is characterized by febrile episodes alternating
with afebrile periods, and lasts for several weeks. Each relapse is
the result of a change in the antigenic structure of the organism:
antibodies already formed are ineffective against the new variants.

Antibiotic sensitivity

Tetracyclines.

LEPTOSPIRA

Two species are recognized: *L. interrogans* and *L. biflexa*. *L. interrogans* contains two important human pathogenic serogroups: *L. icterohaemorrhagiae* and *L. canicola*, of which the most important reservoirs are rats (*L. icterohaemorrhagiae*) and pigs and dogs (*L. canicola*).

Habitat: Leptospires are found in moist environments. *L. biflexa* is a saprophyte present in pools, ditches and streams. *L. interrogans* is harboured in the kidneys of some rodents and domestic animals.

Laboratory characteristics

Morphology: spiral organisms 5–20 × 0.1 μm, with very numerous closely-set coils and hooked ends.

Culture: obligate aerobes; grow in enriched fluid or semi-solid media; optimum temperature is around 30°C.

Identification: serological.

Pathogenicity

L. interrogans is the cause of the zoonotic disease leptospirosis.

Viability: pathogenic strains may survive for days outside the animal body in moist surroundings, as long as they are not acid.

Antibiotic sensitivity

Penicillin, tetracyclines.

23. Mycoplasma

Mycoplasmas are bacteria which lack cell walls. They are bounded by the cytoplasmic membrane and resemble L-forms of bacteria but, unlike them, are independent naturally-occurring micro-organisms.

Table 23.1 lists some of the better-known mycoplasmas and their habitats. T-strain mycoplasmas form minute colonies ('T'=tiny), and are now classified in the genus *Ureaplasma*. Some mycoplasmas with less exacting growth requirements have been assigned to a separate genus, *Acholeplasma*.

Mycoplasmas are a common contaminant of cell lines, their persistence favoured by the presence of penicillin and other antibiotics in the tissue culture media. They are derived from the mouth of those handling the cells, from constituents of the medium, e.g. serum, and from cross-infection between cell cultures.

Laboratory characteristics

Morphology and staining: pleomorphic; several different forms exist, varying from small spherical shapes to longer branching

Table 23.1 Mycoplasmas and related organisms

Genus, species	Habitat
M. pneumoniae	Human respiratory tract
M. orale *M. salivarium*	Human mouth
M. hominis *M. genitalium*	Human genital, and possibly respiratory, tracts
Ureaplasma urealyticum	Human genitourinary tract
Acholeplasma laidlawii	Soil, water

filaments. Gram-negative, but stain poorly with Gram's stain; colonies on agar are best demonstrated after staining by the Dienes' method.

Culture: on semi-solid enriched medium containing 20% horse serum, yeast extract and DNA; incubate aerobically for 7–12 days with CO_2, or in nitrogen with added CO_2. *Observe:* typical 'fried-egg' colonies, embedded into the surface of the medium.

Identification of isolates: by inhibition of growth round discs impregnated with specific antisera, or by immunofluorescence on colonies transferred to glass slides.

Pathogenicity

Mycoplasma pneumoniae

The main pathogenic member of the group: it is a major respiratory pathogen responsible for one form of atypical pneumonia. It also causes febrile bronchitis and milder upper respiratory infections.

Ureaplasma urealyticum (T-strain mycoplasma)

Implicated in, although not the major cause of, nonspecific urethritis, vaginitis and cervicitis. Rarely, can cause respiratory disease in preterm infants due to transfer of infection from the mother.

Mycoplasma hominis

Has been implicated in some cases of gynaecological or post-partum sepsis. An unusual cause of atypical pneumonia.

Antibiotic sensitivity

Sensitive to tetracycline – the drug of choice for treatment – and also to erythromycin.

Mycoplasmas are resistant to antibiotics that interfere with bacterial cell wall synthesis, e.g. penicillin.

Bacterial disease

24. Normal flora

The normal human body has a profuse flora of commensal bacteria, which exist in a symbiotic equilibrium with the host. Many of the commensals are potential pathogens.

Infection may result if this equilibrium is disturbed:

- by some breach of the body's defences
- if a parasite of greater pathogenicity is acquired
- if an organism which is commensal at one site gains access to another where it is not (e.g. *Escherichia coli*, resident in the colon, entering and infecting the urinary tract).

Virtually all 'unequivocal' pathogens may be encountered in healthy carriers.

Bacteriologists need a detailed knowledge of the normal flora, because many specimens cultured in the laboratory yield commensal bacteria as well as those causing infection. The interpretation of the results of culture needs both knowledge and experience.

Change and composition: the normal flora is not static and is subject to constant change: individual components wax and wane.

Beneficial role: the presence of the normal flora prevents other more pathogenic bacteria from gaining a foothold in the body. Gut bacteria seem to be responsible for the normal structure and function of the intestine: they degrade mucins, epithelial cells and carbohydrate fibre and their metabolism produces vitamins, especially vitamin K.

Alteration by antibiotics: broad-spectrum drugs can disrupt the composition of the normal flora by inhibiting sensitive organisms and allowing overgrowth of resistant bacteria. As a rule, the host can cope with these changes, but they occasionally result in serious infection.

Distribution: The internal organs, e.g. bladder, kidneys, bronchi, lungs, CNS, are sterile in health, with the exception of the alimentary tract. Effective local defence mechanisms maintain the sterility of these sites; in addition, complement and antibodies in serum and tissue fluids promote the powerful phagocytic activity of the polymorphonuclear leucocytes.

The main bacterial species which make up the normal flora of the different sites of the body are described below.

RESPIRATORY TRACT

The lower respiratory tract is sterile, but the upper tract is colonized – heavily in the case of the mouth and nasopharynx (Table 24.1). Saliva contains about 10^8 bacteria/ml; gingival-margin debris and dental plaque consist almost entirely of microorganisms.

GASTROINTESTINAL TRACT

The oesophagus has a flora similar to that of the pharynx. The empty stomach is sterile due to gastric acid.

The normal flora of the duodenum, jejunum and upper ileum is scanty but the large intestine is very heavily colonized with bacteria (Table 24.2).

Faeces contain enormous numbers of bacteria, which constitute up to one-third of the faecal weight. The majority of these bacteria seem to be dead. The number of living bacteria in faeces is about

Table 24.1   Main bacteria of the upper respiratory tract

Nose	Staphylococcus epidermidis Staphylococcus aureus Corynebacteria	
Oropharynx	Viridans streptococci Commensal neisseriae Corynebacteria 'Bacteroides' Fusobacteria Spirochaetes Lactobacilli Veillonella and other anaerobic cocci Actinomyces	
	Haemophilus influenzae Streptococcus pneumoniae }	Important potential pathogens
	Less common: Streptococcus pyogenes Neisseria meningitidis	

Table 24.2   Main bacteria of the large intestine

'Bacteroides' (mainly members of the genus *Bacteroides*)
Bifidobacteria
Anaerobic cocci
Escherichia coli
Enterococci
Clostridia
Lactobacilli

Less common inhabitants:
   Klebsiella species
   Proteus species
   Enterobacter species
   Pseudomonas aeruginosa

10^{10}/g, and almost all (99.9%) are anaerobes: the anaerobic environment of the colon is maintained by aerobic bacteria utilizing any free oxygen.

Bifidobacteria and *Bacteroides species* are the dominant anaerobes. Bifidobacteria are Gram-positive bacilli somewhat similar to lactobacilli, but are strict anaerobes; like lactobacilli they are virtually non-pathogenic. *Bacteroides fragilis* is a considerably rarer gut inhabitant than other *Bacteroides species*, but has much greater potential for pathogenicity.

GENITAL TRACT

For anatomical reasons, the female genital tract is much more heavily colonized than that of the male. Normal vaginal secretions contain up to 10^8 bacteria/ml, and 98% of them are lactobacilli. The genital flora is listed in Table 24.3.

Note: The secretions of both male and female genitalia may contain *Mycobacterium smegmatis* – acid-fast bacilli which, if they contaminate urine specimens, can easily be mistaken for tubercle bacilli.

Mycoplasma: Strains of mycoplasma, including T-strains or ureaplasma, which form minute colonies on culture, are commonly present as part of the normal genital flora of both sexes.

SKIN

Skin has a rich resident bacterial flora (estimated at 10^4 organisms/cm^2). It is not evenly distributed: the bacteria exist in microcolonies of 10^2–10^3 organisms.

Table 24.3 Main flora of the male and female genital tracts

Female	
Vulva	*Staphylococcus epidermidis*
	Corynebacteria
	Escherichia coli and other coliforms
	Enterococci
	Yeasts
Vagina	Lactobacilli (known as Döderlein's bacilli)
	'Bacteroides' (especially *Prevotella melaninogenica*)
	Enterococci
	Corynebacteria
	Gardnerella vaginalis
	Yeasts
Male and female	
Distal urethra	*Staphylococcus epidermidis*
	Corynebacteria

Anaerobic organisms predominate, particularly in areas with many sebaceous glands, where anaerobic conditions prevail. In moist skin, e.g. that of the axilla and groin, coliform organisms are often present (Table 24.4).

External auditory meatus

An extension of the skin, and often profusely colonized: the main species found are *Staphylococcus epidermidis* and corynebacteria. Acid-fast mycobacteria are occasionally present in the wax.

Conjunctival sac

Bacteria are scanty: occasionally *Corynebacterium xerosis* and *Staphylococcus epidermidis* are found.

Table 24.4 Main bacteria of the skin flora

Propionibacterium acnes	
Anaerobic cocci	
Staphylococcus epidermidis	
Micrococci	
Corynebacteria	
Less common:	
Staphylococcus aureus	This potential pathogen is present in up to 50% of normal adults
Coliforms	

25. Host-parasite relationship

Infection is the result of breakdown in the host-parasite relationship, and follows when the balance is tipped in favour of the parasite.

The human 'host' *lives in general balance with his environment*. This environment includes numerous bacteria found in all sites, animate and inanimate, with which humans come into contact: most important is their own normal flora.

Bacterial disease is mostly due to organisms which form – at least from time to time – part of the commensal flora. There are exceptions, however – some pathogenic bacteria are never commensal, and are found only in disease.

Selection pressure favours the survival of bacteria with limited pathogenicity which can maintain a symbiotic relationship with their host. Virulent pathogens, which severely incapacitate or kill humans, are denied the opportunity to spread within a community because their host is no longer able to circulate and come into contact with other individuals: human beings are gregarious, but only when they are healthy.

DEFENCE MECHANISMS OF THE HOST

Host factors influence the outcome of host-parasite interaction. Some factors are linked with socio-economic status, e.g. malnutrition, poverty and overcrowding – conditions that also favour the transmission of a virulent pathogen within a community. Some host factors are listed below:

1. *Nutrition*: malnutrition (e.g. vitamin or protein deficiency) predisposes to infection.
2. *Age*: the very young (especially preterm neonates) and the aged are particularly liable to infection.
3. *Gender*: rarely important; occasionally attributable to occupational risks.

155

4. *Race:* sometimes a factor, e.g. black people are more susceptible than white people to tuberculosis.
5. *Occupation:* some occupations (e.g. those associated with inhalation of minerals) are associated with a higher than normal risk of infection with certain microorganisms (such as *Mycobacterium tuberculosis*).
6. *Impairment of the host immune response,* by:
   - treatment, e.g. immunosuppressive, cytotoxic or steroid drugs; radiotherapy
   - disease, e.g. malignancy (especially of the lymphoid system), metabolic diseases (diabetes, renal or hepatic failure).

The host has a number of defence mechanisms with which to counteract bacterial aggression. There are two categories of defence mechanisms:

1. *Nonspecific:* not directed at a particular organism and non-immunological.

2. *Specific:* directed against a particular organism, and dependent on immunological mechanisms. Once established, protection is long-lasking and can be mobilized rapidly due to *immunological memory.*

NONSPECIFIC DEFENCE MECHANISMS

Skin

Skin is a tough layer or integument, which forms an excellent and generally impermeable barrier to invasion of the tissues by organisms from either the normal flora of the skin or the environment. When this barrier is breached, e.g. by a surgical or traumatic wound, infection is frequent.

Normal flora

The normal flora can make it difficult for exogenous pathogens to establish themselves. Substances with antibacterial activity, such as fatty acids, are produced by skin flora from glycerides in sebum and by intestinal anaerobes from the contents of the colon.

The term *colonization resistance* has been used to describe the predominant microflora which imparts resistance to infection. For example, within the gastrointestinal tract the maintenance of a predominantly anaerobic population is beneficial to the host, especially during antibiotic therapy: it is said to prevent super-infection by coliform organisms following either overgrowth of endogenous flora or colonization by exogenous bacteria.

Lysozyme

Lysozyme is an enzyme found in tears and other body fluids, which lyses the mucopeptide of the cell wall of Gram-positive bacteria.

Flushing action

Tears: contain lysozyme: tears keep the surface of the eye sterile.

Respiratory tract mucus: traps bacteria and constantly moves them upwards, propelled by cilia on the cells of the epithelium.

Urine: voiding helps to flush out bacteria that have gained entry to the bladder.

Low pH

Stomach: ingested bacteria are usually destroyed by the low pH of stomach acid; this can, of course, be buffered by food.

Vaginal secretions in young women have acid pH due to lactobacilli, which metabolize glycogen present in the epithelium because of circulating oestrogens: the lactic acid produced prevents access of harmful bacteria.

Phagocytosis

Phagocytosis is a powerful defence mechanism, mediated by scavenger cells which ingest invading organisms and destroy them intra-cellularly by enzyme action.

There are two types of phagocyte:

1. *Neutrophil polymorphonuclear leucocytes ('polymorphs')*: also known as *microphages*. They are produced in the bone marrow and, when mature, circulate in the bloodstream for 6–7 h. These short-lived cells arrive rapidly at the scene of infection, attracted by chemotactic substances elaborated during the inflammatory process. Specific antibody and complement act as *opsonins* – substances which bind to bacteria and increase their susceptibility to phagocytosis.

Polymorphs, part of the early defence against infection, are the 'pus cells' seen in the exudate from acute infections.

2. *Macrophages of the mononuclear phagocyte system.* Produced in bone marrow, they travel as *monocytes* in the blood-stream to become distributed as *free macrophages* – in lung alveoli, the peritoneum and inflammatory granulomas – or *fixed macrophages*, integrated into the tissues – in lymph nodes, spleen, liver (Kupffer cells), CNS (microglia) and connective tissue (histiocytes). Phagocytosis by these long-lived cells can be either nonspecific or promoted by antibody and complement.

Macrophages participate in the resolution of the acute inflammatory response, and they are very important cells in chronic inflammation. In addition, they process bacterial antigens and present them to lymphocytes to stimulate a specific immune response. They are also involved in cell-mediated immunity. Many of these functions are initiated and regulated by a variety of chemical mediators (e.g. the interleukins, tumour necrosis factor) collectively known as *cytokines*.

Phagocytic function can be divided into four stages:

1. *Chemotaxis*: attraction of the phagocyte to the site of the organism.

2. *Attachment (adherence)* of the bacterium, often previously opsonized, to the membrane of the phagocyte.

3. *Ingestion*, in which the phagocytic cell extends small pseudopods to envelop the bacterium: these fuse to form a pouch or *phagosome*. Lysosomes containing hydrolytic enzymes and other bactericidal substances migrate towards the phagosome, and fuse with its membrane to form a *phagolysosome*.

4. *Intracellular killing* of the ingested bacterium: most bacteria are killed within a few minutes of phagocytosis, although the degradation of the bacterial cell may take several hours.

Complement

A family of proteins present in serum: these react together one after another in a cascade, following activation of the first stage by the combination of specific antibody with a bacterial or other antigen: the sequential reaction liberates fragments that attract phagocytic cells by chemotaxis, promote subsequent phagocytosis (opsonization) and induce the changes characteristic of the inflammatory reaction.

SPECIFIC DEFENCE MECHANISMS – THE IMMUNE SYSTEM IN INFECTION

There are two main mechanisms by which the host mounts a specific immune response against bacterial infection:

1. **The humoral (antibody) response**
2. **The cell-mediated response**.

Antibody response

Antibodies are proteins in the bloodstream produced in response to infection by microorganisms. They are specifically directed against the *antigens* of the microorganism or its component parts – which are usually proteins but occasionally carbohydrates. The stimulation of antibody production by antigens is an *immune response*.

When an antigen, e.g. on a bacterium, encounters *B- (bone marrow derived) lymphocytes* in the secondary lymphoid organs (e.g. spleen, lymph nodes), the lymphocytes are activated and transformed into antibody-secreting *plasma cells*. The antigen is presented by macrophages and the involvement of *T-lymphocytes*, especially T-helper cells, is required to initiate the immune response to some antigens.

Structure of antibodies

Antibodies are *immunoglobulins* (Ig) – protein molecules of high molecular weight. Their structure is Y-shaped and consists of an *Fc fragment* (the stem of the Y) and two *Fab fragments* (the arms of the Y). The Fab fragments contain the combining sites for specific antigens and, in antibodies to different antigens, show highly variable amino acid sequences. The Fc fragment of different antibodies, on the other hand, has a relatively constant amino acid composition and is the site for the attachment of complement. In addition, the Fc fragment is recognized by specific receptors in the membrane of phagocytic cells during opsonophagocytosis.

Although there are five types of immunoglobulin, only three are involved in the response to infection. These are:

1. **IgM**: a pentamer of IgG of molecular weight 1.0×10^6 – the first antibody produced: appears approximately 1 week after infection and persists for about 4–6 weeks.

2. **IgG**: a monomer of molecular weight 1.6×10^5 – the main antibody produced: appears about 2 weeks after infection, and persists for long periods of time.

3. **IgA**: molecular weight 1.7×10^5: a monomer in blood, but present as a dimer in body secretions, e.g. saliva, respiratory and alimentary mucus, tears, colostrum. IgA in extracellular fluids (*secretory IgA*) is coupled to a protein *secretory piece*, which is not found on serum IgA.

Mechanism of action of antibodies

Antibodies are a powerful defence mechanism against viruses, because they neutralize viral infectivity. They are much less effective on their own (i.e. without complement) against bacteria, but are nevertheless important in combating bacterial infection, by the following mechanisms:

- *Neutralization of toxins*
- *Promotion of phagocytosis*: antibody-coated bacteria are more readily phagocytosed, i.e. they are opsonized more effectively than those coated with complement alone
- *Bacterial lysis*: certain Gram-negative bacilli, e.g. some strains of *Escherichia coli*, are lysed in the presence of antibody and complement.

Cell-mediated response

Delayed hypersensitivity – or *cell-mediated immunity* – was first described in tuberculosis in the late 19th century. Delayed hypersensitivity develops slowly over 24–48 h, and is especially important in infections due to organisms which persist or multiply intracellularly, such as the bacteria which cause tuberculosis, leprosy and brucellosis, and viruses. In delayed hypersensitivity, the inflammatory lesion is heavily infiltrated with sensitized T-lymphocytes and macrophages.

The overall effect of delayed hypersensitivity is to limit the size of the lesion and to localize the organism within it: although initially protective, there is some risk of unwanted tissue damage.

T-(thymus-dependent) lymphocytes are a population of lymphocytes which have undergone maturation in the thymus. Responsible for cell-mediated immunity, they comprise the majority of the circulating lymphocytes in humans. When sensitized, or primed, T-lymphocytes become activated, and release a variety of cytokines which in turn recruit other inflammatory cells, to mount the cell-mediated immune reaction.

The activities of these cytokines (*lymphokines*) include:

1. *Inhibition of macrophage migration* (this probably localizes the macrophages to the site of infection)
2. *Chemotactic attraction* of lymphocytes, macrophages and polymorphonuclear leucocytes to the site of infection
3. *Increase in capillary permeability*
4. *Mitogenic activity* – stimulation of lymphocytes to transform
5. *IgE production*: mast cell activation.

Other T-lymphocytes, so-called helper and suppressor cells, regulate the immune response. In particular, many, but not all, antigens are thymus-dependent and require the cooperation of T-helper cells for B-lymphocyte activation and antibody production.

AGGRESSIVE MECHANISMS OF THE PARASITE

Bacteria vary in their *pathogenicity*, or ability to produce disease, in humans. *Virulence* is a commonly used but ill-understood term, which indicates the degree of pathogenicity.

Neither pathogenicity nor virulence is easy to measure: it is impossible to do so in human beings for ethical reasons. Experiments in laboratory animals can measure the incidence of disease or death following inoculation of an organism, but the results are not always – and probably not often – analogous to the behaviour of the organism in the human host.

Bacteria as pathogens have two basic mechanisms for producing disease:

- Invasiveness
- Toxin production.

Although bacteria can cause disease which is predominantly invasive or toxic in origin, most infections are due to a combination of both activities.

Invasiveness

Invasiveness is the ability of an organism to spread within the body once it has gained its initial foothold. It depends on the action of *toxins* elaborated by the bacterium, e.g. staphylococcal leucocidin, and on *cell surface components*, which enable it to resist phagocytosis. The latter may be demonstrable as visible capsules (e.g. pneumococcus), or present as part of the cell wall (e.g. the M protein of *Streptococcus pyogenes*, the K antigens of entero-bacteria).

A high degree of bacterial invasiveness is usually associated with severe infection: spread from a local site is often via the lymph channels (*lymphangitis*) to the draining lymph nodes (*lymphadenitis*), and possibly then to the bloodstream (*septicaemia*) – one of the most serious manifestations of infection.

Bacterial toxins

These are of two types: exotoxins and endotoxins.

The main differences between exotoxins and endotoxins are shown in Table 25.1.

Exotoxins

Liberated extracellularly from the intact bacterial cell under genetic control, exotoxins spread via the bloodstream or, sometimes, nerves. They can produce ill effects locally and also at sites far distant from the infective process. A few bacterial diseases (e.g. diphtheria, tetanus) are the result of microorganisms which remain localized at the site of entry but form exotoxins which produce severe, distant effects. Other exotoxins are enterotoxins (e.g. produced by *Staphylococcus aureus*) and the neurotoxin produced by *Clostridium botulinum*.

Table 25.1 Bacterial toxins

	Exotoxins	Endotoxins
Composition	Protein	Lipopolysaccharide
Action	Specific	Nonspecific
Effect of heat	Labile	Stable
Antigenicity	Strong	Weak
Produced by	Gram-positive; some Gram-negative bacteria	Gram-negative bacteria
Convertibility to toxoid*	Yes	No

Toxoid is toxin treated, usually with formaldehyde, so that it loses toxicity but retains antigenicity

Endotoxins

Endotoxins are O antigens, structural components of the cell wall of Gram-negative bacteria, which are liberated only on cell lysis or death of the bacterium. Although differing from each other antigenically, they all produce the same physiological effects.

Aggressins

In addition to exotoxins and endotoxins, some bacteria produce substances, often called *aggressins*, which enable them to withstand the host defences:

- Phospholipase: causes membrane lysis
- Coagulase: deposits fibrin
- Hyaluronidase: dissolves cell-binding material, aids spread.

26. Epidemiology

Epidemiology is the study of the spread of infection. From the point of view of its origin, bacterial disease can be considered in two categories:

1. *Endogenous*: when the organism is derived from the individual's own flora; but *note*: an epidemic organism may first be acquired as part of the normal flora.

2. *Exogenous*: when the organism is acquired from outside sources.

Epidemiology is chiefly concerned with exogenously-acquired infection and the effect of infectious disease on a community or the population at large.

RESERVOIRS AND SOURCES

In most instances, the reservoir and the source of infection are one and the same – but not always: sometimes the source has acquired the infecting organisms from the reservoir. Below are some common reservoirs and sources. *Note*: many of these are inter-related and interdependent.

Human beings

By far the most important source of infection. Human beings act as sources of infection in three main ways:

1. *Active cases of disease*:
Patients suffering from an infectious disease usually shed the causal organism, sometimes in large numbers. However, they may be incapacitated by illness and prevented from circulating in the community.

2. *Inapparent (subclinical) infections*: people with symptomless disease may nevertheless shed the infecting organism: since they

165

continue to circulate in the community, they are unrecognized, and therefore important, sources of infection.

3. *Carriers*: some people – of whom a proportion may have had symptomless infection – become long-term carriers and excretors of pathogenic organisms. Carriers circulate in the general population, and are often undiagnosed.

Animals

Infection from animal sources is an occupational hazard to farm workers, veterinary surgeons and slaughtermen.

Animal products such as meat, milk and hides can be sources of infection of the general population.

Food

An important source of infection: it may be infected at its animal origin (e.g. meat, milk), or later become contaminated when handled by humans. Food may be more than a passive vehicle: pathogenic bacteria can multiply rapidly in some foods, and can also produce toxins if the contaminated food is allowed to remain at a warm environmental temperature. *Cooking* is the best preventive measure.

Water

Britain has a safe and pure water supply, which is normally uncontaminated by sewage. If a sewerage system breaks down, or in countries with inadequate sewers (which includes many tropical or subtropical areas), the water supply is often polluted and waterborne outbreaks of infection can ensue due to faecal bacteria (or viruses).

Soil

Most organisms in soil are non-pathogenic or of very low pathogenicity. However, soil may become contaminated with pathogenic organisms derived from animal faeces or discharges.

Air

Air has a resident flora of bacteria of relatively low pathogenicity. However, a proportion of air bacteria are derived from human beings, who shed organisms from the skin as desquamated scales and from the respiratory tract. Air also contains dust particles (see below).

Dust

Dust is generally contaminated with bacteria shed from human beings and from clothing, furnishings, bed linen and so on. Bacteria in the air (particularly if contained in droplets) are deposited or fall into the dust and, conversely, contaminated dust particles can be swept up into the atmosphere by air currents or movements of personnel.

Fomites

Strictly speaking, these are objects of a porous nature which absorb and can pass on contagion: in practice, any object which can be contaminated with bacteria is regarded as a fomite.

ROUTES OF INFECTION

The route of infection depends largely on the reservoir or source. The main routes are listed below.

Inhalation

A common route of infection, particularly in the case of respiratory tract infections. Spread is by inhalation of droplets of respiratory secretions from someone suffering from active or symptomless infection.

Droplets produced by sneezing and coughing can be:

- *large*: travel only a few feet and contaminate the environment to produce infected dust and fomites
- *small*: droplet nuclei (5 μm or less in diameter) remain suspended in the air: these droplets can be inhaled to reach the respiratory tract directly.

Ingestion

A common mode of spread: organisms derived from faeces can be passed on by the faecal-oral route, usually via contaminated fingers, towels, etc. Gastrointestinal infection can also spread via contaminated drinking water or food.

Contact

Direct contact can spread infection via hands or kissing. Indirect contact, from fomites, usually involves final transfer via the hands.

Sexual transmission

Many infections spread wholly or partially by sexual intercourse – not surprisingly, such diseases usually consist of lesions on the genitalia, and the organisms, which often do not survive well outside the body, are inoculated directly onto the genital (or sometimes rectal or pharyngeal) mucous membranes.

Inoculation

Infection may take place through broken skin due to accidental trauma, animal bites or as a result of surgery. Infection can also be introduced by medical procedures such as catheterization, insertion of prostheses, injection, blood transfusion.

Vector-borne

Arthropod insects and parasites which bite and are blood-sucking, such as mosquitoes, ticks, lice and fleas, are a route of some infections – a common route in tropical countries, but rare in temperate climates like that of Britain.

Transplacental

Some maternal infections can cross the placenta to infect the fetus: less commonly in the case of bacteria than viruses.

OUTBREAKS OF INFECTION

The control and prevention of outbreaks of infectious disease depends on an understanding of reservoirs, sources and routes of transmission, but sometimes even when these are known it is impossible to control infection.

Strain differentiation of organisms from potential sources and cases of infection helps to trace, and often control, outbreaks.

The spread of an infectious disease in a community or institution depends on the following factors:

Number of susceptible hosts

The chance of an outbreak of infection correlates directly with the number of susceptible people. Immediately after an outbreak, the general level and prevalence of antibody is high, i.e. there is good *herd immunity*. With time, the level of antibody wanes and more children – who have never experienced the infection (and therefore have no antibody) – are born into the population. The herd immunity then becomes low, with a relatively large number of susceptible hosts – under these circumstances, the organism can infect again on a large scale.

Note: Many infections are not seen solely in individuals with a low level of, or no, antibody: for example, most people are susceptible to food poisoning, and to staphylococcal wound infection in hospital although the organisms have often been encountered before.

Pathogenicity

Some organisms inherently possess a high capacity to spread (*infectiousness* or *communicability*) or to cause disease (*virulence*). Some organisms, like *Salmonella typhi*, can infect in very small doses; others, like *Salmonella typhimurium*, require large numbers of organisms to establish infection – *S. typhi* is therefore more virulent than *S. typhimurium*. The viruses causing influenza and measles are classic examples of microorganisms with a high capacity to spread.

Route of spread

This factor may determine whether there is an outbreak of infection – for example, a breakdown in the water supply may give faecal organisms from sewage the opportunity to infect large numbers of people via contaminated water. Intravenous drug abuse and blood transfusion with infected blood have caused outbreaks of hepatitis B, and the increase in male homosexual promiscuity was probably an initial factor in the current outbreak of AIDS in the USA. Modern air-conditioning systems, if contaminated with water containing legionellae, can cause outbreaks of air-borne Legionnaires' disease.

Carriers

When there is a relatively high proportion of carriers in a community, this increases the likelihood of an outbreak of infection. Outbreaks of meningococcal meningitis are often preceded by an increase in the proportion of people in the community who carry the organism in their throat.

Climate

Climate may contribute to the incidence of infection. Cold, wet weather increases the number of deaths due to pneumonia and other respiratory disease, whereas hot weather enhances the risk of food poisoning.

MEASUREMENTS IN EPIDEMIOLOGY

Epidemiologists use various measurements by which infection in a community can be assessed. A community may be a family, an institution, a geographical area or the population of an entire country. These measurements include:

Incubation period:

To trace and to contain the spread of an outbreak, it is important to know the incubation period of the infection – particularly if this is relatively long: this can allow time for preventive or containment measures to be instituted.

Incidence or incidence rate:

The number of cases of disease in the community expressed as the number of cases per 1000 people (or 10000, 100000, or per million – whatever is appropriate) in the population concerned. Prevalence is a similar measurement, but usually refers to the incidence in a population within a certain stated time.

Attack rate:

Another way of expressing incidence: this term is used when the rate is applied to a particular defined group, for example, inhabitants of an institution.

Secondary attack rate:

An important statistic for an epidemiologist: the number of secondary cases of infection which appear in the contacts (e.g. family or workmates) of an index case of the disease.

Mortality rate:

The proportion of people in the community who die from the disease, expressed as deaths per 1000, 100000, etc.

Case fatality rate:

The proportion of patients with the disease who die as a result of it: usually expressed as a percentage.

SURVEILLANCE

Measurements of infectious disease are constantly being monitored by epidemiologists and microbiologists. Outbreaks cannot always be prevented, but preventive measures, promptly applied, can successfully halt the spread of an epidemic.

EPIDEMIC DISEASES

Most world-wide *epidemics* or *pandemics* nowadays are viral, but cholera is an exception. In the past 36 years, cholera has spread west from its original focus in the Far East, to South America. Countries with adequate systems for sewage disposal are not at risk from this disease.

EPIDEMIC BACTERIAL DISEASES

Many bacterial diseases remain a major problem for public health authorities. These diseases include salmonella food poisoning, tuberculosis and dysentery. The reservoirs, sources and routes of spread of these diseases are well understood, but it has not proved possible to eradicate them.

Other bacterial diseases, like streptococcal sore throat, are always endemic in the population and wax and wane – often for no apparent reason.

Immunization can radically alter the epidemiology of an infectious disease – indeed, the main purpose of immunization is to do this. Vaccines are generally less effective in the prophylaxis of bacterial diseases than of viral diseases. *Toxoids* are an exception to this, and the prophylaxis of diphtheria and tetanus by toxoids is extremely effective.

EPIDEMIC VIRUS DISEASES

AIDS is the most recent and dramatic example of a virus pandemic. Influenza has not shown a major antigenic shift in its haemagglutinin for many years: when this happens, another pandemic of influenza can be predicted.

Vaccination against smallpox enabled the World Health Organization (WHO) to eradicate a disease that was once a scourge in most countries of the world. Poliovaccine has resulted in the virtual elimination of epidemic paralytic poliomyelitis in many countries, and it is now WHO policy to attempt the eradication of poliomyelitis world-wide.

Live attenuated virus vaccines are the most effective immunizing agents. Killed (or inactivated) virus vaccines are less effective, although they generally give significant protection.

27. Respiratory tract infections

A very important cause of sickness – reckoned to account for a half of general-practitioner consultations and a quarter of all absences from work due to illness.

Route of infection – inhalation. Control of infections acquired by inhalation of infected secretions is well-nigh impossible. More frequent in winter time (October to March): close contact in school, at work and socially allows ready transfer of the causal agents – 'coughs and sneezes spread diseases'. It is now known that spread of the infecting agents, once thought to be exclusively by droplets, can also take place by hand-to-hand transfer of infected respiratory secretions. In family outbreaks, infection is often introduced by the most susceptible member, usually a pre-school or school-age child.

Immunization is only available against a few specific infections, e.g. diphtheria, whooping cough, influenza.

The same clinical syndrome may be produced by a variety of agents, and the same aetiological agent may produce a variety of clinical syndromes.

Respiratory infections can be classified into four groups:

1. Infections of throat and pharynx
2. Infections of middle ear and sinuses
3. Infections of trachea and bronchi
4. Infections of the lungs.

INFECTIONS OF THROAT AND PHARYNX

Sore throat is the commonest symptom, accompanied by a variable degree of constitutional upset. Typical throat appearances for the different aetiological agents are described below, but it is often impossible to decide on the cause of a sore throat by clinical

173

examination alone. Over two-thirds of these infections are caused by viruses – often with sore throat as part of the common-cold syndrome; the remainder are bacterial in origin, almost all due to *Streptococcus pyogenes*.

STREPTOCOCCAL SORE THROAT

Clinical features

Mild redness of tonsils and pharynx may be the only sign, but the classical picture is of infection and oedema involving the fauces and soft palate with exudate – *acute follicular tonsillitis*. Infection is most common in 5–8-year-olds.

In severe cases, the tonsillitis may be complicated by a peri-tonsillar abscess (*quinsy*) and extension of the infection to involve the sinuses and middle ear, producing *sinusitis* and *otitis media*. Systemic illness with fever is the rule and the cervical lymph nodes may be enlarged. *Scarlet fever* is a streptococcal infection – usually involving a sore throat – accompanied by an erythematous rash when the infecting strain of *S. pyogenes* produces erythrogenic toxin in a susceptible (i.e. non-immune) patient – usually a child.

Incubation period: 1–3 days.

Source: infection is acquired from either cases or carriers. After an acute attack, transient carriage for a few weeks is common. Throat carriers outnumber nasal carriers but the latter, who often have an associated sinusitis, are much more effective disseminators.

Treatment

Penicillin is the drug of choice. Therapy should be started parenterally and continued orally for 10 days, to prevent complications and further spread of the organism to contacts. Patients hypersensitive to penicillin are given erythromycin: tetracycline resistance is common.

Late complications of streptococcal infections

Streptococcal infections, usually those causing sore throat, are some-times followed by disease which appears to be immunologically induced. The disease is of two main kinds:

- Rheumatic fever
- Acute glomerulonephritis.

RHEUMATIC FEVER

Clinical features

The acute onset of fever, pain and swelling of the joints, and pancarditis occurs on average 2–3 weeks, but up to 5 weeks, after streptococcal sore throat. The most serious manifestation is involvement of the heart: patients commonly have myocarditis and sometimes, in addition, pericarditis and endocarditis. The disease has been said to 'lick the joints but bite the heart'.

Now relatively uncommon, it was formerly a disease associated with poor living conditions and overcrowding – circumstances that facilitated the spread of streptococcal sore throat. It remains a major problem in developing countries.

Prognosis: rheumatic fever usually clears up spontaneously, although it has a *marked tendency to recur* after subsequent episodes of pharyngitis in those predisposed to the disease: it may follow infection with almost any serotype (Griffith type) of *S. pyogenes*, although certain M types, notably 5, 18 and 24, are particularly associated with institutional outbreaks of the disease.

The main problem is that after the acute phase of rheumatic fever, patients later, often much later, develop, as the result of endocardial involvement, chronic valvular disease of the heart – usually stenosis or incompetence of the mitral or aortic valves.

Pathology: rheumatic fever is a disease of connective tissue which is immunological in origin. The typical lesion is the *Aschoff nodule* – a pale hyaline focus with lymphocytic and macrophage infiltration, and sometimes giant cells: these lesions heal to leave minute focal scars.

Immunology: rheumatic fever may be the result of antibodies, produced against protein and polysaccharide cell wall antigens of *S. pyogenes*, cross-reacting with connective tissue in the heart and elsewhere.

Laboratory diagnosis

The diagnosis can normally be made clinically, but it is useful to check for the continuing presence of *S. pyogenes* in the throat by examining a throat swab, and to seek serological evidence of recent infection.

Serology

Specimen: clotted blood: paired samples should be sent.

Examine: for antibody to streptolysin O (ASO) – a haemolysin produced by *S. pyogenes*. An ASO titre of 200 units or more is regarded as significant: evidence of recent infection requires the demonstration of rising or falling titres in two samples taken a few weeks apart. Tests are available to detect antibody to other streptococcal products, e.g. hyaluronidase, DNAase B – they may be positive when the ASO titre is not raised.

Use of antibiotics

Antibiotics are required to eradicate *S. pyogenes* from the throat. Thereafter, prophylaxis on a long-term basis is mandatory to prevent reinfection, with its risk of precipitating a recurrence. Penicillin is the drug of choice, and administration should be continued until adult life, when the natural incidence of infection falls.

ACUTE GLOMERULONEPHRITIS

Also an immunological complication which may follow streptococcal sore throat or, less often, skin infection, e.g. impetigo. It is particularly liable to follow infection with certain serotypes of *S. pyogenes*: notably, in throat infections, type 12 (the main nephritogenic streptococcus) and, in skin infections, type 49. The latent period between infection and symptoms is shorter than in rheumatic fever.

Clinical features

Acute glomerulonephritis presents 1–3 weeks after a streptococcal throat infection, with haematuria, albuminuria and oedema. The oedema affects the face on waking, causing a characteristic puffy appearance; as the day wears on, this disappears and oedema of the feet and ankles develops. Oliguria is common, and there may be hypertension.

Prognosis: good, especially in childhood – morbidity and mortality increase with age. Although the disease usually clears up spontaneously, it may cause permanent kidney damage and eventually progress to renal failure. Second attacks are uncommon.

Pathogenesis: the disease is the result of an immunological process, but the exact pathogenesis is unclear. Pathologically, there is increased cellularity of the glomeruli, with larger deposits on the outer and smaller deposits on the inner surfaces of the basement membrane. The deposits are immune complexes, thought to be formed by combination of antistreptococcal antibody with either (i) streptococcal antigens already on the basement membrane, or (ii) streptococcal antigens circulating in the blood, later deposited on the membrane after complex formation. The complexes activate complement, with the release of toxic substances, which provoke an inflammatory reaction.

Laboratory diagnosis

Diagnosis is usually on clinical grounds: attempts should be made to confirm past or present streptococcal infection, as described above for rheumatic fever.

Although less common than throat infection as a precipitating cause of the disease, streptococcal impetigo has been responsible for some outbreaks of glomerulonephritis in the USA and in some tropical countries. It should be diagnosed by culture of a swab or sample of pus from the skin lesion.

Complement estimations: the level of C3 in serum is reduced: this has been interpreted as evidence of immune complex formation.

Use of antibiotics

Eradicate *S. pyogenes* if the organism is still present at the site of infection: penicillin is the drug of choice.

DIPHTHERIA

This throat infection is described on page 235.

CANDIDIASIS

Oral thrush due to the yeast *Candida albicans* presents as white patches superimposed on red, raw mucous membrane, which may involve the throat as well as the more common site of the mouth (Fig. 27.1). It is particularly common in babies.

Source: endogenous. In adults, candidiasis may be precipitated by antibiotic treatment, but the patient is often debilitated by disease, e.g. malignancy, diabetes.

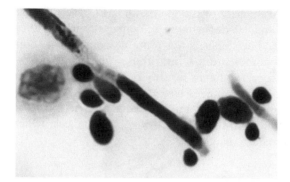

Fig. 27.1   *Candida albicans* in pus (approx. × 1000).

Treatment

Locally applied nystatin, amphotericin B or miconazole. Oral fluconazole is used in immunocompromised patients.

VINCENT'S ANGINA

An *ulcerative tonsillitis*, which causes much tissue necrosis: often an extension of similar disease of the gums and mouth (gingivostomatitis).

Source: endogenous. The causal organisms are a spirochaete *Borrelia vincenti* and a variety of Gram-negative anaerobic bacilli, found in small numbers in the normal mouth (see Fig. 22.3). Overgrowth, to produce disease, is precipitated by dental caries or poor oral hygiene, nutritional deficiency, leucopenia (e.g. in leukaemia) and viral infections (e.g. herpes simplex, infectious mononucleosis).

Treatment

Penicillin and/or metronidazole.

INFECTIOUS MONONUCLEOSIS

Exudative tonsillitis is often the presenting feature of the generalized viral infection due to Epstein-Barr virus – the so-called anginose form of infectious mononucleosis.

Source: oropharyngeal secretions – the kissing disease of young adults.

Treatment

No specific treatment. Antibiotics should be avoided: almost all patients given ampicillin develop a skin rash.

DIAGNOSIS OF THROAT AND PHARYNGEAL INFECTIONS

Diagnosis depends on *isolation* or *demonstration* of the causal bacterium.

Specimen: a well-taken throat swab. Illumination of the throat and depression of the tongue are essential. The swab should be gently rubbed over the affected area, so that it collects a sample of any exudate present.

Gram-stained film: a mixed bacterial flora is always present, and the only findings of value are recognition of Vincent's organisms (Fig. 22.3) and yeasts (Fig. 27.1).

Note: This is the only method of diagnosing Vincent's infection – the causal organisms cannot be isolated by routine culture methods.

Culture: the swab is inoculated onto a variety of media incubated at 37°C for 24–48 h:

1. Blood agar
2. Crystal violet blood agar   – Selective for *Streptococcus pyogenes*, especially if incubated anaerobically
3. Sabouraud's medium   – Selective for *Candida albicans*
4. Loeffler's serum slope   Blood tellurite medium   – For the isolation of *Corynebacterium diphtheriae*; not routine nowadays.

INFECTIONS OF MIDDLE EAR AND SINUSES

Acute infection of the middle ear or sinuses is often due to secondary bacterial invasion following a viral infection of the respiratory tract: this may be a common cold or measles – of which otitis media is a frequent complication.

ACUTE INFECTIONS OF THE MIDDLE EAR AND SINUSES

Clinical features

Otitis media

An upper respiratory infection involving the middle ear by extension of infection up the eustachian tube. Predominantly a disease of infants and children: the main symptom is earache.

On examination, the eardrum is red and the infection may progress to cause bulging, with eventual rupture of the tympanic membrane and discharge of pus from the ear. Recurrent attacks are common.

Sinusitis

Mild discomfort over the frontal or maxillary sinuses due to congestion is a frequent symptom in common colds. Severe pain and tenderness with purulent nasal discharge, however, indicate bacterial infection.

Causal bacteria

Haemophilus influenzae (non-capsulated strains), *Streptococcus pyogenes*, *Streptococcus pneumoniae*, *Moraxella catarrhalis*.

Source

Endogenous spread of organisms from the normal flora of the nasopharynx.

Diagnosis

In the majority of cases of sinusitis and otitis media, specimens from the site of infection cannot be obtained. If the eardrum ruptures or if myringotomy (incision of the tympanic membrane to release pus in the middle ear) is performed, collect a swab of exudate; if drainage or lavage of the sinuses is carried out, material should be collected and cultured in the same way as a sample of pus, on a range of suitable media.

Treatment

Amoxycillin or co-amoxiclav; alternatively, erythromycin.

CHRONIC INFECTIONS OF THE MIDDLE EAR AND SINUSES

Clinical features

Chronic suppurative otitis media

Characterized by suppuration in the middle ear, distorted by chronic pathological changes. Periods of quiescence, when the ear is relatively dry, are followed by exacerbations when there is profuse discharge associated with pain. This is usually a long-standing disease, which can recur at intervals throughout childhood and into adult life.

Chronic sinusitis

Painful sinuses with headache are prominent symptoms; often associated with nasal obstruction and mucoid or purulent nasal discharge.

Causal bacteria

The same as those implicated in acute infections, i.e. infection is usually endogenous, with bacteria from the normal upper respiratory flora. A variety of other organisms may be found, including *Staphylococcus aureus* and a wide range of coliform bacilli. Pseudomonads and proteus are common in chronic ear discharges, and also 'bacteroides'. Detection of these anaerobes requires the careful laboratory examination of a well-taken specimen. The clinical significance of some of these organisms is uncertain.

Diagnosis

Swabs of pus from the ear; lavage specimens from the sinuses – such saline washings are always contaminated by nasal flora. Examine as specimens of pus.

Treatment

Antibiotics often give disappointing results. If prescribed, therapy should be guided by the antibiotic sensitivities of isolated organisms, but treatment may have to be on a 'best-guess' basis. Topical anti-microbials (e.g. neomycin or framycetin, polymyxin, bacitracin) are often given in chronic otitis media because systemic drugs fail to penetrate to the site of infection, but there is conflicting evidence about their efficacy.

INFECTIONS OF TRACHEA AND BRONCHI

Laryngitis, tracheitis and bronchitis are usually associated with or follow a viral infection of the upper respiratory tract.

LARYNGITIS

Clinical features

Hoarseness and loss of voice: in more severe form, *croup* (or acute laryngotracheobronchitis) with croaking cough and stridor. In children, most often associated with parainfluenza virus infection: occasionally due to a rare but important bacterial infection, acute epiglottitis.

ACUTE EPIGLOTTITIS

Clinical features

Severe croup syndrome in children (usually under 5 years of age), which may rapidly progress to respiratory obstruction and death. The epiglottis is inflamed and oedematous.

   Causal bacterium: capsulated strains of *Haemophilus influenzae* (almost always of type b).

   Diagnosis: *H. influenzae* may be isolated from the epiglottis and from blood culture.

Treatment

Parenteral amoxycillin or ampicillin: tracheostomy may be necessary.

   Vaccine: the recent introduction of Hib vaccination in infancy has successfully reduced the incidence of this disease.

BRONCHITIS

Clinical features

A feeling of tightness in the 'tubes'; cough, initially dry and painful, later productive with expectoration of yellow-green sputum, most marked in early morning specimens; variable degree of fever and of constitutional upset. Abnormal chest signs, e.g. rhonchi, are found on auscultation.

Acute bronchitis

Acute bronchitis in a patient with a healthy respiratory tract is often a trivial complication of a viral upper tract infection: the initial viral attack damages respiratory mucous membrane, with paralysis of ciliary movement. Although viral acute bronchitis is usually mild and self-limiting, secondary bacterial infection often supervenes in more severe attacks, especially in patients with chronic respiratory disease such as chronic bronchitis, asthma and bronchiectasis.

Chronic bronchitis

Acute exacerbations of chronic bronchitis are serious events in the course of a major killing disease. Chronic bronchitis is not itself due to infection – aetiological factors include low socio-economic class, urban dwelling (atmospheric pollution) and tobacco consumption, especially cigarette addiction ('smoker's cough'). Exacerbations, however, are associated with bacterial infection. They commonly follow viral respiratory infections or a fall in atmospheric temperature with increase in humidity (together causing foggy weather): all these factors are often present concurrently in winter. During exacerbations, both the volume and the purulence of sputum increase.

Pathology

Pathological changes in chronic bronchitis are: (i) increase in the number of mucus-containing cells in the bronchi, with consequent hypersecretion of mucus; (ii) inflammation, fibrosis, collapse, dilatation and cyst formation in the bronchioles and alveoli. After exacerbations, some changes may resolve but others do not, resulting in progressive irreversible damage.

Causal bacteria and source

1. *Haemophilus influenzae* (usually non-capsulated strains). The closely related organism *H. parainfluenzae* is sometimes isolated, but is of doubtful pathogenicity.

2. *Streptococcus pneumoniae* (pneumococcus).

3. *Moraxella catarrhalis:* disregarded for decades as a potential cause of respiratory infection, but recent reports have drawn attention to its undoubted pathogenic role in some exacerbations of bronchitis.

All three organisms listed above are together present in the upper respiratory tract in health. The secondary bacterial invaders in bronchitis are therefore endogenous. Normal subjects have a sterile bronchial tree, but in chronic bronchitis the bronchi become colonized, especially with *H. influenzae,* even when the disease is quiescent. During exacerbations, the concentration of *H. influenzae* in respiratory secretions increases, along with sputum purulence. Specific antibodies to *H. influenzae,* absent in non-smoking healthy adults, are present in the serum of two-thirds of chronic bronchitics. *H. influenzae* is now regarded as the prime pathogen in exacerbations of chronic bronchitis.

4. *Mycoplasma pneumoniae:* although usually associated with pneumonia, this agent causes a wide spectrum of respiratory disease and is often unrecognized as an aetiological agent in bronchitis. Patients are typically school-age children and young adults.

The source is exogenous and spread is by the respiratory route. Cases are usually sporadic, but there may be family outbreaks and, occasionally, institutional epidemics. The frequency of infection in the community varies from year to year.

Treatment

Acute bronchitis

In previously healthy subjects, acute bronchitis usually subsides in 2–5 days and does not require antibiotic therapy. However, the majority of patients with troublesome, purulent, acute bronchitis are given antibiotics, prescribed on an informed 'best-guess' basis, as for chronic bronchitis.

Chronic bronchitis

Treatment should start as early as possible, and chronic bronchitics should have an emergency supply of antibiotics to take whenever a cold 'goes to the chest': this shortens the duration and reduces the severity of exacerbations but, unfortunately, does not prevent deterioration of respiratory function.

Drugs used must be active against both *H. influenzae* and pneumococci:

- *H. influenzae*: strains resistant to ampicillin/amoxycillin are now not uncommon, and a smaller number are also resistant to tetracycline and co-trimoxazole.
- *Pneumococci*: resistance to penicillin/ampicillin is still rare in Britain, but many strains are now resistant to tetracycline and some also to co-trimoxazole and erythromycin.
- *M. catarrhalis*: most strains produce a β-lactamase, and are therefore ampicillin-resistant.

Short-term (5–7 days) courses of treatment include:

1. *Ampicillin or amoxycillin*: may be bactericidal in action in adequate dosage. Amoxycillin is preferred, because of better absorption in the presence of food and ability to penetrate mucoid sputum: ampicillin only attains bactericidal levels against *H. influenzae* when the sputum is purulent. Co-amoxiclav may be indicated when the infecting strain is shown to be a β-lactamase producer.

2. *Tetracyclines*: bacteriostatic action; uncertain sputum penetration. An advantage is their activity against *M. pneumoniae*.

3. *Co-trimoxazole*: bacteriostatic action; the ratio of sulpho-namide to trimethoprim in the sputum is 4:1 because of poor sulphonamide penetration (compared to the synergistic bactericidal ratio 20:1 found in blood). *Trimethoprim* alone may be prescribed as an alternative.

4. *Erythromycin*: active against almost all pneumococci: *H. influenzae* not fully sensitive but newer macrolides, e.g. *clarithromycin, azithromycin,* possess greater activity. However, erythromycin is effective clinically. *M. pneumoniae* is also sensitive.

5. *Quinolones: ciprofloxacin* and other new quinolones are effective in bronchitis: perhaps surprisingly because, although they are very active against *H. influenzae,* pneumococci are not fully sensitive.

Laboratory examination of sputum is essential if the patient fails to respond to an apparently adequate course of treatment.

Vaccines

Viral

The only vaccine available is that against influenza. Since chronic bronchitics often suffer severe exacerbations after influenza and are at risk of developing secondary bacterial pneumonia, it is recommended that they be vaccinated annually. The vaccine contains inactivated virus of currently circulating A and B strains, and achieves protection of the order of 70%.

Bacterial

Polyvalent pneumococcal polysaccharide vaccines are now available. They may be of value in preventing pneumococcal pneumonia in this 'at risk' group.

Diagnosis

See 'Diagnosis of bacterial chest infections' on page 195.

CYSTIC FIBROSIS

This inherited defect leads to the production of abnormally viscid mucus, which blocks tubular structures in many different organs: the most disabling obstructive changes affect the lungs, and chronic respiratory infection is a major problem. Due to improved management, more infants and children with this disease, transmitted as an autosomal recessive trait, survive to adult life than did formerly.

Causal bacteria

1. *Staphylococcus aureus* and *Haemophilus influenzae* initially, tending to be replaced by:

2. *Pseudomonas aeruginosa*: the strains involved produce an extracellular alginate polysaccharide, which adheres to bronchial mucus, increasing respiratory obstruction. Isolates from sputum form mucoid colonies on culture.

3. *Burkholderia cepacia* (formerly *Pseudomonas cepacia*): recently recognized as an important cause of rapid clinical deterioration; can be acquired readily by direct or indirect person-to-person contact.

Treatment

Determined by bacteriological findings. Ciprofloxacin, although not recommended for children, is a useful antipseudomonal drug. Long-term administration may be required.

PERTUSSIS (WHOOPING COUGH)

Clinical features

An acute tracheobronchitis of childhood.

Onset is insidious – initially a catarrhal stage with common-cold symptoms, which lasts about 2 weeks, followed by a stage of paroxysmal coughing (2 weeks); residual cough persisting for a month or more is a common sequel.

Paroxysmal cough is a diagnostic feature: it consists of repeated violent exhalations with a distressing, severe inspiratory whoop. There is expulsion of tenacious, clear bronchial mucus and vomiting is common (Fig. 27.2).

Fatality is low, but morbidity may be high: there is a significant risk of developing subsequent chronic chest disease, e.g. bronchiectasis. Most acute deaths are in infants during the first year of life, especially in the first 6 months.

Causal bacterium

Bordetella pertussis (types 1,3; 1,2,3; and 1,2). During the 1970s and early 1980s, type 1,3 was responsible for most infections, then

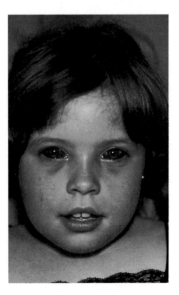

Fig. 27.2   Pertussis: subconjunctival haemorrhages due to spasms of severe coughing. (Photograph by Dr A. K. R. Chaudhuri.)

for a few years type 1,2 predominated before type 1,3 – now responsible for about two-thirds of cases – became common again. This is explained by the sharp decline in vaccine uptake followed by greatly increased acceptance: vaccine immunity protects best against strains containing agglutinogen 2.

B. parapertussis causes mild whooping cough, and is relatively rare in Britain.

A similar syndrome may be caused by adenoviruses (types 1, 2 and 5) and by *Mycoplasma pneumoniae*.

Epidemiology

Following the decline in the acceptance of immunization in the mid-1970s, there were three epidemics of whooping cough in the UK: between 1977 and 1979, 1981 and 1983, and 1985 and 1987. The 1989–1991 and 1994 outbreaks were much smaller, due to the improvement in vaccine uptake, which is now about 90%.

Incubation period: 1–3 weeks: often about 10 days.

Source: patients – most infective during catarrhal stage, becoming non-infective at end of paroxysmal stage.

Spread: airborne, via droplets.

Diagnosis

Isolation, from infected clinical cases: this is not easy and diagnosis is usually based on symptoms. Organisms are much less numerous after the catarrhal stage (i.e. when typical symptoms develop) and in immunized patients.

Specimen:
- Pernasal swab: passed gently along the floor of the nose, to sample nasopharyngeal secretions.
- Cough plate: held in front of mouth during a paroxysm of coughing: superseded by pernasal swabbing.

Inoculate: charcoal blood agar – the preferred medium – or Bordet – Gengou medium.

Incubate: 3–5 days at 35–36°C.

Observe: moist 'mercury-drop' colonies.

Identification: by slide agglutination with specific antisera.

Serology

Rising titres of antibody in *paired* serum specimens may be diagnostic in children over 1 year old. Antibodies are usually detected by an ELISA method. This may give evidence of infection when the opportunity for bacterial isolation has been missed. Interpretation of results is especially difficult in fully or partially immunized children.

Treatment

Antibiotics are only of value if given within the first 10 days of infection, i.e. during the catarrhal stage, when the diagnosis may not be suspected. If secondary pneumonia develops, it should be treated appropriately, guided by the antibiotic sensitivity of the causal organism when this is known.

Administration of erythromycin to the patient reduces the duration of infectivity, and this drug is a successful chemoprophylactic when given to close contacts (e.g. siblings).

Vaccination

This is discussed on page 412.

INFECTIONS OF THE LUNGS

PNEUMONIA

The most severe and life-threatening of respiratory infections, in which there is exudate in the alveolar spaces. Although antibiotic therapy has transformed the prognosis for many patients, pneumonia remains a significant cause of death – in infancy, in the elderly and in immunocompromised patients.

Clinical features

Onset: sometimes abrupt, sometimes insidious when due to the extension of a pre-existing respiratory infection.

Symptoms: fever, rigors, malaise; respiratory symptoms include shortness of breath, rapid shallow breathing, cyanosis, cough, sometimes pleural pain; sputum may be tenacious and rusty initially, later becoming purulent.

Clinical investigation

Investigate for signs of consolidation of lungs, i.e. dullness on percussion, reduced air entry, moist rales. There is usually polymorphonuclear leucocytosis. Assess respiratory function.

Radiology: indicates the site and extent of the consolidation.

Classification

Pneumonia may be classified as follows:

1. *Lobar (or segmental) pneumonia*: in which the consolidation is limited at least initially to one lobe or segment of the lung: the main type of pneumonia seen in previously healthy people.

2. *Bronchopneumonia*: usually bilateral: the consolidation is scattered throughout the lung fields, although it is mainly concentrated at the bases. The most common form of pneumonia, seen principally in the elderly and in patients with debilitating or chronic respiratory disease such as chronic bronchitis, bronchiectasis.

3. *Primary atypical pneumonia*: patchy consolidation of the lungs, in which the walls of the bronchioles are thickened by an interstitial mononuclear cell infiltrate and the lumina contain exudate.

4. *Legionnaires' disease*: a severe pneumonia, first recognized in 1976 amongst members attending an American Legion convention.

Causal agents

Table 27.1 lists the main organisms associated with the different types of pneumonia.

Streptococcus pneumoniae (pneumococcus)

The main cause of pneumonia.

Source: human respiratory tract.

Spread:

- Exogenous: droplet transmission of virulent strains (incubation period 1–3 days).
- Endogenous, due to downward spread of pneumococci from the flora of the nasopharynx.

Treatment: recommended drugs: penicillin, macrolides, e.g. erythromycin. For penicillin-resistant strains: cefotaxime or vancomycin.

Table 27.1 Causes of pneumonia

Pneumonia	Main causal organisms
Lobar pneumonia	*Streptococcus pneumoniae*
Bronchopneumonia	*Streptococcus pneumoniae* *Haemophilus influenzae* Rarely: *Staphylococcus aureus*, coliforms *Mycoplasma*
Primary atypical pneumonia*	*Mycoplasma pneumoniae* *Coxiella burneti* *Chlamydia psittaci* *Chlamydia pneumoniae*
Legionnaires' disease*	*Legionella pneumophila*

* These are multisystem diseases, which affect other organs as well as the lungs.

Haemophilus influenzae

Often underestimated as a cause of pneumonia: in infants, usually due to capsulated strains; in adults it is often, but not always, a complication of chronic respiratory disease. *Note*: in pneumonia following exacerbations of chronic bronchitis, the pneumococcus is the commonest bacterial cause.

Treatment: recommended drugs: ampicillin/amoxycillin, coamoxiclav. Other effective drugs: cefotaxime, co-trimoxazole, ciprofloxacin.

Staphylococcus aureus

A relatively uncommon cause of bronchopneumonia: probably most often seen in hospital patients; sometimes complicates influenza. The cause of severe secondary bacterial pneumonia: an increasing problem in intravenous drug abusers. Often fulminating and rapidly fatal.

Treatment: recommended drug: cloxacillin, often combined with rifampicin or fusidic acid. Very few infecting strains are penicillin-sensitive. Other effective drug: vancomycin.

Coliforms

Coliforms, e.g. *Escherichia coli*, *Proteus species*, *Klebsiella species*, *Pseudomonas species* are rare causes of bronchopneumonia. Their isolation from sputum often indicates merely colonization of the respiratory tract, e.g. after a course of antibiotic, and must be interpreted cautiously. As a cause of pneumonia, they are most often encountered in hospital patients, especially the immuno-compromised or those on support ventilation under intensive care.

Friedländer's bacillus: a klebsiella of uncertain taxonomy; has been described as a cause of a rare pneumonia with much tissue destruction.

Treatment: recommended drugs: cefotaxime, perhaps combined with an aminoglycoside.

Mycoplasma pneumoniae

Formerly known as Eaton agent: responsible for most cases of primary atypical pneumonia. Overall, second only to the pneumococcus as the commonest recognized cause of pneumonia: school-age children and young adults are the group most frequently affected. Radiological changes are often out of proportion to the relatively mild degree of illness – fever and unproductive cough – and the few clinical signs.

Incubation period: 1–3 weeks.

Spread: respiratory (droplet) spread to involve individuals, families and sometimes institutions (e.g. schools, military camps). The prevalence peaks every 4 years: high levels of infection were recorded in the winter of 1994–95.

Treatment: recommended drug: tetracycline. Other effective drug: erythromycin.

Coxiella burneti

Responsible for the acute febrile disease Q fever: up to half of the patients have pneumonia – usually a patchy consolidation. The disease is a zoonosis, acquired from domestic animals – usually cattle and sheep – by the inhalation of infected dust, straw etc.

Treatment: recommended drug: tetracycline. Other effective drug: erythromycin.

Chlamydia psittaci

The causal agent of ornithosis and psittacosis in birds: may infect humans via inhalation of dried bird droppings. Produces an acute influenza-like illness, with patchy pneumonia.

Treatment: recommended drug: tetracycline. Other effective drug: erythromycin.

Chlamydia pneumoniae

Recently recognized. Spreads from person to person: no known animal association. Usually causes mild respiratory infections, but can be responsible for pneumonia. Antibodies are detectable in childhood and are found increasingly with age, indicating that infection must be common.

Treatment: as for *Chlamydia psittaci* infection.

Legionella pneumophila and related species

The result of infection varies from asymptomatic seroconversion, to nonspecific febrile illness (*Pontiac fever*), to pneumonia. The pneumonia, *Legionnaires' disease*, is now being increasingly recognized in middle-aged smokers, who are often in poor general health.

Symptoms: initially influenza-like, with abrupt onset. The illness may progress to a severe pneumonia, with purulent, sometimes blood-stained, sputum and sometimes with respiratory failure. Other prominent features are mental confusion, acute renal failure and gastrointestinal symptoms.

Source: environment: usually associated with water, in which the organism can survive for long periods.

Spread: by contaminated aerosols, e.g. via air-conditioning systems, water from storage tanks through showers and taps, etc. Person-to-person droplet spread has not been recorded.

Epidemiology: the majority of cases are sporadic, with the route of infection unconfirmed. Outbreaks are usually associated with large buildings (e.g. hotels, hospitals), and the origin can often be traced to a source within their complex water systems.

Treatment: recommended drug: erythromycin. Other effective drugs: rifampicin, ciprofloxacin. These may be given in combination.

Viruses

Pneumonia in infants is predominantly due to respiratory syncytial virus. Primary influenzal pneumonia in previously healthy adults is a rare, but exceedingly severe, complication of influenza, and is almost invariably fatal. However, viruses on their own are not usually responsible for pneumonia except in immunocompromised patients, who are especially susceptible to infection with cytomegalovirus. Antibiotic treatment is therefore indicated for all patients diagnosed as having pneumonia.

Treatment

The treatment of pneumonia is governed by the clinician's experience and personal preference, and knowledge of what the infecting agent and its antibiotic sensitivity are likely to be. As a rule, treatment has to be started before laboratory results are available and even after investigation the cause of pneumonia in some patients is never identified.

The penicillins are the drugs of first choice: in patients with lobar pneumonia, when the infecting organism is likely to be *S. pneumoniae* alone, prescribe penicillin; for bronchopneumonia, give ampicillin or amoxycillin, because *H. influenzae* may also be involved. If there is anxiety about antibiotic resistance, use a cephalosporin (e.g. cefuroxime, cefotaxime).

In patients who either present with a *severe* undiagnosed community-acquired pneumonia or fail to respond to initial therapy, a cephalosporin plus erythromycin should be given: flucloxacillin may be added if staphylococcal pneumonia is suspected. Treatment should be changed if laboratory investigation indicates a more appropriate antibiotic.

In hospital-acquired pneumonia, consider the possibility that the causal organism is a coliform (give an aminoglycoside and/or extended-spectrum β-lactam). If aspiration pneumonia is suspected (see below), the causal organism may be an anaerobe (give clindamycin).

TUBERCULOSIS

Although tuberculosis is not considered in this chapter (see Ch. 37), in any long-standing chest infection the possibility of tuberculosis must *always* be considered.

ASPIRATION PNEUMONIA AND LUNG ABSCESS

Aspiration pneumonia follows inhalation of vomit, or sometimes a foreign body, by an unconscious patient.

The causal organisms are commensals of the upper respiratory tract – principally *S. pneumoniae*, but 'bacteroides' are also involved in the majority of cases.

Lung abscess is nowadays rare. It is usually due to obstruction of a bronchus or bronchiole, e.g. by an inhaled foreign body, or to suppuration developing within an area of pneumonic consolidation. The infecting organisms are similar to those listed above – namely *S. pneumoniae* and anaerobic bacteria of the upper respiratory flora.

Diagnosis: the isolation of anaerobic organisms requires the examination of aspirated specimens. They are seldom isolated from sputum.

Treatment: recommended drugs: penicillin and metronidazole or clindamycin.

EMPYEMA

Literally, pus in the pleural space and nowadays a rare complication of pneumonia, or sometimes tuberculous. It is usually due to *S. pneumoniae* or *S. aureus*, with upper respiratory anaerobes sometimes implicated.

Laboratory diagnosis requires aspiration.

Treatment involves drainage and removal of the infected fluid, and appropriate antibiotic therapy.

DIAGNOSIS OF BACTERIAL CHEST INFECTIONS

Diagnosis involves:

1. *Isolation of causal pathogen* from sputum or, less commonly, from the aspirate of a pleural effusion, lung abscess or area of pneumonic lung. Aspiration samples may be collected by the trans-tracheal route, via a fine catheter introduced through the cricothyroid membrane. It is more usual, however, to take specimens during bronchoscopy and broncho-alveolar lavage (BAL) in which saline is injected through a bronchoscope, and then aspirated to sample an affected area of lung – produces a specimen useful in making an accurate diagnosis in difficult cases of pneumonia, particularly in immunosuppressed patients. *Blood cultures* should also be taken, since the infecting bacterium may be present in the blood of up to one-third of patients with pneumonia.

2. *Detection of bacterial antigen* in sputum or urine.

3. *Serology*: demonstration of specific antibody in patient's serum is only useful in cases of atypical pneumonia (see below).

Isolation of pathogen from sputum

Specimen: early morning sputum: likely to be the most purulent.

Collection: try to minimize salivary contamination – but the presence of some oropharyngeal flora is inevitable.

Transport: send to laboratory without delay: in transit, delicate organisms (e.g. *H. influenzae*) die; robust bacteria (e.g. coliforms) multiply and overgrow.

Laboratory examination

Macroscopic: note naked-eye appearance.

Microscopic:

1. *Gram film*: observe amount of pus, squamous epithelial cells (indicating buccal contamination) and nature of the bacterial flora: if this is very mixed, it is probably not significant, but the presence of a predominant organism may allow an immediate provisional diagnosis. Figure 8.2 shows a typical Gram film of sputum from a patient infected with both pneumococci and *H. influenzae*.

2. *Ziehl–Neelsen or auramine film*: examine for acid- and alcohol-fast bacilli. If present, a presumptive diagnosis of tuberculosis can be made. This examination is not always carried out nowadays because of the decline in the incidence of tuberculosis, but should always be done in the case of immigrants or in areas where tuberculosis is still common (e.g. large cities), or if there is any clinical reason to suspect tuberculosis (e.g. patient suffering from AIDS).

Culture

Bacteria are not distributed evenly throughout sputum: select a purulent portion. Alternatively, homogenize the specimen by treatment with a liquefying agent: such treatment allows semi-quantitative culture and may make evaluation of the results easier.

Inoculate:

- Blood agar: observe for presence of predominant organism and assess respiratory flora.
- Chocolate agar with bacitracin: selective for *H. influenzae*.

Incubate:

- Blood agar, and chocolate agar with bacitracin, at 37°C in air with 5–10% carbon dioxide: this atmosphere is necessary for the primary isolation of some strains of *H. influenzae* and *S. pneumoniae*.
- Blood agar at 37°C anaerobically with 5–10% carbon dioxide: this is not done routinely, although *S. pneumoniae* grows better under these conditions – indicated if infection with non-sporing anaerobes is suspected, e.g. in lung abscess or aspiration pneumonia.

Assessment of culture results: may be difficult, because of contamination from the oropharyngeal flora. Viridans streptococci, neisseriae, coagulase-negative staphylococci, commensal coryne-bacteria, etc. are normally regarded as upper respiratory tract commensals. Small numbers of haemophilus and pneumococci in a mixed growth may be part of the normal flora; larger numbers, especially if other bacteria are scanty, are regarded as pathogens.

The oropharynx of patients who have received antibiotics often becomes colonized with coliform organisms and yeasts, and under such circumstances, undue significance should not be placed on their isolation.

Culture for Mycobacterium tuberculosis: not a routine examination nowadays, but should be carried out if indicated clinically. Submit three samples collected on successive days for culture on Löwenstein–Jensen medium for 6–8 weeks.

Detection of bacterial antigen in sputum or urine

Pneumococcal capsular antigens can be detected by a variety of methods. A positive result may be obtained when culture of the same specimen failed to isolate *S. pneumoniae*, usually because the patient had received antibiotics before the sputum was collected.

In some patients with Legionnaires' disease, a rapid diagnosis can be made by the demonstration of *L. pneumophila* in respiratory secretions using direct immunofluorescence. Legionella antigen may be detected in urine by an ELISA test.

Direct immunofluorescence has also been used as a method of detecting *C. pneumoniae* in sputum.

Serological tests

The atypical pneumonias (see Table 27.1) and Legionnaires' disease are difficult to diagnose by isolation of the causal organism, but note that methods for the culture of *Legionella pneumophila* have improved recently (see page 139) and isolation from respiratory secretions should be attempted: for this purpose, BAL fluid is a particularly good specimen. However, all suspected cases of these infections should be investigated serologically, i.e. by detection of antibody in patient's serum. These infections are often diagnosed by stationary high titres, although it is better to demonstrate a fourfold, or greater, rising titre in paired 'acute' and 'convalescent' specimens, collected a few weeks apart. The tests used are complement fixation, immunofluorescence and ELISA.

28. Diarrhoeal diseases

Diarrhoea is still a major cause of morbidity and infant death in developing countries, largely due to inadequate sewage disposal and contaminated water. Most, but not all, cases of diarrhoea are due to infection – bacteria, viruses and protozoa cause diarrhoea, but this chapter deals mainly with bacteria.

Host: the young are most susceptible to diarrhoeal disease, and poor general health and nutrition also predispose to it.

Bacteria: factors such as the size of the infecting dose; enterotoxin production; ability to adhere to gastrointestinal epithelium; and ability to invade the gut wall affect the ability of organisms to infect the gut and cause diarrhoea.

Epidemiology: prevention largely depends on sanitation (i.e. adequate disposal of sewage), clean food and a safe water supply. Personal hygiene (i.e. washing hands after defecation) is a remarkably effective means of preventing faecal-oral spread. The storage of food at room temperature *must* be avoided: this permits rapid bacterial multiplication and, with some bacteria, the formation of toxins. Note that although refrigeration prevents bacterial multiplication, the bacteria are *preserved*, not killed, at 4°C.

INVESTIGATION OF DIARRHOEA

Patient's history

Particular note should be taken of:

- clinical symptoms, duration, etc.
- recent foreign travel
- food history, including symptoms amongst other consumers of suspect food
- probable incubation period.

Specimens for laboratory examination

- Faeces (rectal swab if none available)
- The suspected food: strenuous efforts should be made to obtain samples: this is often difficult, as it has usually all been eaten or discarded
- Vomit
- Blood culture: in severe cases – especially the very young and the elderly.

Other investigations

Other investigations which are especially important in an outbreak include:

- food-handling practices in the kitchen concerned
- faecal samples from kitchen staff.

The main enteropathogenic bacteria, with some characteristics of the epidemiology of the diseases they causes, are listed in Table 28.1.

Table 28.1   Causal organisms and some features of the epidemiology of diarrhoeal diseases

Organism	Usual source	Common route, source of infection
Campylobacter species	Animal gut	Poultry, meat, milk
Salmonella species	Animal gut	Poultry and eggs, meat, milk
Shigella species	Human gut	Faecal–oral or food, fomites
Escherichia coli	Human gut	Faecal–oral or food, water, fomites
Staphylococcus aureus	Septic lesions on food handlers	Cooked meats, dairy products
Clostridium perfringens	Animal gut	Stews, meat pies
Bacillus species	Environment (soil)	Rice
Clostridium difficile	Human gut	Overgrowth of strains already in colon, also faecal–oral
Yersinia enterocolitica	Uncertain	Faecal–oral, personal contact
Vibrio cholerae	Human gut	Water, food

Causes of diarrhoeal disease

The main bacterial causes of diarrhoea in Britain are:

- Campylobacter
- Salmonella
- Shigella
- *Escherichia coli*
- *Staphylococcus aureus*
- *Clostridium perfringens.*

The diseases these organisms cause are described below.

An important cause of diarrhoea in hospital patients is *Clostridium difficile*, and this is considered later in this chapter along with the less common causes of diarrhoea. Cholera, once epidemic in Britain and still a major problem in the Third World, is described at the end of the chapter.

COMMON BACTERIAL CAUSES OF DIARRHOEAL DISEASE IN BRITAIN

CAMPYLOBACTER

This organism is now recognized as a major cause of diarrhoea – in fact, now the commonest in Britain. It requires a high temperature for growth and its frequency and importance were only appreciated when special methods of culture and temperature of incubation were introduced.

Campylobacters are small vibrio-like organisms. The main cause of human infections are *C. jejuni* and *C. coli*.

Clinical features

There are two kinds of clinical presentation, but as in most intestinal infections, symptoms vary from mild (or even symptomless) to a severe illness with prostration:

- With flu-like prodromal symptoms: fever, headache, backache, limb aches, nausea and abdominal pain; after 24 h, sometimes longer, diarrhoea develops.
- Without prodromal symptoms: acute onset of abdominal pain and diarrhoea.

Incubation period: 3-10 days.

Symptoms: Diarrhoea: often severe, with blood and mucus in stools: up to 20 stools a day may be passed, and there may be faecal incontinence.

Abdominal pain is a prominent feature. Septicaemia, with fevers, rigor and malaise, is sometimes seen in severe cases, confirming the invasiveness of the causal organism.

Duration: often several days, and relapses are common.

Pathogenesis

Typically an enterocolitis: infection involves the ileum but is not restricted to the small intestine, and there is often colitis also.

Histology: there is some suggestion from the results of gut biopsy that campylobacters are invasive and penetrate beyond the mucosa.

Diagnosis

Specimen: faeces.

Culture: on selective medium (containing antibiotics to which campylobacters are resistant) at 43°C.

Observe: typical colonies.

Identification: by morphology: curved, slender Gram-negative bacilli, with characteristic darting motility, positive oxidase reaction and other features.

Treatment

Usually self-limiting. Erythromycin reduces the duration of excretion and can relieve symptoms, but should be reserved for severe cases. An alternative drug is ciprofloxacin.

Epidemiology

Source of infection: farm animals – especially poultry – are probably the major source of human infection; milk and water have been incriminated in outbreaks; dogs and cats have also been reported as sources of campylobacters.

Route of infection: eating contaminated food, but note that campylobacters do *not* multiply in food. Although uncommon, there can be faecal–oral spread, especially between children.

Sporadic infections seem to be the rule in the UK, but infections are so common that it may be that outbreaks are missed, due to lack of reliable typing methods.

Control

Food and personal hygiene. Control of infection in animals is not practicable, not least because the organisms are carried symptomlessly and do not harm the animals concerned (usually poultry).

SALMONELLA

Formerly the commonest cause of diarrhoea in Britain – and still with a high incidence. Diarrhoea due to salmonella is, by tradition, called food poisoning – although this term is somewhat misleading.

The incidence of salmonella infection increased dramatically in the UK during the late 1980s: this increase was partly due to the emergence of *S. enteritidis* phage type 4, and its appearance as the commonest cause of 'incidents' in poultry flocks.

There are more than 1500 serotypes of salmonella, but only about 14 are important or common causes of infection. In recent years the commonest serotype has been *S. enteritidis*. Other common salmonellae are *S. typhimurium* and *S. virchow*. *S. typhi* and *S. paratyphi A, B* and *C* classically cause enteric fever, a septicaemic febrile illness in which diarrhoea is a late symptom (see Ch. 29). *S. paratyphi* is intermediate in its pathogenicity, and can cause either mild enteric fever or a primarily diarrhoeal illness.

Habitat: domestic animals, especially poultry.

Clinical features

Asymptomatic infections and cases with only mild gastrointestinal disturbance are not uncommon.

Incubation period is short: around 12-36 h.

Main symptoms are acute onset of abdominal pain and diarrhoea, sometimes with fever and vomiting. Dehydration may require correction, especially in babies.

Septicaemia sometimes develops in severe cases, and is more common with certain serotypes (e.g. *S. dublin, S. virchow, S. cholerae-suis*).

Pathogenesis

Site of infection is the small or large intestine.

Many strains produce enterotoxins similar to those of toxigenic strains of *E. coli*. Other salmonellae invade the mucosa of the small intestine – like shigellae.

Diagnosis

Isolation

Specimen: faeces.

Culture: on MacConkey (indicator) medium and selective and enrichment media.

Observe: pale, non-lactose-fermenting colonies on MacConkey medium or typical morphology on other media.

Identification: initially by biochemical tests; then serologically to determine H and O antigens.

Treatment

Antibiotics are contraindicated except in septicaemic cases: they do not affect symptoms, and may prolong convalescent carriage of the organism; they also contribute to the emergence of antibiotic-resistant strains.

Treatment is rarely necessary: rehydration may be required in babies: oral isotonic fluid replacement can be life-saving in infants with diarrhoea.

Epidemiology

Food derived from domestic animals and poultry is the main *source* – usually meat contaminated from viscera at slaughter. There have been numerous outbreaks due to the contamination of eggs. Infection is transmitted from infected hens via the oviduct to the egg. Poultry- and egg-associated infection caused record numbers of food poisoning cases in the UK in the late 1980s. Occasional outbreaks due to contaminated milk, and sometimes therefore to cheese, have also been reported.

Food, especially meat and offal, is often contaminated in the raw state. If it is then inadequately cooked and stored for some time at a warm room temperature, surviving salmonellae can multiply. Alternatively – and perhaps more commonly – salmonellae from raw meat can contaminate other cooked foods by common use of kitchen tools and work-surfaces, with subsequent multiplication during storage.

Eggs: are often either lightly cooked or eaten raw in sauces, desserts etc. Thorough cooking remains the best method of avoiding food poisoning.

Outbreaks of salmonella food poisoning are common: they often involve communal catering, e.g. weddings, large dinners, etc., but may also be a problem in hospitals, especially in mental or geriatric units.

Control

Difficult – control is clearly unsuccessful at present. It depends on:

1. Control of infection in domestic animals – especially intensively-reared poultry flocks.

2. Good farming and abattoir practice; control of animal feed-stuffs; restricted prescribing of antibiotics – especially to calves, because indiscriminate use results in selection of multiply-resistant bacteria, which can then spread to human populations.

3. Cooking to a temperature (i.e. boiling point) at which vegetative bacteria are killed.

4. Rigorous hygiene in the kitchen, e.g. separation of cooked and raw foods, prompt and effective refrigeration of cooked food, thorough thawing of frozen poultry and meat before cooking.

5. Good personal hygiene among food handlers.

6. Exclusion of known human excretors from food handling.

SHIGELLA

Shigellae cause bacillary dysentery – 'the commonest of the un-preventable diseases'. A world-wide problem, and an important cause of death and morbidity in young children, especially in developing countries.

The four species of *Shigella* are:
- *S. dysenteriae*
- *S. flexneri*
- *S. sonnei* (one serotype: the main cause of dysentery in Britain)
- *S. boydii*.

All the species except *S. sonnei* contain several distinguishable serotypes.

Clinical features

Incubation period: 1–9 days.

Symptoms: diarrhoea with blood, mucus and often pus in the stools, which varies from a severe life-threatening disease to a mild or symptomless infection.

Shiga dysentery

Due to *S. dysenteriae*: a severe, even life-threatening disease found only in tropical countries, with fever, abdominal pain and diarrhoea. The disease sometimes becomes septicaemic, indicating that, unlike other shigellae, *S. dysenteriae* has invasive properties. *S. dysenteriae* produces a powerful *neurological exotoxin*, but this probably does not play a role in Shiga dysentery. An enterotoxin and a cytotoxin are also produced: their role is uncertain, but they may be partly responsible for the organism's invasiveness.

Dysentery due to other shigellae

This is generally a milder disease, which varies from asymptomatic excretion to a prostrating attack of diarrhoea with abdominal pain and (usually minimal) fever. The stools may contain blood, mucus and pus, but blood is unusual in cases of Sonné dysentery.

Sonné dysentery due to *S. sonnei*, is world-wide. The disease is commonest in young children, and outbreaks in nursery schools are not uncommon. The disease is usually mild but in a few cases dehydration ensues, requiring emergency treatment. Epidemics of Sonné dysentery are also frequent in mental hospitals, and the infection may be difficult to eradicate.

S. flexneri was formerly quite common in Britain – still common overseas, mainly in tropical countries.

S. boydii is rare in Britain but is common in the Middle and Far East.

Diagnosis

Isolation

Specimens: stools, rectal swabs.

Culture: MacConkey (indicator), selective, and enrichment media.

Observe: pale (non-lactose-fermenting) colonies, but note: *S. sonnei* is a late lactose fermenter and may produce pale pinkish colonies.

Identification: by biochemical tests, then serologically.

Treatment

Antibiotics are rarely necessary for Sonné dysentery: the more severe disease should be treated systemically, depending on the sensitivity of the organism isolated (multiply antibiotic-resistant strains are common). Antibiotics tend to prolong the excretion of shigellae.

Epidemiology

Reservoir of infection: is the human gut: symptomless infections are common, with excretion of the organism in the faeces. After an acute attack, some patients excrete shigellae for a considerable time (i.e. for weeks, sometimes months). Patients with acute dysentery are the most dangerous sources of infection, doubtless due to the large numbers of shigellae excreted during the acute phase of the disease.

Route of infection is faecal–oral, either directly or via con-taminated equipment, towels and lavatory seats (in nursery schools). Shigellae can remain viable for long periods of time in cool, moist environments.

Spread: 'food, flies, fomites' are the classical means of spread of dysentery; contaminated water can also be a source of infection.

Dysentery waxes and wanes in incidence over long periods of time: after two decades of high incidence which started in 1950, the disease waned in Britain in the late 1970s and early 1980s. This periodicity appears to be unrelated to improved sanitation or other public health measures. 1992 saw a dramatic rise in cases of Sonné dysentery in the UK, but with a return to lower levels in succeeding years.

Control

Good sanitation with safe water; adequate sewage disposal. A high standard of personal hygiene is important – especially in children – but almost impossible to achieve in conditions of poor housing and poverty.

ESCHERICHIA COLI

Although *E. coli* is part of the normal commensal gut flora, certain strains can be a cause of diarrhoea. Several mechanisms of enteric pathogenicity have been discovered in these strains (see Ch. 9), but the picture is confusing because not all the strains associated with disease have these mechanisms.

E. coli diarrhoea

Mainly seen as three types of disease:

1. *Infantile gastroenteritis*: largely confined to babies under 2 years of age
2. *Travellers' diarrhoea*: mostly in adults recently arrived in a foreign country
3. *Haemorrhagic colitis and haemolytic uraemic syndrome*: more serious infections, now being recognized with increasing frequency in the UK.

Less common diarrhoeal diseases caused by *E. coli* are mentioned in separate sections below.

INFANTILE GASTROENTERITIS DUE TO *E. COLI*

Cause: generally enteropathogenic (EPEC) strains, e.g. serogroups 055, 0111, and also sometimes by enterotoxigenic (ETEC) strains, e.g. serogroups 06, 078 (see Ch. 9).

Note: Rota and other viruses are also important causes of infantile gastroenteritis.

Clinical features

Acute diarrhoea, after an incubation period which varies from 1 to 3 days: the diarrhoea may lead to dehydration (Fig. 28.1) and acid-base imbalance.

Hypernatraemia is a particular problem, because of the dispro-portionate loss of water relative to sodium from the extracellular spaces.

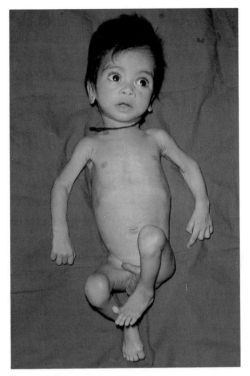

Fig. 28.1   Child with gastroenteritis. (Reproduced with permission from Abbott Laboratories *Slide Atlas of Infectious Diseases*, 1982, Gower Medical Publishing, London. Photograph by Professor H. Lambert.)

Pathogenesis

Not well understood. Some infecting strains produce enterotoxins, but most EPEC strains do not produce toxins and are non-invasive: many show strong adherence to intestinal epithelium – an important pathogenic mechanism.

Diagnosis

Isolation

Specimens: faeces.
    Culture: MacConkey medium.

Observe: pink (lactose-fermenting) colonies, and pick several for further tests.

Identification: serologically.

Treatment

Rehydration, with correction of fluid loss and of electrolyte and acid-base imbalance. Antibiotic therapy is of doubtful value, although it may be useful in severe cases.

Epidemiology

Infection is sporadic in the community in Britain: previously the main problem in this country was outbreaks in institutions and nurseries.

Overseas in countries with poor sanitation and housing, the disease is a major cause of infant mortality. Flies probably play a part in transmitting the infection.

Transmission: faecal–oral, perhaps sometimes via food or contaminated milk.

Control

Scrupulous hygiene in nurseries and neonatal units is necessary.

Outbreaks are controlled by: *prompt isolation* of cases and contacts; *screening* of staff to detect carriers of the epidemic strain; *closure* of the unit to new admissions.

Overseas, control is only possible when clean water, sanitation and adequate housing can be provided.

TRAVELLERS' DIARRHOEA (TURISTA)

Also known as 'Delhi belly', 'Montezuma's revenge', 'Tokyo two-step', etc.

Cause: generally the enterotoxigenic strains of *E. coli* (ETEC). There are more than 100 'O' serogroups: important examples are 06, 078 (see Ch. 9). Most cases are not investigated bacteriologically.

Clinical features

Diarrhoea, abdominal pain and vomiting: usually self-limiting and of a few days' duration; occasionally protracted.

Route of infection: via contaminated food and drinks; polluted water is the usual source of infection.

Pathogenesis

ETEC produce *heat-labile toxin (LT)* or *heat-stable toxin (ST)*, or both. They also possess *colonization factors*, which facilitate attachment of the organism to the epithelium of the small intestine.

Diagnosis

Laboratory facilities are often not available at tourist resorts: information about the cause of this major problem to the tourist industries of many countries has come from a few research studies.

Control

Public health measures, e.g. clean water supply; caution in diet by travellers.

HAEMORRHAGIC SYNDROMES

Two important and sometimes life-threatening syndromes associated with bleeding tendency are due to strains of *E. coli* which produce toxins that have a cytopathic effect on Vero (monkey kidney) cells. There are two Vero cytotoxins, VT1 and VT2 which are antigenically distinct from each other. Vero cytotoxin-producing *E. coli* strains are known as **VTEC**.

Serogroup: By far the commonest VTEC is serogroup 0157: 66 phage types of this serogroup can be distinguished.

Haemorrhagic colitis

A syndrome seen in children and adults, both in outbreaks and as sporadic infections. Deaths have been reported, especially in outbreaks amongst the elderly in residential homes.

Haemolytic uraemic syndrome

Seen mainly in children, both as outbreaks and as sporadic cases. Children have a diarrhoeal prodrome, followed by uraemia, thrombocytopenia and haemolytic anaemia.

The syndrome is associated with various serogroups, notably 0157 – but others, some of which are classified as enteropathogenic (EPEC strains) are occasionally involved.

Uraemia due to VTEC is one of the commonest reasons for renal dialysis in children, and has a significant (although low) case fatality rate.

Epidemiology

Cattle are often carriers of serogroup 0157, and the main source of infection is *beef*.

Several large outbreaks have been traced to hamburgers, and meat patties, inadequately cooked at barbecues, are another source. A large outbreak in Scotland, with several deaths amongst the elderly, was due to meat pies.

ENTEROINVASIVE *E. COLI* (EIEC)

EIEC cause a disease like shigella dysentery in all age groups, and share the same invasive pathogenic mechanisms as shigellae. They are atypical in the laboratory in that they do not ferment lactose.

They belong to several serogroups, e.g. 0124, 0164.

OTHER OUTBREAKS OF DIARRHOEA DUE TO *E. COLI*

Outbreaks in *adults* have been reported: for example, a large-scale outbreak of cheese-borne food poisoning has been attributed to *E. coli*.

The laboratory investigation of faeces for specific serotypes of *E. coli* is impractical in sporadic cases of diarrhoea.

STAPHYLOCOCCUS AUREUS

A classic cause of toxic food poisoning, which is due to the ingestion of food contaminated with the enterotoxin of *S. aureus*. The disease is very rapid in onset, because it is due to preformed toxin in food.

Cause: about 40% of *S. aureus* strains produce several heat-stable enterotoxins – A, B, C, D, E. There are three types of enterotoxin C. Enterotoxin-producing strains mostly belong to phage group III.

Clinical features

Symptoms: acute onset of nausea and vomiting within a few hours of eating the contaminated food, sometimes followed by diarrhoea. Self-limiting and rarely severe; dehydration is occasionally a problem in the uncommon severe case.

Pathogenesis

Preformed toxin is ingested in contaminated food and has a local action on the gut mucosa. The toxin resists temperatures that kill *S. aureus*, so food may contain toxin but no viable staphylococci.

Diagnosis

Isolation

Specimens: the suspect food, vomit or faeces.
   Culture: for *S. aureus* on ordinary media or a selective medium.
   Identification: by commercial slide test; later, by phage typing to correlate identity of strains from food and patients.

Demonstration of enterotoxin

In culture filtrate from a strain of *S. aureus* isolated from food or vomit. Examine immunologically, by reverse passive latex agglutination.

Treatment

The disease is short and self-limiting, so treatment is unnecessary.

Epidemiology

Source of infection: usually a staphylococcal lesion on the skin, especially of the fingers of a food handler.
   Route of infection: ingestion – enterotoxin-producing strains of *S. aureus* multiply in the food and liberate toxin. The toxin is relatively heat-stable and, unless the food is thoroughly heated afterwards, retains activity.
   Food: usually, cooked food is involved – although contamination most often takes place after initial cooking. Cold cooked meat is often implicated. Unless food is correctly stored at 4°C, staphylococci can multiply in the warm conditions of the

kitchen, with consequent toxin production. Other foods which have been involved include milk and milk products, e.g. creams and custards.

Outbreaks: the international nature of staphylococcal food poisoning is vividly illustrated by a large outbreak in Japanese air travellers, who became ill while en route from Tokyo to Denmark after eating ham contaminated by a food handler in Alaska.

Control

Food hygiene: exclusion of handlers with septic lesions; prompt refrigeration of food after preparation.

CLOSTRIDIUM PERFRINGENS

Diarrhoea or food poisoning due to *C. perfringens* is fairly common, and is due to the contamination of food by spore-bearing (and therefore heat-resistant) anaerobic organisms.

Classically, non-haemolytic strains of *C. perfringens* which have particularly heat-resistant spores are involved, but β-haemolytic strains with relatively heat-labile spores are also implicated.

Clinical features

Onset is acute: between 8 and 24 h after eating contaminated food. The predominant symptoms are diarrhoea and abdominal pain: vomiting is rare. The illness is self-limiting.

Pathogenesis

Heat-resistant spores of C. perfringens survive 100°C for 30 min. During cooling after cooking, the spores germinate into vegetative bacilli. These multiply rapidly if food is stored at room temperature (the temperature range for growth of *C. perfringens* is 15–50°C) and if there are anaerobic conditions (e.g. some deep meat pies).

Following ingestion of food contaminated with vegetative *C. perfringens*, sporulation takes place in the small intestine – with liberation of a *heat-labile enterotoxin*, which acts mainly on the membrane permeability of the small intestine.

Diagnosis

Strains which cause food poisoning also form part of the normal flora in 5–30% of the population, so that laboratory diagnosis of an individual case is difficult. However, there are many different serotypes of *C. perfringens*, and isolation of the same serotype in large numbers from the victims of an outbreak of food poisoning and from the suspect food (when available) is strong presumptive evidence that it is the cause.

Isolation

Specimens: faeces from as many as possible of the patients involved in the outbreak; samples of suspected food.

Culture: aminoglycoside blood agar, anaerobically.

Observe: typical colonies, β-haemolytic or non-haemolytic.

Identification: by Nagler reaction; serotype in a specialist reference laboratory for epidemiology.

Detection of enterotoxin

In stools, by reverse passive latex agglutination test.

Treatment

Sometimes, rehydration. Antibiotic therapy is unnecessary.

Epidemiology

C. perfringens is often present in large numbers as a commensal in the animal and human intestine; it is also ubiquitous in the environment.

Control

Food hygiene: adequate cooking of meat and meat products, with prompt refrigeration if stored before consumption.

LESS COMMON BACTERIAL CAUSES OF DIARRHOEA

BACILLUS SPECIES

Diarrhoea due to these relatively non-pathogenic organisms is typically associated with Chinese restaurants, because of their frequent use of rice.

Bacillus species are aerobic, spore-forming Gram-positive bacilli, often found in soil and the air and dust of the environment. *B. cereus* is the principal cause of this form of food poisoning, but members of the subtilis group (e.g. *B. subtilis, B. pumilus* and *B. licheniformis*) are increasingly implicated.

Clinical features

There are two distinct types of illness:

- *Short incubation period*: 1–2 h, with nausea and vomiting, often followed by diarrhoea: associated with bulk-prepared rice. This is by far the more common type.
- *Longer incubation period*: 6–16 h, with sudden onset of abdominal pain and diarrhoea: associated with soups and sauces.

Pathogenesis

The disease is due to an enterotoxin produced by *Bacillus* species.

Diagnosis

Isolation

Specimens: suspected food, vomit, faeces.
  Culture: on ordinary media.
  Observe: significant numbers of the typical 'curled hair' colonies.

Treatment

The disease is self-limiting.

Epidemiology

Source: *Bacillus* species and their spores are widespread in soil, and cereals are commonly contaminated with them.
  Route of infection: some spores survive cooking – if storage is at a warm temperature, there is germination into vegetative bacilli, which multiply and produce toxin.

Control

Food hygiene: correct storage of cooked food; reheating should be rapid.

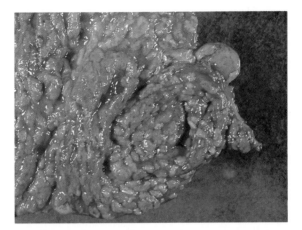

Fig. 28.2   Pseudomembranous colitis. Segment of large bowel with typical pseudomembranous plaques. The plaques consist of fibrin and polymorphs and are the characteristic gross and microscopical lesions in the condition. (Photograph by courtesy of Dr Hugh Gilmour, Pathology Department, University of Edinburgh.)

CLOSTRIDIUM DIFFICILE

Diarrhoea is a common side-effect of oral antibiotic therapy, probably as a result of disturbance of the normal intestinal flora due to the antibacterial action of the drug. This diarrhoea is usually mild and self-limiting. However, antibiotic therapy – particularly in the elderly in hospitals – can cause severe diarrhoea, which is occasionally fatal. This diarrhoea is due to *Clostridium difficile*.

C. difficile is acquired as part of the intestinal flora, most often as a result of cross-infection, either from other patients who are excretors or from contamination in the environment. Antibiotic or other therapy allows *C. difficile* to proliferate and produce toxins. In severe cases, the disease may take the form of fulminant pseudomembranous colitis (Fig. 28.2).

Clindamycin (now rarely used in Britain) was particularly associated with this form of diarrhoea but other antibiotics, notably ampicillin and cephalosporins, can also cause it.

C. difficile can also cause diarrhoea in the absence of antibiotic therapy, and is carried by 3–5% of healthy people.

Clinical features

Varies from mild diarrhoea to the life-threatening disease pseudomembranous colitis: the diarrhoea can be very profuse (up to

20 stools per day); abdominal discomfort, fever and leucocytosis are often present. Sometimes fatal – especially in the vulnerable elderly.

Pathogenesis

Toxin production within the colon. *C. difficile* produces two toxins:

- *Toxin A: an enterotoxin*: responsible for the gut symptoms
- *Toxin B: a cytotoxin*: has a cytopathic effect in cell cultures; a useful marker for identification, since it is always associated with toxin A.

Diagnosis

Clinically, a high index of suspicion is necessary.

Proctosigmoidoscopy: may show the characteristic membrane, or isolated areas of white or yellow material adhering to the colonic mucosa: these areas should be biopsied for histological examination; the rectum is sometimes unaffected.

Laboratory diagnosis

Demonstration of toxin

In *faecal filtrate*, by testing for cytotoxic effect on cells in tissue culture (e.g. Vero or human embryo lung cells). The toxic effect is neutralized by antiserum to *Clostridium sordellii*, which cross-neutralizes *C. difficile* cytotoxin in tissue culture.

Isolation

Isolation of *C. difficile* from faeces on selective media, with subsequent demonstration of toxigenicity.

Treatment

Oral vancomycin or metronidazole.

Epidemiology

Outbreaks of infection have been reported in elderly patients in long-stay wards, and are often associated with contamination of the ward environment by *C. difficile*. Many cases in hospital patients are sporadic.

CLOSTRIDIUM SEPTICUM

C. septicum can cause *neutropenic enterocolitis*, a rare disease seen in neutropenic patients (e.g. associated with cytotoxic therapy for leukaemia): it is sometimes associated with septicaemia.

Neonatal necrotizing enterocolitis, an important and life-threatening complication in preterm babies, is not antibiotic-associated and no bacterial cause has been established.

YERSINIA

Yersinia are not a common cause of diarrhoea in Britain, but have been reported as important enteric pathogens in Europe (especially Belgium and Scandinavia) and North America (particularly Canada). The causal organism is *Y. enterocolitica*.

Clinical features

Acute gastroenteritis, with abdominal pain and fever; as a rule, resolves without treatment in 1–3 weeks. Yersiniosis may mimic appendicitis, and the disease can cause acute terminal ileitis and mesenteric lymphadenitis.

Infection may progress to septicaemia – usually in debilitated patients. Reactive polyarthritis is a recognized complication (see p. 314).

Diagnosis

Isolation

Specimens: faeces, blood cultures or mesenteric lymph nodes (if specimens of these are available).

Serology: demonstration of a rising antibody titre.

Treatment

Tetracycline, aminoglycosides, co-trimoxazole or chloramphenicol.

Treatment is of doubtful value since the disease is usually self-limiting: however, systemic yersiniosis carries a high mortality – despite antibiotic therapy.

Epidemiology

Reservoir of infection: pigs.

Spread: probably via the faecal–oral route, directly person-to-person or from animals by contaminated food and water. However, most cases are sporadic and their epidemiology is uncertain.

Note: *Y. pseudotuberculosis* is a zoonosis: infection in humans takes the form most often of mesenteric adenitis, causing abdominal pain that can mimic appendicitis. It rarely causes diarrhoea. The organism is widespread in birds and wild animals, especially rodents and other small mammals.

VIBRIO PARAHAEMOLYTICUS

This organism is a rare cause of infective diarrhoea, transmitted by shellfish. *V. parahaemolyticus* is a marine bacterium, found in warm coastal waters and in fish and shellfish.

Clinical features

Symptoms: acute onset of vomiting and diarrhoea, usually 8–24 h after eating raw seafood – especially imported shellfish.

Epidemiology

More prevalent in warmer months. Most common in the Far East, where raw fish is a delicacy: cases in Britain have been due to imported seafood, although the organism exists in British sea waters.

LISTERIA MONOCYTOGENES

Outbreaks of gastroenteritis due to this organism have been described, mainly in the USA.

CHOLERA

Cholera is caused by *Vibrio cholerae* O1, and also by non-O1 type 139.

In 1961, the world experienced the start of the seventh pandemic of cholera, which has persisted and spread over the succeeding 36 years: the six previous pandemics were during the

19th and early 20th centuries. Glasgow Royal Infirmary is built on the site of mass cholera graves from the epidemic of 1849. The factors which determine the onset of epidemic spread are unknown.

In 1991, cholera broke out in an epidemic in Peru, later to spread to neighbouring countries in South America and to Mexico.

Late in 1992, a new epidemic of cholera appeared in Bengal due to non-O1 type 139, and spread – causing many deaths in the Indian sub-continent.

Clinical features

Acute onset, after an incubation period of from 6 h to 5 days, of abdominal pain and diarrhoea – the diarrhoea is typically of exceptional severity, progressing to the continuous passage of 'rice-water' stools. Vomiting, dehydration, acidosis and collapse may follow. Some cases are much less severe, with only mild diarrhoea.

Two forms of disease are recognized:

- *Severe classical cholera*
- *Milder cholera, associated with the O1 El Tor biotype.*

Pathogenesis

V. cholerae produces a potent *exotoxin*, very similar to the LT enterotoxin of ETEC, which is plasmid-coded. The toxin stimulates the activity of the enzyme adenyl cyclase, which raises the concentration of cyclic AMP in cells – this causes an increase in the flow of water and electrolytes into the bowel lumen. The fluid lost has relatively high concentrations of bicarbonate and potassium.

V. cholerae is not invasive and does not penetrate the gut mucous membrane, although adhesion to gut epithelium plays a part in its pathogenicity.

Diagnosis

Isolation

Specimen: faeces.
  Culture: on alkaline selective medium.
  Observe: typical colonies.
  Identification: by slide agglutination, with polyvalent antiserum.

Treatment

Correction of dehydration by intravenous administration of fluid and electrolytes, to restore the acid-base balance: mortality can be reduced from more than 50% to nil with fluid replacement treatment.

Tetracycline, given orally or intravenously, may help to limit the duration of diarrhoea and reduce fluid loss.

Epidemiology

Reservoir of infection: is the human gut.

Spread is faecal–oral, usually via contamination of the water supply with sewage, but sometimes via food contaminated by flies or unclean hands.

Symptomless carriers are common in epidemics – for example, the case:carrier ratio may reach 1:100 – and they form an important source of infection.

Pandemic: since 1961, the milder (El Tor) form of cholera has gradually spread through the Far East to reach Africa and beyond: air travel has probably increased the risk of importation of the disease into cholera-free areas. The current epidemic in South America is due to the El Tor biotype. Poorly cooked seafood from contaminated estuarine waters probably played a role in its spread.

Control

Good sanitation, with a clean water supply and adequate sewage disposal, together with personal hygiene (i.e. hand washing after defecation) are effective methods of controlling the spread of cholera. Unfortunately, in many areas of the world these methods are simply not practicable. Carriers and cases should, if possible, be isolated.

Vaccination

A vaccine, containing heat-inactivated organisms, is available: this confers protection of the order of 50–60%. A live attenuated vaccine has also been developed, and been shown to be effective in early trials. There is no protection against the non-O1 strain 139.

WHIPPLE'S DISEASE

A rare multisystem disorder, usually affecting middle-aged Caucasian males.

Pathology: many organs – but especially the small intestine, heart and CNS – are infiltrated with macrophages.

Causal organism: an actinomycete, *Tropherema whippelii*: not yet cultured, but demonstrated within macrophages and numerous other cell types.

Clinical features

Usually of gradual onset, with low-grade fever.

Symptoms include chronic diarrhoea, progressing to malabsorption with steatorrhoea, abdominal pain, weight loss, and arthralgia. Anaemia is common, and there may be neurological signs and symptoms.

Diagnosis

Microscopy of small bowel biopsy.

Treatment

Co-trimoxazole, for 1 year.

NON-BACTERIAL INFECTIVE DIARRHOEA

It must never be forgotten that diarrhoea is often due to infection with non-bacterial agents. The more important of these are listed, with some of their characteristics, in Table 28.2.

Table 28.2   Non-bacterial causes of diarrhoea

Agent	Disease	Diagnosis	Treatment
Viruses			
Rotavirus	Diarrhoea	Electron microscopy of stools; ELISA for antigen in stools	Symptomatic
Adenovirus	Diarrhoea	Electron microscopy of stools	Symptomatic
Astrovirus	Diarrhoea		Symptomatic
Small round structured viruses	Diarrhoea		Symptomatic
Protozoa			
Entamoeba histolytica	Amoebic dysentery	Microscopy of stools; serology	Metronidazole
Giardia lamblia	Giardiasis	Microscopy of duodenal aspirate and stools	Metronidazole
Cryptosporidium	Diarrhoea	Microscopy of stools	Symptomatic
Cyclospora	Diarrhoea	Microscopy of stools	Symptomatic

29. Enteric fever

Enteric fever includes typhoid and paratyphoid fevers. Both are due to salmonellae which are markedly more pathogenic and invasive than those which cause food poisoning. Paratyphoid fever is generally a milder disease than typhoid fever.

The causal organism of typhoid fever is *Salmonella typhi*. *S. paratyphi A, B* and *C* cause paratyphoid fever. *S. paratyphi B* is still sometimes seen in Britain; *S. paratyphi A* and *C* are found in tropical countries.

Note: this chapter refers to both typhoid and paratyphoid fevers except where otherwise indicated.

TYPHOID FEVER

Clinical features

Cause: *S. typhi*

  Incubation period: 14–21 days; sometimes longer.

  Symptoms: a septicaemic, febrile illness with headache, toxaemia, dullness, and apathy. Rose-coloured spots (which contain the infecting organism) are often seen, as a sparse rash on the trunk. Splenomegaly is sometimes present together with some soft abdominal swelling and discomfort generally. Leucopenia is common. Diarrhoea is a late symptom, usually in the third week of illness.

  Duration: untreated, about 4 weeks: symptoms clear up in around 3–4 days with antibiotic therapy.

  Complications: relapse, intestinal perforation and haemorrhage are the most serious; rarely, periostitis, myocarditis, pneumonia.

  Relapse is common, with recrudescence of symptoms about a week after the end of the primary illness.

  Carriers: around 2–5% of patients with typhoid fever become chronic carriers, due to persistent infection of the gall bladder:

this results in *S. typhi* being discharged into the gut and excreted in the faeces.

Pathogenesis

S. typhi invades firstly the alimentary tract by ingestion then via the lymphatic system and the thoracic duct into the bloodstream. This first septicaemic phase leads to infection of the reticulo-endothelial system and the gall bladder. Infection of the gall bladder causes the discharge of organisms into the intestine, with heavy infection of the *Peyer's patches* and septicaemia – and the onset of symptoms.

PARATYPHOID FEVER

Cause: S. parayphi A, B and C

Clinically, a milder febrile illness than typhoid fever, and of shorter duration and incubation period. Transient diarrhoea and symptomless infection are common.

Carriers: patients become carriers less frequently than after typhoid fever.

Diagnosis

Isolation

Specimens: faeces, blood, and urine. Blood culture is positive in over 80% of patients in the first week of illness.

Culture: Blood and urine: MacConkey medium (enrichment and selective media are not necessary). Blood culture is positive in over 80% of patients in the first week of illness. *Faeces*: use indicator medium (for non-lactose-fermenting colonies), and selective and enrichment media.

Identification:
- Biochemical reactions (API test). *Note: S. typhi*, unlike other salmonellae (including *S. paratyphi*) produces no gas on fermentation of sugars.
- Serological: preliminary identification with salmonella polyvalent H and O antisera; final identification: send to Reference Typing Laboratory.

Phage typing: useful in identifying different strains of *S. typhi* (and also of *S. paratyphi B*) for epidemiological investigation into the source of outbreaks.

Serology

The classic test is the *Widal test*: agglutination test for antibodies to flagellar H antigens and somatic O antigens of *S. typhi*, and *S. paratyphi A* and *B*, but the results are difficult to interpret, especially if the patient has been immunized with typhoid vaccine. Diagnosis is best made by isolation of the infecting organism.

Treatment

Acute disease

1. *Chloramphenicol*: effective, but resistance is now a problem: can, rarely, have serious side-effects.
2. *Co-trimoxazole*: less good than chloramphenicol, but has less serious side-effects.
3. *Ciprofloxacin*: may become the drug of choice, especially with the emergence of multi-resistance involving other antibiotics – but care needed with children.

Carriers

It is notoriously difficult to eradicate *S. typhi* from the gall bladder. Antibiotic therapy is effective in curing some carriers, but in a proportion, the infection persists and they become long-term permanent carriers. Early trials of ciprofloxacin have given promising results.

Epidemiology

Habitat: the human gut.

Source of infection: carriers or cases who excrete the organism: excretion in faeces – less commonly in the urine – continues for about 2 months after the acute illness.

Route of infection: ingestion of water or food, contaminated by sewage or via the hands of a carrier. Direct case-to-case spread is rare.

Infecting dose: small numbers of *S. typhi* can cause typhoid fever – hence water-borne infection is common, despite the dilution of organisms. Larger doses are required to infect in paratyphoid fever.

Sporadic cases are now rare in Britain, but infection is endemic in many tropical areas, e.g. Africa, Asia, Latin America.

Outbreaks are often explosive – sometimes involving large numbers of people. There are two main types of outbreak:

- *Water-borne*: in which sewage containing organisms from a carrier pollutes drinking water, e.g. the outbreaks in Croydon in 1937 and in Zermatt in 1963.
- *Food-borne*: in which food becomes contaminated via polluted water or via the hands of carriers. 'Typhoid Mary', possibly the most famous carrier, worked as a cook in the USA and caused numerous outbreaks there in the early years of this century.

  Typhoid and paratyphoid bacilli multiply readily in most types of food.

Tinned food may become contaminated during canning – the large outbreak in Aberdeen in 1964 was due to a tin of corned beef which had been cooled in sewage-contaminated water; bacteria entered the can through tiny holes in the metal casing.

Shellfish often grow in estuaries, where the water may be polluted by sewage: if eaten uncooked, they may cause infection – in the past, a significant source of typhoid, but not paratyphoid, fever.

Milk or cream products, contaminated through handling by carriers, have caused outbreaks of both typhoid and paratyphoid fever.

Other foods, e.g. meat products, dried or frozen eggs, dried coconut, have been responsible for infection as a result of contamination by handlers who were carriers.

Animals: *S. paratyphi B*, unlike *S. typhi*, occasionally infects cattle; this has caused some outbreaks amongst humans, but much less commonly than infection from human sources.

Control

Public health. The most effective way of controlling typhoid and paratyphoid fevers is provision of a clean water supply, adequate arrangements for sewage disposal and supervision of food processing and handling.

Carriers are refractory to treatment, they must not be employed in food preparation. When instructed in personal hygiene (i.e. washing hands after defecation), carriers are rarely a danger to family and close contacts.

Vaccination

Two effective typhoid vaccines are available: the oral live vaccine (Ty 21a) and the injectable Vi capsular polysaccharide vaccine (see Ch. 46).

30. Gastritis and peptic ulcer

Although spiral bacteria were observed in the human stomach a century ago, it was not until 1982 that the organism now known as *Helicobacter pylori* was isolated from a gastric biopsy. Infection with *H. pylori* is considered an important causal factor in peptic ulceration – a view supported by the beneficial response to anti-biotic treatment.

Clinical associations

Infection results in a chronic gastritis (type B or non-autoimmune gastritis), which is often life-long. Although the gastritis is usually asymptomatic, it is strongly associated with duodenal ulcer (present in 90% of cases), and less markedly with gastric ulcer (present in 65% of cases).

Long-term gastritis is a recognized risk factor in gastric carcinoma, and is implicated in about 60% of cancers involving the antrum and body of the stomach. It is even more closely associated with the much rarer tumour, primary malignant lymphoma.

Epidemiology

H. pylori has been demonstrated in saliva, dental plaque and faeces.

There is no evidence that the infection is a zoonosis – it is probably spread from person to person by the oral–oral and/or faecal–oral route.

This common, world-wide, infection affects both males and females. Infection is commoner in developing countries and in lower socio-economic groups is developed countries, indicating that poor living conditions are a predisposing factor. Infection may be acquired in childhood: in developed countries, the prevalence of infection increases with increasing age. Serological studies indicate an infection rate of 20% at 20 years of age, rising to 50% at age 50.

The majority of those infected do *not* develop peptic ulcers, and remain symptom-free.

Pathogenesis

H. pylori is found associated with, but not invading, gastric-type epithelium in the stomach (particularly the antrum). It is also sometimes found in the duodenum, but only if there is ectopic gastric epithelium – a common finding in patients with duodenal ulceration.

The organism survives under a layer of mucus. Its intense urease activity produces ammonia from the urea in gastric juice, which neutralizes the bactericidal action of gastric acid. The organism induces an acute then chronic, inflammatory cell infiltrate within the mucosa, which later atrophies. Gastritis results in a dramatic increase in the release of gastrin, which in turn causes excess acid secretion. The reason for this is uncertain: gastrin production may be stimulated by a rise in mucosal pH, due to ammonia formed by bacterial urease activity, or by cytokines released in the inflammatory response. With the development of gastric atrophy there is progressive reduction in the secretion of acid, and eventually complete achlorhydria.

Although gastritis caused by *H. pylori* is associated with peptic ulcers, the mechanism linking the pathologies is uncertain and *H. pylori* infection must not be considered the only causal factor in peptic ulceration. However, gastritis does reduce the resistance of the epithelium to ulceration and the longer-term atrophic changes, with metaplasia, predispose to cancer.

Infection provokes an antibody response, but this is not protective.

Diagnosis

Three main methods: each has a diagnostic accuracy greater than 90%:

1. *Endoscopy and biopsy*: the samples removed are examined by:
   - histology
   - culture: isolation of *H. pylori* enables antibiotic sensitivity of infecting strain to be determined

- direct urease test: a positive result makes an immediate diagnosis.

This method is invasive and expensive.

2. *Serology*: usually an ELISA test, to detect IgG antibody. This method allows large numbers of samples to be screened at low cost, but antibody levels take many months to fall after successful treatment.

3. *Breath test*: patient swallows ^{13}C- or ^{14}C-radiolabelled urea, which is split by *H. pylori* urease into ammonia and CO_2: detection of radiolabelled carbon in expired air (blown into a bag by the patient) makes the diagnosis. The test becomes negative rapidly after successful treatment.

Treatment

The indication for treatment is a peptic ulcer with evidence of infection. Eradication of infection allows healing of the ulcer, and this greatly reduces recurrence – which is usually due to relapse, rather than reinfection.

All regimens use a combination of drugs: complexity of treatment may result in poor patient compliance. Give *two antimicrobial agents for two weeks* – choose from tetracycline, metronidazole, amoxycillin, clarithromycin, bismuth compounds along with *a gastric antisecretory drug for a longer period* – choose either an H_2-receptor antagonist (eg. cimetidine, ranitidine) or a proton pump inhibitor (eg. omeprazole).

Success rates of around 90% have been reported.

31. Diseases due to toxins

Bacteria elaborate both exotoxins and endotoxins, and the production of these is a main pathogenetic mechanism in bacteria. Some diseases are characterized by lesions and symptoms which are primarily due to the effects of circulating toxin, distant from the site of bacterial multiplication.

Toxin may circulate via the bloodstream or, in some diseases, via the peripheral nerves.

Four main bacterial diseases are of this type:

- Diphtheria
- Tetanus
- Botulism
- Toxic shock syndrome.

DIPHTHERIA

Cause: Corynebacterium diphtheriae.

A severe disease, in which the primary site of infection is the throat: if untreated, there is a high case fatality rate.

Clinical features

Incubation period: 2–5 days.

Local symptoms: sore throat, due to inflamed fauces, with greywhite membrane, due to serocellular exudate caused by locally-produced toxin. Formerly, death was often due to suffocation caused by obstruction of the airways by membrane. Diphtheria sometimes affects the nose – usually causing milder disease.

Distant symptoms: due to circulating exotoxin: are of two types:
- *Cardiotoxic*: exotoxin affects the heart to cause heart failure – a common cause of death in diphtheria.

- *Neurotoxic*: exotoxin acts on nerves to cause cranial and peripheral nerve paralysis.

Pathogenesis

Classically, a disease with toxic effects at sites distant from the focus of primary infection. But note, severe effects are also due to exotoxin produced locally with formation of a suffocating membrane in the throat. Gravis strains of *C. diphtheriae* (see Ch. 13) cause the most severe disease, mitis strains a milder form.

Diagnosis

Isolation

Specimen: throat swab.
 Culture: on Loeffler or tellurite media.
 Observe: typical grey-black colonies on tellurite medium composed of bacteria with distinct microscopic morphology using Neisser's stain.
 Note: Because of the rarity of the disease in the UK, many laboratories no longer routinely culture throat swabs for *C. diphtheriae*.

Demonstrate toxin production

Production of toxin (see p. 102) can be demonstrated by:

- Elek plate in vitro (toxin-antitoxin lines of precipitation in agar gel)
- Guinea pig inoculation in vivo:
 Observe: for death, with gelatinous oedema at site of inoculation, and adrenal haemorrhage: one animal of two tested should be injected with antitoxin, to demonstrate protection.

Treatment

Antitoxin: inject on suspicion of the diagnosis of diphtheria.
 Antibiotics: penicillin or erythromycin.
 Tracheotomy: may be necessary to relieve laryngeal obstruction.

Epidemiology

About 50 non-toxigenic and three toxin-producing strains are isolated annually in the UK. Diphtheria is now rare in well-vaccinated developed countries, although occasional solitary cases and small outbreaks are seen, usually due to infection imported from abroad. In 1991–1994, the former Soviet Union experienced a large epidemic of infection involving several thousand cases, apparently due to inadequate immunization programmes and increased population movement.

Source of infection is respiratory secretions from the throat – and also the nose – of cases and symptomless carriers. Spread is facilitated by close contact. Most at risk are those in poor health and those living in bad housing conditions.

TETANUS

Due to *Clostridium tetani*, tetanus follows contamination of wounds. The toxin produced is one of the most powerful known.

Tetanus is a very rare disease in the UK (fewer than 10 notified cases each year), although the wounds from which it can develop are common, and may be trivial.

Clinical features

Incubation period: 5–15 days.

Symptoms: severe and painful muscle spasms: the masseter muscles are often affected, causing 'lockjaw' (the familiar name for tetanus) and 'risus sardonicus' the characteristic facial grimace produced by spasm of the facial muscles. Because the extensor muscles of the body are more powerful than the flexors, as the spasms progress the body becomes arched in *opisthotonus*, with only the patient's head and heels touching the bed (Fig. 31.1).

Death is due to exhaustion, asphyxiation or intercurrent infection, and the case fatality rate is still high despite intensive therapy. The elderly are particularly at risk.

Pathogenesis

C. tetani produces a protein exotoxin, although this is mainly released by bacterial lysis. It has two components:

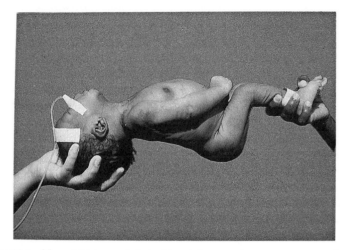

Fig. 31.1   Neonatal tetanus. Infant with opisthotonus due to extensor muscle spasm. (Reproduced with permission from Abbott Laboratories *Slide Atlas of Infectious Diseases*, 1982, Gower Medical Publishing, London. Photograph by Dr T. F. Sellers Jr.)

- *Tetanospasmin*: acts on synapses, to block the normal inhibitory mechanism that controls motor nerve impulses
- *Tetanolysin:* lyses erythrocytes.

Spread: C. tetani does not spread beyond the wound but the toxin, absorbed at the motor nerve endings, travels via the nerves to the anterior horn cells in the spinal cord.

Site: wounds of the face, neck and upper extremities are more dangerous than those of the legs and feet: they are associated with more severe disease and a shorter incubation period.

Tetanus neonatorum, in which the umbilical stump is the portal of entry, is still common in rural areas of Asia, Africa and South America (Fig. 31.1).

Diagnosis

The diagnosis is often clinical: attempts at bacteriological confirmation frequently fail.

Specimen: swab or exudate from wound.

Direct Gram film: examine for characteristic Gram-positive bacilli with round terminal spores – 'drumsticks' (see Fig 18.2).

Culture: on blood agar and aminoglycoside blood agar, anaerobically, and in Robertson's meat medium.

Observe: typical translucent spreading colonies.

Identification: by biochemical tests, and demonstration of the exotoxin by the inhibition of haemolysis on blood agar by specific antitoxin – confirm by demonstration of mouse pathogenicity and its prevention by antitoxin.

Treatment

Supportive: artificial ventilation, with muscle relaxants to control spasms; excision of wound.

Antitoxin: large doses intravenously, to neutralize toxin.

Antibiotics: penicillin or tetracycline, to prevent further toxin production.

Epidemiology

Source: faeces of animals, especially horses: *C. tetani* is hardly ever found in human faeces. Wounds become contaminated with spores which, in anaerobic conditions, germinate to produce vegetative bacilli which form toxin.

World-wide in distribution, but the incidence is much higher in the Third World – where it is an important cause of death.

Classically, tetanus is associated with severe wounds contaminated with soil or dust, similar to those that precede gas gangrene. Today in countries with good medical services, prophylactic measures prevent patients with such wounds developing the disease. Rather surprisingly, tetanus now often follows minor injuries disregarded by the patient, e.g. a small penetrating wound from a splinter of wood. In a few reported cases in the UK, no wound could be found.

Prevention

Official policy in Britain is for active immunization in childhood, with formol toxoid in the Triple Vaccine.

In casualty departments, a common problem is wound contamination with soil or dust and therefore, potentially, with *C. tetani*. The wound must first be thoroughly cleansed and then:

- If previously fully immunized, give a booster dose of tetanus toxoid. If the wound is dirty and more than 24 hours old, human antitetanus immunoglobulin must also be administered.

- If non-immune or if the previous immunization history is uncertain, give human antitetanus immunoglobulin and start a full course of tetanus toxoid.

When active and passive immunization need to be given at the same time, interference between toxoid and antitoxin must be minimized by the administration of vaccine and antiserum into different arms.

Penicillin (usually a mixture of short- and long-acting varieties) has been recommended on its own as prophylaxis, but its value is not proven. Nevertheless, in practice it is common to give penicillin to the wounded, not only as part of the scheme to prevent tetanus but also in an attempt to avoid pyogenic infection.

BOTULISM

A rare but severe food-borne disease, due to ingestion of a bacterial toxin preformed in food; diarrhoea is not a symptom.

Causal organism: *Clostridium botulinum*, types A, B and E (rarely, types C, F and G).

Clinical features

Incubation period: usually 12–36 h.

Symptoms: neurological: the toxin acts by inhibiting acetyl-choline release at neuromuscular junctions, to cause signs and symptoms such as oculomotor and pharyngeal paralysis, vomiting, constipation, thirst, dryness of mouth, vertigo; sometimes difficulty in speaking.

Prognosis: often fatal: death is due to respiratory failure.

Pathogenesis

C. botulinum is a spore-forming anaerobe, which forms an exceedingly powerful exotoxin. It is found in soil, water and sludge. If spores contaminate food in anaerobic conditions, germination follows and the vegetative bacilli multiply, with production of toxin during storage at room temperature. Spore germination and toxin formation are inhibited by a low pH, so are not usually a problem in acid fruits. The toxin is sensitive to heat and is destroyed by cooking.

Diagnosis

1. *Demonstration of toxin*

Specimen: suspected food; patient's serum and faeces.
 Demonstrate toxin: by inoculation of mice.
 Observe: for paralysis and death.
 Identification: test mice protected by antitoxins to toxin types A, B and E: protection by the corresponding antitoxin identifies the toxin present.

2. *Isolation*

Specimen: suspected food, patient's faeces.
 Culture: after pasteurization of the food to destroy non-sporing bacteria, anaerobic culture at 35°C.
 Identification: of isolated suspect colonies.

Treatment

Antibiotics are of no value. Treatment is supportive, with artificial ventilation, etc. and the administration of antitoxin to neutralize absorbed toxin.

Epidemiology

Table 31.1 shows the habitat, geography and the kind of food associated with the three types of *C. botulinum* that cause human disease. The disease is extremely rare in Britain, but there was a small outbreak in Birmingham in 1978 due to tinned Alaskan salmon contaminated with type E toxin. In 1989, a sizeable outbreak of botulism in Britain was caused by the contamination of hazel-nut purée with *C. botulinum* type B: the toxin was ingested in hazel-nut yoghourt.
    Person-to-person spread does not occur.

Control

Amateur canning and preservation of food should be avoided. Commercial canning and pickling processes should be carefully controlled: a temperature that will kill the heat-resistant spores of *C. botulinum* is essential, e.g. 120°C for 20 min.

Table 31.1   Main medically important types of *Clostridium botulinum*

Type	Habitat	Geography	Usual source of infection
A	Soil	USA Former USSR	Home-preserved vegetables, meat, fish
B	Soil	Europe USA	Meat, especially pork
E	Soil, sea water, sludge	Japan Canada Alaska	Raw or tinned fish

INFANTILE BOTULISM

Rare in this country, but not uncommon in the USA. It is due to the ingestion of *C. botulinum* spores, not preformed toxin.

Causal organism: *C. botulinum*, usually type A or B. The spores are sometimes found in contaminated honey.

Clinical features

Affects infants, often when mixed feeding starts, causing constipation, failure to thrive, cranial palsies and even sudden death.

Pathogenesis

After colonization of the gut, the bacteria multiply and produce toxin: the subsequent absorption of toxin leads to symptoms.

Diagnosis

Isolation: of *C. botulinum* from stools.
Demonstration: of *C. botulinum* toxin in stools or (rarely) serum.

TOXIC SHOCK SYNDROME (TSS)

Clinical features

Fever, collapse, diarrhoea and vomiting, with a diffuse erythematous macular rash, followed by skin desquamation. The patient is often severely ill and there is a significant mortality, with multisystem involvement and hypotension (or 'shock').

Patients are mainly menstruating women who use tampons, especially the super-absorbent varieties marketed in the 1980s.

These encourage the growth of *Staphylococcus aureus*, present as a commensal in the vagina. TSS occasionally complicates other forms of staphylococcal sepsis, usually of the skin, in both men and women.

Pathogenesis

Due to circulating toxins, in particular TSST-1 (toxic shock syndrome toxin-1), formerly known as enterotoxin F.

Diagnosis

Isolation from vagina, tampon or other infected site, of a strain of *S. aureus* producing TSST-1.

Treatment

Flucloxacillin.

SCALDED SKIN SYNDROME

Also called Ritter–Lyell disease, this is characterized by extensive skin desquamation due to the local production of epidermolytic toxin by *S. aureus*. It is considered on page 264.

SEPTIC (ENDOTOXIC) SHOCK

A severe disease, not due to circulating exotoxin but associated with Gram-negative bacteraemia. Endotoxins – or the O surface antigens – of Gram-negative bacilli are responsible for this severe and often fatal shock syndrome (see p. 280).

32. Urinary tract infections

Urinary tract infections remain a major clinical problem, over 50 years after the introduction of antimicrobial chemotherapy: many consultations in general practice are because of urinary infections.

Urinary infection is defined as *bacteriuria*, i.e. the multiplication of bacteria in urine within the renal tract: a concentration of greater than 10^5 organisms/ml (10^8/l) is regarded as significant bacteriuria.

Pyuria is the presence of pus cells (polymorphs) in the urine: it usually – but not always – accompanies bacteriuria.

Infections of the urinary tract may involve:

- bladder: *cystitis*
- kidney: pelvis – *pyelitis*; parenchyma – *pyelonephritis*
- urethra: *urethritis*.

It is difficult to distinguish between pyelitis and pyelonephritis, and it is probably better to refer to both as pyelonephritis. Urethritis is considered in Chapter 39.

Clinical features

Cystitis: the classical symptoms are dysuria, frequency, urgency, suprapubic pain, and sometimes haematuria. Episodes of cystitis greatly outnumber those that involve the kidney.

Pyelonephritis: the signs are loin pain and tenderness, rigors and fever.

Chronic pyelonephritis causes general ill-health and malaise, with nocturia.

Children: symptoms are often nonspecific, e.g. failure to thrive in infants, febrile convulsions in toddlers, unexplained fever in older children.

Women: urinary infection is predominantly a disease of women (sex ratio 10:1).

245

Symptoms of infection, usually those of cystitis, are surprisingly common. Only a minority of women who experience frequency and dysuria consult their doctor, and of those who do, only about two-thirds have infected urine. Of the remainder, some will subsequently develop significant bacteriuria but others never have bacteriuria – although pyuria may be present. The cause of their symptoms, which may be recurrent, is unclear and this condition is referred to as the 'urethral' or 'dysuria-pyuria' syndrome.

Symptomless urinary infection, or 'covert bacteriuria', is, conversely, also not uncommon: it can be detected in 5% of adult women, 1–2% of girls and 0.3% of boys (in whom it is often associated with abnormality of the renal tract). In pregnancy it is associated with a high risk of developing pyelonephritis.

Screening to detect symptomless or covert bacteriuria has been advocated in schoolchildren and pregnant women.

Causal organisms

Escherichia coli is the cause of 60–90% of urinary infections. Certain serotypes of *E. coli* are particularly common in urinary infection (e.g. 02, 04, 06, 07, 018, 075): this is probably because they are often present in the colon, rather than because of inherently high pathogenicity for the urinary tract. However, some strains are reputed to be more invasive than others. *Factors associated with virulence* include: the possession of K (capsular) antigens, which inhibit phagocytosis and the bactericidal effect of normal human serum; and the ability to adhere to uro-epithelium, due to specialized fimbriae.

Staphylococcus saprophyticus is an important cause of infection, related to sexual activity in women under 25 years old. It is detected in 30% of such infections, but surprisingly is seldom isolated from faeces and the anogenital region of young women.

Proteus mirabilis: responsible for 10% of infections.

Klebsiella species: often multiply antibiotic-resistant.

Enterococcus faecalis: often found accompanying infection with coliforms.

Fastidious Gram-positive bacteria (e.g. lactobacilli, streptococci, corynebacteria), which require incubation for 48–72 h in the presence of 7% CO_2 for isolation. Routine urine culture fails to grow these organisms, but when they have been detected by appropriate methods, it is claimed that they are associated with pyuria and symptoms, of infection. Infection with them may be one cause of the urethral syndrome.

Pseudomonas aeruginosa ⎫ especially after catheterization
Staphylococcus aureus   ⎭ or instrumentation.

Mycobacterium tuberculosis: renal tuberculosis is described in Chapter 37.

Acute uncomplicated urinary infection is usually due to one type of organism.

Chronic infection is often associated with more than one type of organism.

Source, route and factors influencing urinary infection

Source: the reservoir of urinary pathogens is the flora of the colon.

Route of infection is ascending via the urethra from the perineum.

Female preponderance is probably due to the shortness of the female urethra: turbulence of urinary flow during micturition may result in bacteria entering the bladder.

Colonization of the periurethral area with potential pathogens is said to be a necessary prerequisite for infection: this may be prevented by the bactericidal activity of urethral and vaginal secretions.

Sterility of urine is maintained by 'flushing' (i.e. from the frequent and complete emptying of the bladder and constant in-flow of newly formed urine), by antibody and nonspecific antibacterial substances in urogenital secretions, and by local defence mechanisms in the bladder wall.

Residual urine: after micturition the bladder should be empty – residual urine enables bacteria to multiply, and predisposes to infection.

Sexual intercourse, especially within the previous 48 h, is correlated with infection and the onset of symptoms in young women – possibly due to retrograde 'milking' of the urethra during coitus ('honeymoon cystitis').

Incompetence of the vesicoureteric valve, due to congenital abnormality or inflammation of the bladder wall, causes reflux of urine into the kidney pelvis during micturition; this may lead to pyelitis and pyelonephritis.

The risk of infection is also greatly increased by abnormalities of the renal tract which cause *obstruction* and *stasis* in the tract, e.g. congenital structural abnormalities, urinary calculi, neurogenic bladder, prostatic enlargement.

Diagnosis

Specimen: a mid-stream specimen of urine (MSSU), collected to avoid contamination from perineum or vagina; in babies, use a strategically-placed self-adhesive plastic bag – but suprapubic needle aspiration of the full bladder may be necessary. A catheter specimen of urine (CSU) is excellent, but catheterization to obtain urine for laboratory examination cannot be justified because of the risk of introducing infection.

Transport: bacteria multiply in urine, so specimens must be submitted to the laboratory within 2–4 h of collection. If this is not possible, do one of the following:

- Refrigerate the specimen at 4°C
- Use container with boric acid, a bacteriostatic preservative, to give a final concentration in urine of 1.8%
- Use a dip-slide coated on both sides with culture medium and inoculated by dipping into the freshly-voided urine: can be read even after several days' delay.

Direct examination:
- *Wet film*: for the presence of pus cells and bacteria: erythrocytes and casts should be noted.
- *Gram film*: not often required: sometimes useful for immediate presumptive identification of causal bacteria. Figure 32.1 shows a typical Gram film of the urinary deposit in an acute infection due to Gram-negative bacilli.

Culture: semi-quantitative culture on media such as CLED or MacConkey agar (to prevent swarming of proteus).

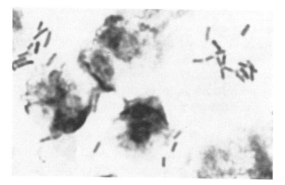

Fig. 32.1 Urinary deposit: coliform infection (approx. × 1000).

Observe and count the number of colonies obtained (Fig. 32.2):

- More than 10^5 bacteria/ml: evidence of urinary infection: carry out sensitivity tests with appropriate antibiotics.
- Between 10^4 and 10^5 bacteria/ml: significance doubtful: further specimens should be obtained.
- Less than 10^4 bacteria/ml: regard as contaminants (unless the patient is on treatment for a known urinary infection).

Note: One cause of pyuria without bacteriuria is *renal tuberculosis*. When there is no obvious cause for pyuria without bacteriuria (e.g. recent urinary infection), three entire early-morning specimens should be examined for *Mycobacterium tuberculosis*.

Detection of site of infection within urinary tract

A number of laboratory tests, none foolproof, have been proposed to distinguish between renal and bladder bacteriuria. Kidney involvement is said to be likely when:

1. Renal concentration efficiency is reduced: tested by water deprivation.
2. Excess of β_2 microglobulin is present in urine.
3. Antibodies to the infecting organism can be detected in serum.
4. Antibody-coated bacteria can be demonstrated in the urine by immunofluorescence microscopy.

Treatment

Acute uncomplicated infections

Numerous suitable oral antibiotics are available, all are excreted in the urine in high concentration:

- Trimethoprim
- Co-trimoxazole
- Ciprofloxacin
- Nitrofurantoin.

A short (3-day) course is usually adequate: in fact, a single dose may be effective.

β-lactam antibiotics (e.g. ampicillin, co-amoxiclav, cephalexin) are, in general, less effective.

Pyelonephritis or chronic recurrent infections: parenteral therapy with an aminoglycoside or β-lactam, e.g. cephalosporin,

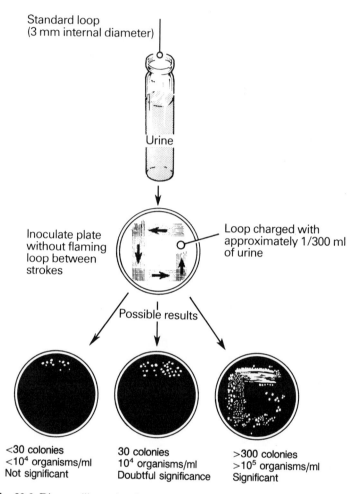

Standard loop
(3 mm internal diameter)

Urine

Inoculate plate
without flaming
loop between
strokes

Loop charged with
approximately 1/300 ml
of urine

Possible results

<30 colonies
<10⁴ organisms/ml
Not significant

30 colonies
10⁴ organisms/ml
Doubtful significance

>300 colonies
>10⁵ organisms/ml
Significant

Fig. 32.2 Diagram illustrating the semi-quantitative culture of urine specimens.

aztreonam may be required. The efficacy of β-lactams given parenterally is not in doubt.

Cure rate of acute infections is around 90%, but 50% of the infections recur within a year and about 10% of patients have repeated recurrences, most likely if infection involves the kidney.

Relapse: recurrence within 1 month of stopping treatment is usually due to relapse, i.e. recrudescence of infection with the same organism: evidence of therapy failure.

Reinfection: later recurrence is often a result of reinfection with a different organism.

Recurrent infections often require long-term suppressive treatment with low doses of trimethoprim or nitrofurantoin. Because there may be underlying abnormality of the urinary tract further investigations may be required, e.g. intravenous urography and other more sophisticated tests.

Prognosis

In adults, bacteriuria, with or without symptoms, is a relatively benign condition and permanent or progressive renal damage is rare.

In children under 5 years of age, the prognosis is much worse: bacteriuria with vesicoureteric reflux often results in progressive renal damage, with scar formation and impairment of kidney growth. Some of these children go on to develop chronic pyelonephritis – which accounts for 20% of end-stage renal failure. Reflux resolves spontaneously in most children as they grow older.

In children with chronic pyelonephritis, renal scarring may be reduced by antibiotic treatment of acute episodes and prophylaxis against recurrence with long-term trimethoprim: this is essential if reflux is present.

HOSPITAL URINARY INFECTION

A particular problem in urological wards.

80% of hospital-acquired urinary tract infections are associated with urethral catheterization.

Catheterization: the risk of infection after a single catheterization – even if carefully carried out – is about 5%: almost all patients with an indwelling catheter develop infection.

Septicaemia: one quater of septicaemias in hospital patients originate from urinary tract infection.

Source of infection

Endogenous: from contamination of the patient's urethra or perineum by bacteria from the colonic flora.

Exogenous: due to cross-infection with bacteria from the infected urinary tract of another patient: transmission is by instruments (e.g. cystoscopes, catheters) or by hands of doctors and nurses.

Prevention

Strict attention to aseptic technique: use of disposable plastic catheters; introduction of antiseptics into the urethra before instrumentation. Careful handwashing and drying between patients is *essential*.

Indwelling catheters should be attached to a closed drainage system, to prevent retrograde bacterial spread into the bladder from the collection bag.

Short-term antibiotic prophylaxis to reduce the risk of septicaemia may be given at the time of operations on, or the removal of catheters from, an infected urinary tract.

33. Meningitis

Bacterial meningitis (classically, 'pyogenic' or polymorphonuclear meningitis) is a much more severe disease than viral meningitis (classically 'aseptic' or lymphocytic), and untreated is almost always fatal. Even with antibiotic therapy, bacterial meningitis remains a serious cause of morbidity and mortality and is a bacteriological emergency requiring urgent diagnosis and treatment.

Clinical features

Symptoms: severe headache with malaise and fever – the onset is often abrupt. Vomiting, photophobia and convulsions are sometimes seen, and patients often show irritability and are lethargic, with drowsiness progressing to unconsciousness.

Signs of meningeal irritation: neck and spinal stiffness; pain and resistance on extending the knee when the thigh is flexed (Kernig's sign). 'Meningism' (signs of meningeal irritation without meningitis) may be a feature of other types of severe infection: the diagnosis of meningitis has to be differentiated from meningism, subarachnoid haemorrhage and cerebral abscess.

Age: although meningitis is largely a disease of infancy and childhood, the disease is encountered throughout life.

Neonatal meningitis: the characteristic clinical features of meningitis are usually absent – the only presenting features being that the baby is obviously unwell, with failure to feed and, often, vomiting. The condition is much more common in premature than in full-term babies.

The elderly and the immunocompromised: typical clinical signs and symptoms of meningitis may again be absent; mental confusion is sometimes a prominent feature.

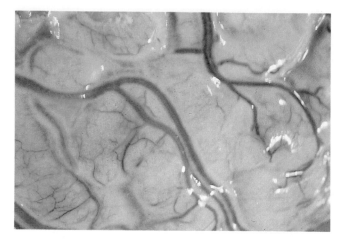

Fig. 33.1   Surface of brain in pneumococcal meningitis. *Note*: Congested meningeal vessels with purulent exudate, best seen within the sulci.

Sequelae

There are extensive pathological changes within the CNS (Fig. 33.1) and, despite appropriate antibiotic therapy, neurological sequelae can follow in survivors. The commonest sequela is deafness; other, rarer, neurological sequelae include encephalopathy, cranial nerve palsies, and obstructive hydrocephalus.

CAUSAL ORGANISMS

The most common causal organisms are:

- *Neisseria meningitidis* (meningococcus)
- *Haemophilus influenzae*
- *Streptococcus pneumoniae* (pneumococcus)
- *Mycobacterium tuberculosis*.

Neisseria meningitidis (meningococcus)

The main cause of meningitis in Britain: affects all ages, but most common in infants, children and young adults. In the UK, group B strains are responsible for the majority of infections, but group C strains have become more common in recent years. In 1995–6, 40% of isolates were group C and 50% group B; before that, the proportions were 26% group C and 70% group B. The other five serogroups (see Ch. 16) are usually found in carriers rather than in cases. The disease is endemic, and sometimes epidemic.

Meningococcal septicaemia: is a dangerous early manifestation of meningococcal meningitis. It has a high mortality rate, and is associated with adrenal haemorrhages, causing sudden collapse (Waterhouse–Friderichsen syndrome). During the meningo-coccaemia a characteristic petechial rash, rare in other types of meningitis, is common.

Incubation period of meningitis: short: around 3 days.

Source: the reservoir is the human nasopharynx.

Spread: via infected respiratory secretions from carriers and cases (i.e. 'droplet spread'). Carriage rate in normal populations is about 10–25%: this may rise to 50% or more in household contacts of sporadic cases and during epidemics in closed communities, e.g. institutions, military camps.

Route of infection: from nasopharynx, probably via the blood-stream, to the meninges.

Treatment: penicillin is the drug of choice: cefotaxime or chloramphenicol are alternatives. Sulphonamide penetrates the CSF well, but its effectiveness has diminished due to the frequency of sulphonamide-resistant strains.

Chemoprophylaxis: use for *close* contacts of a patient, e.g. members of the same household, possibly contacts in school, to eradicate the organism from the nasopharynx. Rifampicin is the drug of choice: alternatives are ceftriaxone (by injection only) or ciprofloxacin (not for children).

Vaccine: N. meningitidis type B is unfortunately non-immunogenic. Effective vaccines are available for types A and C.

Haemophilus influenzae

A common cause of meningitis in infants and pre-school children aged 1 month to 4 years. The causal strains are capsulated and almost always of serological type b. Spread to the meninges is from the nasopharynx, probably via the bloodstream.

Treatment: chloramphenicol penetrates readily to the CSF, and is the drug of choice. Ampicillin or cefotaxime are alternatives.

Chemoprophylaxis of close contacts: rifampicin.

Vaccine: Hib vaccine has now been introduced for the immunization of infants (see Ch. 46) and has caused a dramatic fall in the incidence of the disease.

Streptococcus pneumoniae (pneumococcus)

Although not uncommon in children, this is the usual cause of meningitis in the middle-aged and elderly, especially in patients who are in poor general health. This type of meningitis is often the sequela to pneumococcal infection of the middle ear, sinuses or lungs; fracture of the base of the skull, communicating with the nasopharynx, is another risk factor.

Case fatality rate: is high, despite appropriate antibiotic therapy – around 20%.

Treatment: penicillin: but note that a small proportion of *S. pneumoniae* are now penicillin-resistant: if resistant, use cefotaxime.

Mycobacterium tuberculosis

Seen in people of all ages – but most common in children – and at any stage after the primary infection. Now rare in developed countries: about 100 cases per year in England and Wales. Typically lymphocytic (aseptic) meningitis, although polymorphs are present in the early stages.

Treatment: triple therapy with isoniazid, rifampicin and pyrazinamide: include ethambutol and streptomycin if resistance suspected. Continue isoniazid and rifampicin for 12 months, with pyrazinamide for the first 2 months. Steroids are given with the antibiotics to reduce the inflammatory response.

Rare causes of meningitis

- *Listeria monocytogenes*: mainly seen in infants, the elderly and immunocompromised patients; often, but not always, a lymphocytic meningitis.
- *Cryptococcus neoformans*: meningitis due to this yeast is rare in previously normal people, but is found in immunocompromised patients, e.g. those with leukaemia or lymphoma.
- *Leptospira interrogans*: a lymphocytic meningitis.

Neonatal meningitis: a serious form of meningitis: mainly due to Gram-negative bacilli such as *Escherichia coli*, *Klebsiella* species and *Proteus* species, but also to *L. monocytogenes* and β-haemolytic streptococci of Lancefield group B (usually acquired from the mother's vagina). Premature (low birth-weight) babies are at greatest risk, especially if there has been a prolonged interval between rupture of the membranes and delivery.

Treatment of neonatal meningitis: if due to coliform bacilli: give gentamicin with ampicillin, or a β-lactamase-stable cephalosporin. Chloramphenicol is of limited value. If due to listeria: give gentamicin with ampicillin.

Group B β-haemolytic streptococcal meningitis in babies is best treated with penicillin and gentamicin in combination.

Gentamicin penetrates the blood-brain barrier poorly, and may be given intrathecally or intraventricularly as well as systemically.

Diagnosis

Laboratory diagnosis of bacterial meningitis depends on examination of the CSF. Table 33.1 lists the results of CSF examination in meningitis compared to that in the other two most important diseases in the differential diagnosis – subarachnoid haemorrhage and cerebral abscess.

Red blood cells may be present in a normal CSF due to accidental damage to a blood vessel during lumbar puncture (universally known as a 'bloody tap'): in such cases the supernatant fluid after centrifugation is clear, whereas in subarachnoid haemorrhage it is stained yellow to orange (xanthochromic).

Isolation

Specimens: CSF obtained by lumbar puncture; blood.
  Examination of CSF:

- in a counting chamber, for white blood cells and erythrocytes
- Gram film of centrifuged deposit, for bacteria and cells
- if indicated, Leishman film of centrifuged deposit, to differentiate polymorphonuclear leucocytes from lymphocytes
- if indicated, Ziehl–Neelsen film of centrifuged deposit, for tubercle bacilli.

  Culture of CSF:

- centrifuged deposit onto blood agar and chocolate agar, and into glucose broth and cooked meat broth: incubate plates in air plus 5% CO_2
- if indicated, Löwenstein–Jensen medium, for culture for tubercle bacilli.

Table 33.1 Findings in cerebrospinal fluid

	Causal microorganisms	Appearance	Cells/mm^3	Microbiology	Protein	Glucose
Normal	–	Clear, colourless	0–5 lymphocytes	Sterile	150–450 mg per litre	2.8–3.9 mmol per litre
Bacterial meningitis	Neisseria meningitidis Haemophilus influenzae Streptococcus pneumoniae	Turbid	500–20 000, mainly polymorphs, few lymphocytes	Bacteria in Gram-stained deposit. Growth on culture	Markedly raised	Reduced or absent
Viral (aseptic) meningitis	Enteroviruses Mumps virus	Clear or slightly turbid	10–500, mainly lymphocytes	Viruses rarely isolated from CSF. Diagnose by stool culture (enteroviruses) or serology (mumps)	Normal or slightly raised	Normal
Tuberculous meningitis	Mycobacterium tuberculosis	Clear or slightly turbid	10–500, mainly lymphocytes, polymorphs in early stages	AAFB in ZN-stained deposit – often scanty. Growth on LJ culture	Moderately raised	Usually reduced
Cerebral abscess	Streptococcus milleri Bacteroides species, Staphylococcus aureus, Proteus species	Clear or slightly turbid	0–500, mainly polymorphs, some lymphocytes	Organisms often not present in CSF	Normal or raised	Normal
Subarachnoid haemorrhage	–	Turbid, often blood-stained; supernatant yellow–orange	Large numbers of red blood cells	Sterile	Markedly raised	Normal

AAFB: acid- and alcohol-fast bacilli; ZN: Ziehl–Neelsen; LJ: Löwenstein–Jensen.

Blood culture: positive in over 40% of patients with meningitis due to *N. meningitidis*, *H. influenzae* or *S. pneumoniae*.

Demonstration of bacterial antigen

Of value when meningitis has been partially treated and no infecting organisms can be seen or cultured: bacterial antigen is detected immunologically by latex agglutination or Phadebact coagglutination for *N. meningitidis*, *H. influenzae* type b and pneumococci.

Antibiotic treatment

Before the results of laboratory tests are available, if meningitis is suspected give penicillin immediately: this may be life-saving in the case of meningococcal septicaemia.

The treatment of meningitis of known cause is covered in the corresponding sections above.

Meningitis of unknown cause

When many polymorphs are present in the deposit of the CSF, but no bacteria have been detected and there is no growth on culture, treatment must be empirical. This state of affairs is usually the result of inadequate treatment, given outside hospital before the patient is admitted. Broth cultures may give a positive result after a few days' incubation when cultures on solid media remain negative.

On a *'best-guess'* basis, give either chloramphenicol or a β-lactamase-stable cephalosporin. The triple therapy of penicillin, sulphonamide and chloramphenicol – once very popular – is used less often nowadays.

34. Sepsis

The term *'sepsis'* covers numerous and diverse purulent infections, some trivial and others serious. These include:

- superficial skin infections
- cellulitis
- necrotizing fasciitis
- wound infections
- peritonitis
- abscesses
- septicaemia.

These diseases are amongst the most common encountered in medicine. The causes are numerous and often involve many different bacteria. Bacteriology laboratories, therefore, have an important role in the diagnosis and treatment of these infections.

SKIN INFECTION

The skin is an efficient barrier to infection and, provided that it is not breached, usually prevents invasion by either resident commensal or exogenous bacteria. Nevertheless, skin infections are common, probably because minor skin trauma is a part of everyday life.

The main forms of skin sepsis are shown in Table 34.1.

Clinical features

Boils, carbuncles, styes, sycosis barbae

With the exception of carbuncles, skin infections are uncomfortable and unsightly rather than serious. Carbuncles are rarely seen nowadays except in diabetics, who have a predisposition to

Table 34.1   Skin infections

Infection	Site	Causal organism
Boil	Hair follicle	*Staphylococcus aureus*
Carbuncle	Multiple hair follicles	*Staphylococcus aureus*
Stye	Eyelash follicle	*Staphylococcus aureus*
Sycosis barbae	Shaving area	*Staphylococcus aureus*
Impetigo	Cheeks, around mouth	{ *Streptococcus pyogenes* / *Staphylococcus aureus*
Erysipelas	Face, sometimes limbs	*Streptococcus pyogenes*
Pemphigus neonatorum	Infant's skin	*Staphylococcus aureus*
Toxic epidermal necrolysis	Infant's skin	*Staphylococcus aureus*
Acne vulgaris	Face and back	*Propionibacterium acnes*

develop septic lesions: they are associated with considerable malaise and systemic disturbance.

Below are listed some characteristics of these skin infections:

1. Due to *Staphylococcus aureus*, mainly of phage groups I or II.

2. Tend to be recurrent – appearing in crops at the same site, often over weeks or months.

3. Infection is usually endogenous and due to a strain carried in the nose and on the skin.

4. Generally more common in males than females: seen in previously healthy young males surprisingly often. *Sycosis barbae* is a chronic infection of the skin of the shaving area, and consists of a septic pustular rash: almost certainly spread by the minor trauma inflicted on skin and hair follicles by a razor, and seen only in males (Fig. 34.1).

Treatment: boils and styes do not require antibiotic therapy – in any event, this does not prevent recurrences. Severe infections like carbuncles should be treated with penicillin if the causal strain is sensitive; otherwise, with a different antistaphylococcal drug such as flucloxacillin. Sycosis barbae should be treated with topical antibiotics, e.g. cream containing neomycin and bacitracin, fusidic acid or mupirocin.

Carriage sites: application to the nostrils of creams containing topical antibiotics such as neomycin or bacitracin can suppress (but rarely eradicate) the nasal carriage of *S. aureus*. Mupirocin is generally effective against MRSA (methicillin-resistant *S. aureus*). The regular use of hexachlorophane soap reduces overall skin carriage.

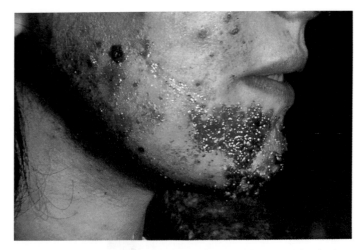

Fig. 34.1 Sycosis barbae. Staphylococcal infection of the skin of the shaving area. (Photograph by Dr A. Lyell.)

Impetigo

A disease of young children, in which vesicles appear on the skin around the mouth: later they become purulent, with characteristic honey-coloured crusts. Nowadays most often due to *S. aureus*, but *Streptococcus pyogenes* can also cause impetigo (Fig. 34.2).

Outbreaks are not uncommon in schools, where infection is spread by contact, shared towels and contaminated fomites.

Glomerulonephritis has been described following impetigo due to *S. pyogenes*, especially Griffith type 49.

Treatment: antibiotics topically, e.g. tetracycline, chloramphenicol, bacitracin, mupirocin (reserve for MRSA); systemic antibiotics are rarely required for this superficial infection.

Erysipelas

A spreading infection due to *S. pyogenes*, presenting as a red, indurated and sharply demarcated area of skin; oedema often develops, causing a characteristic 'orange-skin' texture to the skin, and the patient may be acutely ill, with high fever and toxaemia. A rare disease nowadays.

Treatment: penicillin.

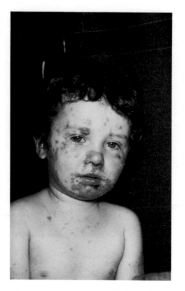

Fig. 34.2   Impetigo. (Photograph by Dr W. C. Love.)

Neonatal skin sepsis

Neonates are especially susceptible to infection, and *S. aureus* can become epidemic in neonatal nurseries – with outbreaks of pustules, sticky eyes, boils and abscesses. Neonates readily become carriers, in the nose, skin and umbilical stump.

Two severe infections associated with skin splitting are sometimes seen in neonates and infants: both are due to staphylococci of phage group II, which produce an epidermolytic toxin which causes skin splitting and desquamation:

- *Pemphigus neonatorum*: in which the skin splitting is focal or localized in large vesicles or bullae: a more serious disease than the neonatal infections listed above, but it responds well to antibiotic treatment.
- *Toxic epidermal necrolysis*, also called *Ritter–Lyell's disease* or, more descriptively, 'scalded skin syndrome': a serious disease in which large areas of the skin desquamate, leaving a red weeping surface which resembles a scald (Fig. 34.3). Seen predominantly in neonates, but also in young children and occasionally in adults: usually responds to antibiotic treatment with full recovery.
  Treatment: flucloxacillin.

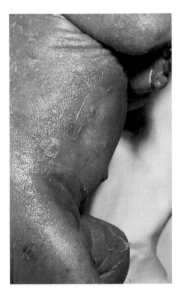

Fig. 34.3   Ritter–Lyell's disease: 'scalded skin' produced by epidermolytic toxin of *Staphylococcus aureus*. (Photograph by Dr W. C. Love.)

Acne vulgaris

A common and disfiguring skin disease of adolescence: it sometimes persists into adult life, leaving residual pitting or scarring. Acne is probably not primarily an infectious disease, but bacteria play a cofactor role in its pathogenesis.

Propionibacterium acnes (and *P. granulosum*) can regularly be isolated from inflamed comedones (whiteheads). These bacteria may induce an inflammatory reaction in the skin by the production of lipase, which liberates irritant fatty acids from lipid in the sebum within sebaceous glands.

Treatment: topical erythromycin, tetracycline, clindamycin. In severe cases: tretinoin or other non-antibacterial drugs.

Note: bacteriology plays no part in diagnosis.

Diagnosis of skin infections

Isolation

Specimens: swabs from lesions: pus, exudate.

Direct Gram film: observe for bacteria, noting especially the arrangement of any Gram-positive cocci (see Figs 7.1 and 8.1).

Culture: blood agar.
Observe: typical colonies.
Identification: as appropriate for the organisms isolated.

CELLULITIS

An infection of subcutaneous tissue. There are two main clinical and bacteriological forms.

Acute pyogenic cellulitis

Due to *Streptococcus pyogenes*. Presents as a red, painful swelling, usually of a limb; commonly associated with lymphangitis and lymphadenitis, involving local draining lymph glands (Fig. 34.4).
    Treatment: penicillin.

Anaerobic cellulitis

Rare – sometimes due to non-sporing anaerobes (e.g. 'bacteroides') or clostridia, but more usually a synergistic infection with both aerobic and anaerobic bacteria. The aerobes produce reducing or anaerobic conditions, which enable the anaerobes to multiply.

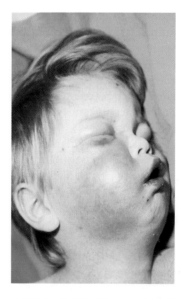

Fig. 34.4   Acute streptococcal cellulitis. (Photograph by Dr A. K. R. Chaudhuri.)

Causal organisms: a combination of aerobes (coliforms, *P. aeruginosa*, *S. aureus*, *S. pyogenes*) and anaerobes (most often 'bacteroides' or anaerobic cocci; rarely, clostridia).

Clinically: redness, swelling and oedema around a primary wound (which may be traumatic or surgical): usually situated on the abdomen, buttock or perineum, or less commonly the leg.

NECROTIZING FASCIITIS

A serious infection, most often due to *S. pyogenes* but sometimes to a mixture of organisms such as streptococci, staphylococci, coliforms, 'bacteroides' and fusiform bacilli. Two main syndromes are recognized, but clinically their features overlap.

Necrotizing fasciitis

Originally described as 'streptococcal gangrene': the external appearance of the skin is initially normal, while the infective-ischaemic process spreads along the fascial planes causing extensive necrosis. Later the overlying skin, deprived of its blood supply, discolours – becoming painful and red, and finally numb and necrotic. The patient is severely ill with fever, toxaemia and shock. *S. pyogenes* is the most common cause of the infection.

Treatment: wide excision of the skin to expose the entire area of necrosis, with general supportive measures including appropriate antibiotics.

Progressive bacterial synergistic gangrene

Usually due to mixed infection with aerobic and anaerobic organisms; often follows surgery. The overlying skin becomes purplish and there may be central necrosis (Fig. 34.5). When the infection involves the peno-scrotal area it is known as 'Fournier's gangrene'.

Treatment: surgery, with appropriate antibiotics.

WOUND INFECTION

Minor wounds are commonplace in everyday life and, naturally, some become infected. The commonest cause is *S. aureus*; most heal without antibiotic treatment.

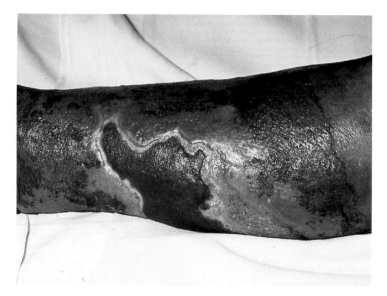

Fig. 34.5   Progressive bacterial gangrene due to *Streptococcus pyogenes* and *Bacteroides* species. (Photograph by Dr D. H. M. Kennedy.)

HOSPITAL WOUND INFECTION

'*Every operation in surgery is an experiment in bacteriology.*'

(Lord Moynihan, 1920).

Clinically, hospital wound infection is a more serious problem than infection of minor wounds because the majority of surgical patients have wounds which involve not only skin and subcutaneous tissue but also muscle and deeper tissues, e.g. bone, peritoneum and viscera.

Clinical features

Surgical wound infection starts with reddening of the wound edges, usually with pus formation. Sometimes pus gathers below the suture line in the deeper layers of the wound, to form a *wound abscess*: as a rule, this eventually discharges to the surface through the sutured incision.

Patients may develop fever, but systemic disturbance is often minimal. However, infection impairs and delays healing and therefore prolongs hospitalization and significantly increases the cost of treatment.

Complications:
- *Dehiscence*: the wound may break down completely, sometimes with exposure of viscera, and needs to be resutured.
- *Spread of infection to:*
    - *local tissues*, e.g. the peritoneum in the case of abdominal wounds
    - *blood*: causing septicaemia.

Causes: the main bacterial causes of surgical wound infections are shown in Table 34.2.

Sources

Endogenous infection: many wound infections are due to organisms carried on the patient's skin, e.g. *S. aureus*, or in the gut, e.g. coliforms, 'bacteroides'. During hospitalization, before surgery, the patient may become colonized with antibiotic-resistant bacteria from the environment which later cause wound infection: this represents endogenous infection from a hospital source.

Exogenous infection of wounds can be acquired during operation, from the surgeon or other theatre personnel.

Mixed infection: surgical wounds are often infected with more than one bacterial species (except in the case of *S. aureus*, which is usually present in pure culture). For example, it is common to find more than one species of coliform together with enterococci, *Bacteroides species* or *C. perfringens*: this flora is known to bacteriologists as *faecal flora*, and is the usual cause of abdominal wound sepsis. Note that the presence of *C. perfringens* does not imply that gas gangrene is about to supervene.

Table 34.2   Main bacterial causes of surgical wound infection

Bacteria	Species	Most common site
1. Aerobic	*Staphylococcus aureus*	Any wound
	Escherichia coli	Any wound but especially abdominal, urological and gynaecological
	Proteus species	
	Klebsiella species	
	Enterococci	
	Pseudomonas aeruginosa	Urological; burns
2. Anaerobic	*Bacteroides fragilis*	Abdominal and gynaecological
	Prevotella melaninogenica	
	Anaerobic cocci	
	Clostridium perfringens	

Pseudomonas aeruginosa is not commonly found in the human bowel: it is a particular problem where there are breaches of mucosa, e.g. after prostatectomy, or with skin ulcers, e.g. bed sores. It is usually acquired exogenously from contamination of the environment, e.g. water, fluids, ventilators, humidifiers, even antiseptic solutions, and is often highly antibiotic-resistant.

Diagnosis of wound infection

Isolation

Specimens: swab of pus, exudate, or tissue from wound.
  Direct Gram film: observe for organisms present.
  Culture: blood agar, CLED or MacConkey agar, aerobically; blood and aminoglycoside blood agar, anaerobically; Robertson's meat medium.
  Observe and identify: bacteria isolated by standard tests.

Treatment

Antibiotics appropriate for the bacteria isolated, but may not be necessary in the absence of generalized symptoms.
  Sepsis syndrome and septic shock (see p. 280), especially the latter, need prompt appropriate therapy, together with supportive measures to control the circulatory collapse in septic shock.

Factors affecting surgical wound sepsis

The following factors increase the likelihood of wound infection:

- operations involving opening of the bowel
- presence of drains, catheters, venous lines or other foreign bodies
- long operations
- large wounds with considerable tissue trauma
- obesity.

Incidence: the sepsis rate of surgical wounds therefore varies:
  Low: in clean elective surgery, e.g. hernia repairs, 'cold' orthopaedic operations: around 1%.
  High: in operations, and particularly emergency surgery, in a contaminated site (e.g. large bowel): around 15%.

Prevention

Difficult and complex: needs rigid observance of aseptic and antiseptic technique, both in preparation for and during operation. Many patients are colonized before operation with organisms which subsequently infect their wounds: the risk of this increases with length of stay in hospital.

Theatre: surgeons and assistants must wear gowns to prevent the dispersal of bacteria shed from the body surface, and masks to trap respiratory secretions; surgeon's hands and patient's skin must be disinfected before operation; surgeon and assistants must wear gloves. Infection acquired at operation is most often due to bacteria entering the wound, either from the patient's commensal flora or from the skin of the surgeon and assistants. Theatres should be kept free from dust and have positive-pressure ventilation to prevent air and dust being sucked in from outside; they should be sited away from main thoroughfares in the hospital.

Ward: bacteria abound in hospital wards: patients with discharging wounds should be isolated to prevent the dissemination of pathogenic bacteria; floors must be kept clean and free of dust; blankets, nowadays made from cellular cotton and not wool, must be regularly washed at a sufficiently high temperature to kill vegetative bacteria.

Antibiotic prophylaxis: if carefully chosen, antibiotics given before operation and for a short time afterwards can reduce the incidence of wound infection after certain operations: especially indicated when heavy soiling of the wound edges is unavoidable, e.g. in colonic surgery.

SPECIAL TYPES OF WOUND INFECTION

Burns

Extensive burns have a large moist exposed surface, which is usually being prepared for a skin graft and is always heavily colonized with bacteria – surprisingly, this often does not prevent the graft from taking.

Two organisms present particular problems in burns units:

- *Streptococcus pyogenes*: a highly dangerous organism in a burns unit: not only affects the patient's general well-being, e.g. by causing septicaemia, but also causes the graft to fail.

- *Pseudomonas aeruginosa*: has a particular propensity to persist in a burns unit: it can be difficult to eradicate from both individual patients and the environment of the unit; of relatively low invasive powers.

Complications: bacteraemia – the invasion of the bloodstream by bacteria from the burn – is a dangerous but not uncommon complication of infected burns.

Orthopaedics

Wound infection is a problem in orthopaedic surgery, in which healing of bone by first intention is important for future weight-bearing and movement. Infection may be acquired by local contamination during surgery, or by blood-borne spread. *Staphylococcus aureus* is the principal cause.

Joint replacement: has revolutionized the mobility of elderly patients with arthritis, but about 1–5% of these operations fail due to low-grade chronic infection, which causes the prosthesis to work loose: most often due to *Staphylococcus epidermidis*.

Indwelling catheters

Widely used nowadays in hospital practice: provide an important opportunity for a focus of infection because they involve a wound together with the presence of a foreign body in the tissues. The usual route of infection is by colonization of the catheter with skin commensals and their subsequent shedding into the blood or other tissues or fluids. Catheters may be arterial or venous, e.g. Hickman lines, cannulae, and infection is especially likely if the catheter is in situ for long periods, e.g. for total parenteral nutrition, in the peritoneum (for continuous ambulatory peritoneal dialysis) or urinary catheters. (See also Ch. 42.)

Causes: S. epidermidis; less often, coliforms, S. aureus, yeasts.
Diagnosis: by blood or other fluid culture; culture of catheter tip.

Tracheostomies

Tracheostomies are widely used in hospitals, especially in intensive care units. The wounds have a marked tendency to become colonized with coliforms – which are often multiply-antibiotic resistant – from the resident hospital flora. Low-grade pathogens like *Acinetobacter* and *Serratia* species can be particularly difficult to eradicate. It is often uncertain whether the presence of these and other coliforms in tracheal secretions actually harms the patient.

Puerperal sepsis (including septic abortion)

Formerly due mainly to *Streptococcus pyogenes*, the important causes nowadays are streptococci of Lancefield group B, *Prevotella melaninogenica* and anaerobic cocci; still a severe disease which requires prompt treatment.

Clostridium perfringens is a rare but dangerous cause of puerperal sepsis.

Clostridial wound infection

Wound infection primarily due to anaerobic clostridia usually takes the form of gas gangrene (see below). It differs clinically from the infections described above in that it is *not purulent* and therefore is not, strictly speaking, a form of sepsis. Clostridial wound infection could also be considered as a disease due to toxins.

GAS GANGRENE

A rare disease in peacetime, but a scourge amongst wounded armies in the field – notably during the First World War.
   Causal organisms:

- *Clostridium perfringens* (65% of cases)
- *Clostridium novyi* (20–40% of cases)
- *Clostridium septicum* (10–20% of cases).

More than one species are often present.

Clinical features

A spreading gangrene of the muscles, with profound toxaemia and shock. There is oedema, with blackening of the tissues and a foul-smelling serous exudate, and crepitus (palpable crackling or bubbling) can often be detected under the skin due to gas production by the clostridia (Fig. 34.6).

Severity: a serious disease with a high case fatality rate, often requiring wide excision or amputation.

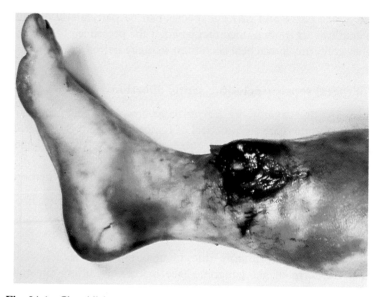

Fig. 34.6   Clostridial gas gangrene, complicating a compound fracture. (Photograph by Professor J. G. Collee.)

Pathogenesis

Due to contamination of wounds by dirt and soil which contain clostridia derived from animal faeces: infection is favoured by extensive wounding with the presence of necrotic tissue, blood clot and foreign bodies – all of which produce anaerobiasis. Vascular damage may also impair blood supply to the site.

Gas gangrene is encountered following major trauma; occasionally, it complicates operations on the bowel (*C. perfringens* is a normal bowel inhabitant), mid-thigh amputation or vascular surgery on an ischaemic limb.

Clostridia produce powerful toxins which themselves cause tissue damage – and so anaerobiasis – and thus enhance spread of the infection.

Diagnosis of gas gangrene

Isolation

Specimens: exudate, tissue.

Direct Gram film: observe for typical Gram-positive bacilli – spores may or may not be seen. In clinical material, *C. perfringens* is usually capsulated but does not form spores.

Culture: blood agar and aminoglycoside blood agar, anaerobically; Robertson's meat medium.

Observe: typical colonies.

Identification: *C. perfringens* – Nagler reaction; identification of other clostridia may be difficult: largely based on biochemical reactions and toxin production.

Treatment

Surgical: by wide excision or amputation of affected tissue.

Antibiotics: large doses of penicillin, perhaps with metronidazole in addition.

Antitoxin: widely used in wartime; of doubtful value.

Hyperbaric oxygen, to reduce anaerobiasis in tissues, has been reported to be effective. This supportive treatment requires special apparatus.

PERITONITIS

A serious form of sepsis: often a complication of abdominal surgery and of diseases that cause perforation of the gastrointestinal tract, e.g. peptic ulcer, diverticulitis, acute appendicitis, Crohn's disease; perforated typhoid ulcer is still a cause of death in enteric fever.

Causal organisms: usually a mixed infection with faecal flora, i.e. coliforms, enterococci, *Bacteroides fragilis*, sometimes *Clostridium perfringens*.

CAPD: peritonitis is a serious and not uncommon complication of continuous ambulatory peritoneal dialysis for renal failure (often due to *S. epdermidis*).

Clinical features

The patient's condition deteriorates markedly, with fever, toxaemia and shock; there may be tenderness on palpation of the abdomen and the absence of bowel sounds due to paralytic ileus.

Diagnosis

A specimen of peritoneal exudate is examined in the same way as pus from a wound.

Treatment

Appropriate antibiotics: it is usually necessary to start therapy before sensitivity results are available. A suitable combination would be: amoxycillin, gentamicin and metronidazole. Alternatively: a cephalosporin, e.g. cefuroxime or cefotaxime; ciprofloxacin; or imipenem with cilastatin. If *S. epidermidis*, consider rancomycin.

Therapy should be reviewed as soon as the results of sensitivity tests are known.

ABSCESSES

An important form of sepsis, and sometimes very difficult to diagnose. Abscesses, both obvious and cryptic, are an important part of the work of hospital bacteriology laboratories.

An *abscess* is a collection of pus within – often deeply within – the body, walled off by a barrier of inflammatory reaction with fibrosis. It is therefore often impossible to treat abscesses satisfactorily by antibiotics alone: surgery and drainage are also necessary.

Abscesses can form in almost any tissue or organ of the body, but some sites are much more common than others: these are listed in Table 34.3.

Tuberculosis commonly causes abscesses but these are 'cold', i.e. not accompanied by pain, redness or an acute inflammatory response: they are discussed in more detail in Chapter 37.

Clinical features

Abscesses may be clinically obvious or cryptic.

Clinically obvious abscesses include those at sites such as breast, axilla, peritonsillar (quinsy), perianal, ischiorectal and Bartholin's glands: there is painful swelling with local inflammation, fever and often some degree of systemic upset. Brain abscess commonly presents with the signs of a space-occupying lesion, most often in the temporal lobe (Fig. 34.7).

Cryptic abscesses can be exceedingly difficult to diagnose and, unfortunately, are relatively common. Many abdominal and pelvic abscesses are of this type: the patient presents with vague, progressive ill health and fever and, although obviously toxic, there are no definite localizing signs.

In addition to the clinical history, however, there may be *other clues*. For example, a subphrenic abscess may be detected radiologically: a positive blood culture helps to confirm a diagnosis of sepsis, but does not localize it – a computed tomography (CT) scan may do this, but in some cases laparotomy

Table 34.3   Abscesses – some common sites

Site	Route of infection, predisposing factors	Bacteria usually responsible
Subcutaneous tissues, e.g. finger pulp, palmar space	Penetrating wounds	*Staphylococcus aureus*
Axilla	Extension of superficial infection via lymphatics to axillary lymph nodes with suppuration	*Staphylococcus aureus*
Breast	Breast-feeding – infected from infant	*Staphylococcus aureus*
Peritonsillar (quinsy)	Streptococcal sore throat	*Streptococcus pyogenes*
Intra-abdominal e.g. appendix, subphrenic, paracolic	Appendicitis: abdominal sepsis; peritonitis due to any cause	Faecal flora *Streptococcus milleri*
Ischiorectal	Direct from rectum	Faecal flora
Perianal	Infected hair follicle round anus	*Staphylococcus aureus* Faecal flora
Pelvic	Abdominal or gynaecological sepsis	Faecal flora Genital flora
Tubo-ovarian (pyosalpinx)	Gynaecological sepsis; gonorrhoea	Genital flora *Neisseria gonorrhoeae*
Bartholin's gland	Local spread	Genital flora *Neisseria gonorrhoeae*
Perinephric	Extension of acute pyelonephritis	Coliforms
Cerebral	Otitis media; sinusitis Haematogenous	*Streptococcus milleri* 'Bacteroides' *Staphylococcus aureus*, *Proteus* species
Hepatic	Ascending cholangitis; portal pyaemia	Faecal flora *Streptococcus milleri*
Lung	Aspiration pneumonia; bronchial obstruction with collapse (e.g. tumour) *Staphylococcus aureus* pneumonia	Oropharyngeal flora *Staphylococcus aureus*

Note: The anaerobic members of the commensal flora ('Bacteroides', anaerobic cocci, etc.) can also play a role in abscess production – usually in conjunction with other organisms.

is required – and should be carried out if there is a high degree of clinical suspicion.

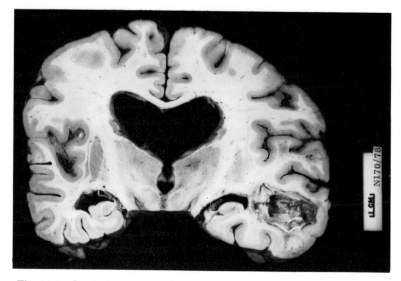

Fig. 34.7   Cerebral abscess. Section of brain with an abscess in the right temporal lobe, secondary to suppurative otitis media. (Photograph by Professor J. Hume Adams.)

Pathogenesis

Abscesses are localized but do not necessarily form at the site of primary infection: there may be tracking of pus, leading to a purulent collection at a site some distance from the original infection – e.g. subphrenic and pelvic abscesses.

Metastatic abscesses: occasionally, multiple abscesses form as a result of blood-borne or 'pyaemic' spread of infected thrombi: such abscesses are found in many sites. *Portal pyaemia*, in which the source is intra-abdominal sepsis (often the appendix), results in liver abscesses.

Diagnosis

Isolation

Specimens: pus (which may have to be collected at operation or by aspiration); blood.

Culture: on blood agar aerobically and anaerobically; Robertson's meat medium. Incubation may have to be continued for some days.

Observe: bacterial colonies or growth.

Identification: by tests appropriate for the bacteria isolated.

Treatment

Antibiotics are rarely sufficient on their own: if the abscess does not discharge spontaneously (which can have serious effects), surgical intervention and drainage may be necessary. This should be done under appropriate antibiotic cover: the drugs to be administered depend on the site of the abscess and, therefore, the likely infecting bacteria (see Table 34.3).

SEPTICAEMIA

Literally, 'sepsis of the blood'. In the past, two terms have been used to describe the presence of organisms in the bloodstream:

- *Bacteraemia*: originally used in the case of a patient with positive blood cultures but no signs of clinical infection; often asymptomatic and transient, and usually of minor or no clinical relevance.
- *Septicaemia*: patient has positive blood cultures, and clinical evidence is suggestive of infection.

Nowadays it is not useful clinically to distinguish between these two terms.

Septicaemia is usually a complication of a localized infection, e.g. pyelonephritis, peritonitis, cholangitis, pneumonia, osteomyelitis, abscesses of internal organs. It is also a basic feature of generalized infections e.g. enteric fever, brucellosis.

Causal organisms: the organisms that cause septicaemia and the underlying infections or associated clinical conditions are shown in Table 34.4. In about 95% of cases a single infecting organism is responsible for an episode of septicaemia.

Note: Infective endocarditis is also associated with septicaemia, and is described in Chapter 35.

Clinical features

The signs and symptoms are variable – sometimes minimal, sometimes severe and rapidly progressive. The predominant signs may be those of the underlying disease (e.g. pneumonia, peritonitis).

The presenting feature is usually a worsening of the patient's condition with fever, rigors, tachycardia, tachypnoea, cyanosis, hypotension; in elderly patients there may be confusion, agitation or behavioural changes.

Table 34.4 Bacteria commonly causing septicaemia

Predisposing factor	Causal organisms*
Abdominal sepsis (peritonitis, hepatobiliary infection, abscess, etc.)	Coliforms 'Bacteroides' Enterococci *Streptococcus milleri*
Infected wounds, burns, pressure sores	*Staphylococcus aureus* *Streptococcus pyogenes* Coliforms 'Bacteroides'
Gynaecological sepsis (puerperal infection, pelvic abscess, salpingitis, etc.)	Coliforms Enterococci 'Bacteroides' *Streptococcus pyogenes* Lancefield group B streptococci
Urinary tract infection	Coliforms Enterococci
Osteomyelitis Septic arthritis	*Staphylococcus aureus*
Pneumonia	*Streptococcus pneumoniae*
Meningitis	*Streptococcus pneumoniae* *Neisseria meningitidis* *Haemophilus influenzae*
Meningitis in neonates	Coliforms Lancefield group B streptococci
Food poisoning	*Salmonella* species (not *S. typhi* or *S. paratyphi*) *Campylobacter jejuni*
Drip sites, shunts, intravascular catheters	*Staphylococcus aureus* *Staphylococcus epidermidis* Coliforms
Intravenous drug abuse	*Staphylococcus aureus*
Splenectomized patients	*Streptococcus pneumoniae*
Immunosuppressed patients	Coliforms *Staphylococcus aureus* *Pseudomonas aeruginosa* *Streptococcus pneumoniae*

SEPSIS SYNDROME AND SEPTIC SHOCK

The *sepsis syndrome* is defined as clinical evidence suggestive of infection together with signs of a systemic response to infection, e.g. tachypnoea, tachycardia, fever (or hypothermia). The sepsis syndrome results from microorganisms initiating a cascade of reactions causing the sequential release of endogenous mediators. Among the mediators induced, the cytokines, tumour necrosis factor α (TNFα), interleukin-1 (IL-1) and interleukin-2 (IL-2) are of particular importance. A central mediator does not seem to exist, although TNFα is often proposed.

Septic shock occurs when the sepsis syndrome progresses to severe hypotension and tissue anoxia, leading to multiple organ failure (e.g. heart, lungs, liver, kidneys). Septic shock has a poor prognosis, despite antibiotics and supportive therapy: mortality is often higher than 50%. Septic shock is usually a complication of septicaemia with Gram-negative bacilli and, occasionally, Gram-positive bacteria. Research has focused on the role of endotoxin present in the membrane of Gram-negative bacteria. Endotoxin can activate the complement system, cause intravascular coagulation and release vasoactive substances and various cytokines. Septic shock is sometimes called *endotoxic shock*.

Diagnosis

Blood culture

More than one culture may be required (see Chapter 5 for detail of method). When septicaemia is suspected in a severely ill patient, two or three separate sets of cultures should be taken from different veins at intervals of about 5 min – whenever possible, before antibiotics are administered.

Observe: early signs of growth, usually nowadays in a 'Bactec' or similar automated sampling equipment.

Subculture: to blood agar, aerobically and anaerobically.

Identification: as appropriate for the organism isolated.

Treatment

Control of infection may need surgical intervention (e.g. to drain an abscess, resuture a ruptured viscus). Antimicrobial therapy is also required, and should be bactericidal; administered intravenously; and in prompt and adequate dosage. Table 34.5 lists some of the antimicrobial drugs of choice: in practice, combinations are often used.

Septic shock: in addition to antibiotic therapy, special resuscitative measures, with fluid replacement, inotropic support and artificial ventilation are necessary. Newer approaches to therapy include monoclonal antibodies to endotoxin and TNF.

Table 34.5 Antimicrobial therapy in septicaemia

Organism	Antimicrobial drugs
Streptococcus pneumoniae *Streptococcus pyogenes* *Streptococcus milleri* *Neisseria meningitidis*	Penicillin
Staphylococcus aureus *Staphylococcus epidermidis*	Flucloxacillin or vancomycin, often with gentamicin
Coliforms	Gentamicin or cefotaxime
Pseudomonas aeruginosa	Gentamicin and/or ceftazidime
Enterococci	Ampicillin or vancomycin
'Bacteroides'	Metronidazole

35. Infective endocarditis

Infective endocarditis is an infection of the endocardium – most commonly affecting the heart valves, and sometimes the endocardium around congenital defects. The infection was formerly known as bacterial endocarditis: the change in nomenclature recognizes that organisms other than bacteria can cause it.

Mortality: before antibiotics were available the disease was always fatal: progressive damage to the heart valves led to cardiac failure and death – even nowadays, the case fatality rate is around 30%.

Table 35.1 Causes of infective endocarditis

Organism		Percentage of cases
Bacteria		
Streptococcus sanguis		
Streptococcus bovis	Viridans or	
Streptococcus mutans	non-haemolytic	50–60
Streptococcus mitior	streptococci	
Enterococci		
Staphylococcus aureus		20–30
Staphylococcus epidermidis		
Other bacteria		5–10
(e.g. corynebacteria,		
Haemophilus species, coliforms)		
Fungi		
Candida albicans		Rare
Aspergillus species		
Rickettsia, chlamydia		
Coxiella burneti		Rare
Chlamydia psittaci		

Causal Organisms

These have changed over the years. Viridans streptococci remain the most common, but staphylococci are now a major cause (Table 35.1).

Clinical Features

The disease used to be described as 'acute' or 'subacute', based on the progression of the untreated disease.

Acute form: followed a fulminant course, with fever, toxicity and death, usually within a few days or weeks: commonly associated with infection with *Staphylococcus aureus, Streptococcus pneumoniae* or *Streptococcus pyogenes*.

Subacute form: was a more chronic disease which progressed slowly: usually caused by viridans streptococci, and resulted in death after about 3 months.

This terminology is now no longer used: it is preferable to assess the disease in terms of the causative microorganism and the underlying pathology.

Signs and symptoms: classically fever, malaise, weight loss, cardiac murmur, anaemia, splinter haemorrhages (i.e. under the finger nails), haematuria, petechiae, splenomegaly. Nowadays these classical features are rarely seen fully developed: most patients who present with significant malaise and fever are diagnosed at an early stage.

Clinical course: unless adequately treated (and even in some patients apparently so treated) there is progressive damage to the heart valves, leading to cardiac failure and death.

Pathogenesis

Although most patients are known to have pre-existing cardiac disease, a substantial proportion – about one-third – have had previously normal hearts or undiagnosed abnormalities.

Cardiac and other abnormalities which predispose to infective endocarditis are:

- *Rheumatic valvular disease*: e.g. stenosis or incompetence of the mitral and aortic valves following rheumatic fever
- *Congenital defects*: e.g. bicuspid aortic valve, septal defects, patent ductus arteriosus, coarctation of the aorta
- *Intracardiac prostheses*: usually, replacement of diseased heart valves with prosthetic valves

- *Degenerative cardiac disease:* e.g. calcific aortic stenosis
- *Drug abuse*: addicts who take drugs intravenously have a high risk of endocarditis – often with atypical clinical features. Involvement of the tricuspid valve is particularly common: usually due to *S. aureus*.

Formerly an infection of adolescence and young adult life, the mean age of patients in developed countries is now over 50 years, due to the increasing importance of degenerative disease and the decreasing incidence of rheumatic heart disease.

Pathology

Infective endocarditis usually occurs at the site of a predisposing heart lesion or congenital defect, where the velocity of blood is such as to cause turbulence, resulting in damage to the surface of the endocardium. On such roughened surfaces, usually of the mitral or aortic valves, thrombi of fibrin and platelets form. Circulating microorganisms colonize the avascular thrombi and convert them into infected *vegetations*: the end result is

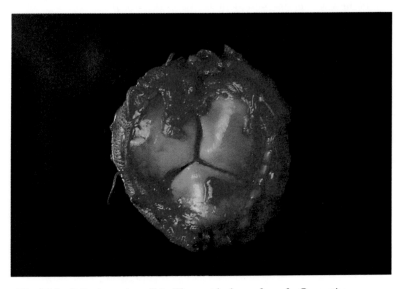

Fig. 35.1 Infective endocarditis. The ventricular surface of a Carpentier Edwards aortic valve, explanted 5 weeks postoperatively because of prosthetic valve endocarditis caused by *Staphylococcus epidermidis*. Vegetations are seen attached to all three cusps. (Reproduced with permission from *Current Medicine 4*, Churchill Livingstone.)

destruction of the valve (Fig. 35.1). As a rule, only a single valve is affected.

Infection of endocardial thrombi results from:

- *Transient, asymptomatic bacteraemia*: usually with organisms derived from the normal flora, particularly that of the mouth – which explains the frequency of viridans streptococci as a cause of infective endocarditis. Although this type of bacteraemia is common after dental surgery (e.g. extractions), a history of recent, significant dental treatment is surprisingly uncommon. Other predisposing procedures include surgery on the gastrointestinal and genitourinary tracts – including even minor manipulations such as endoscopy or catheterization.
- *Septicaemia*: less common, usually part of a generalized infection with more virulent organisms (such as *S. aureus*, *S. pneumoniae*).

Vegetations: organisms are shed from these into the bloodstream – often over long periods of time. Minute thrombi are also dislodged, to give rise to distant embolic manifestations of the disease: cerebral emboli are an important complication.

Immune complexes can also form, and may produce vasculitis and glomerulonephritis.

Prosthetic valve endocarditis

An important complication of cardiac surgery. *Early-onset* endocarditis has a high mortality: the infection is acquired at operation, when it is usually due to staphylococci. *Late-onset* endocarditis may be acquired in the same way as that of natural valves, and although the infecting organisms reflect the normal microbiological pattern of the disease (Table 35.1), coagulase-negative staphylococci are a frequent cause. The distinction between early-onset and late-onset endocarditis is becoming less clear-cut.

Diagnosis

Close collaboration between the microbiologist and the clinician is essential: prompt diagnosis and early treatment are imperative.

Blood culture

The corner-stone of diagnosis and important for the subsequent treatment of the patient: repeated cultures may be necessary to isolate the causal organism, e.g. two to six, if possible taken over 48 h. Take blood cultures before the start of antibiotic treatment: however, in seriously ill patients therapy should not be delayed until blood culture results are available.

Observe: early signs of growth.

Subculture: to blood agar, aerobically and anaerobically.

Identification: as appropriate for the organism isolated.

Echocardiography

This is a useful investigative technique and complementary diagnostic aid: it can detect vegetations on heart valves. Diagnostic sensitivity varies, and is dependent on the echocardiographic technique used, the size of the vegetations and the stage of the infection.

Antibiotic sensitivity tests

The usual disc diffusion method of testing is generally considered to be inadequate in infective endocarditis. The following tests should be carried out:

- *Minimum inhibitory concentration* of potentially useful drugs, both singly and in combination.
- *Minimum bactericidal concentration* must also be determined, because it is important to achieve a bactericidal level of antibiotic in the blood (rather than merely a bacteriostatic level).

Culture-negative endocarditis

In 10% of cases, no organisms can be grown from blood cultures. This may be due to:

- infection with *Coxiella burneti* or *Chlamydia psittaci*: perform serological tests to confirm or exclude these diagnoses
- recent antibiotic therapy: repeat blood cultures over a few days, in absence of chemotherapy
- infection with fastidious organisms, difficult to grow in ordinary media (e.g. bacterial L-forms, nutritionally-exacting streptococci): repeat blood cultures using special media if these are suspected
- the disease being in a phase in which organisms are not shed into the bloodstream: repeat blood cultures.

Treatment

Depends on adequate – and this usually means high – dosage with an antimicrobial drug: two drugs in combination are often preferred.
   The antibiotic regimen selected must be:

- bactericidal
- parenteral (at least initially)
- continued for several weeks.

High doses of bactericidal drugs are necessary, because the aim of therapy is to eliminate the organisms from their sites enmeshed in the relatively avascular vegetations. Some of the antibiotic regimens used are shown in Table 35.2.

Laboratory monitoring of therapy

- *Estimation of the antibiotic level* in patient's serum: rarely necessary if large doses are being given intravenously, but may be indicated when there is a switch to oral therapy. Also used to avoid overdosage with toxic drugs (e.g. aminoglycosides).
- *Estimation of the bactericidal activity* of the patient's serum against the causal organism: although of little prognostic value, a poor result (e.g. no killing at a 1 in 8 dilution of a 'peak' serum sample) indicates that the antibiotics chosen, their dose and route of administration should be reconsidered.
- *Measurement of C-reactive protein* is useful in monitoring the response to treatment, and also in detecting intercurrent infections and complications.

Table 35.2   Antibiotic regimens for infective endocarditis

Causal organism	Antimicrobial drugs
Viridans streptococci	Penicillin or cephalosporin, plus gentamicin
Enterococci	Penicillin or ampicillin plus gentamicin*
Staphylococcus aureus	Flucloxacillin plus gentamicin
Staphylococcus epidermidis	Vancomycin plus gentamicin and/or rifampicin
Fungi	Amphotericin B plus 5-fluorocytosine or fluconazole
Coxiella burneti *Chlamydia psittaci*	Tetracycline

*Although enterococci are not sensitive to either penicillin or gentamicin alone, this combination is usually bactericidal and, in practice, effective.
Note: Vancomycin is also a useful drug for infections due to streptococci and *Staphylococcus aureus*, especially in patients hypersensitive to the penicillins.

Surgery

Replacement of damaged valves is now accepted as part of the management of cases of infective endocarditis; it is often life-saving.

Prophylaxis

Although not of proven value, 'at risk' patients (e.g. those with valvular or congenital heart disease) should be given prophylactic antibiotics – oral amoxycillin or, if hypersensitive to penicillins, oral clindamycin or parenteral vancomycin – before dental procedures. Prior to surgery or instrumentation on the gastrointestinal or urinary tract, parenteral ampicillin with gentamicin is an appropriate prophylactic combination.

In addition, much more emphasis should be placed on improving oral hygiene, by encouraging all people to seek regular routine dental care.

36. Pyrexia of unknown origin

Fever results when the release of endogenous pyrogens (e.g. interleukin-1, tumour necrosis factor) raises the setting of the thermoregulatory centre in the hypothalamus. This is usually due to an inflammatory cause, most often infection. In young children, a trivial virus infection may result in significant fever – whereas in the elderly, severe infection may be accompanied by only a minimal temperature elevation.

Cause of fever is usually easy to diagnose – febrile episodes of short duration are almost always due to infection.

Pyrexia of unknown origin, popularly known as PUO, is a clinical entity in which the patient has a fever that is:

- significant (a temperature over 38°C)
- persistent (for at least 1 week – usually longer, often 3 weeks)
- without a readily identifiable cause.

Cause: is often due to a relatively common disorder with an atypical presentation, lacking the expected localizing features, but is sometimes caused by an illness that is not easy to diagnose.

Diagnosis can be exceedingly difficult – in some cases it is never made, and the patient may recover spontaneously.

The principal types of disease which can be responsible for PUO are shown in Table 36.1.

INFECTION

The most important cause of PUO: with a stringent definition, infection accounts for 40% of cases; with less rigid criteria (i.e. lower grade fever of shorter duration), it is responsible for at least 70% of cases.

Bacterial infections which can present as PUO are listed in Table 36.2.

Table 36.1   Causes of pyrexia of unknown origin

Cause		Percentage of cases
Infections		40
Neoplasms	Especially lymphoma and leukaemia, but also other forms of cancer, e.g. hypernephroma, hepatoma, disseminated malignancy	20
Connective tissue diseases	Systemic lupus erythematosus, polyarteritis nodosa, temporal arteritis	20
Others	For example: (i) Granulomatous diseases – Crohn's disease, sarcoidosis (ii) Drug-induced fevers (iii) Malingering ('factitious fever')	20

Other infectious causes of PUO include:

- *Viral diseases endemic in the UK*: infectious mononucleosis (glandular fever), hepatitis, others such as enterovirus, cytomegalovirus infections, childhood fevers with atypical presentation.
- *Q fever*: due to the rickettsia-like organism, *Coxiella burneti*: most common in males in agriculture.

Table 36.2   Bacterial diseases commonly presenting as pyrexia of unknown origin

Cause	Disease – special features
Systemic infections	
Infective endocarditis	Infection of heart valves
Tuberculosis	Pulmonary, non-pulmonary (e.g. bone, renal) or cryptic miliary
Enteric fever	Usually acquired abroad
Brucellosis	Usually acquired abroad
Leptospirosis	Occupational association
Localized sepsis	
Hepatobiliary sepsis	Cholecystitis, cholangitis, liver abscess
Intra-abdominal abscess }	Usually follow intestinal or gynaecological
Pelvic abscess	sepsis; sometimes postoperative
Renal infections	Chronic pyelonephritis; perinephric abscess
Sinusitis	
Dental infection	Apical dental abscess
Bone sepsis	Osteomyelitis

- *Psittacosis*: due to *Chlamydia psittaci*: suspect if the patient keeps parrots, budgerigars or pigeons.
- *Protozoal diseases*: malaria, amoebiasis (with liver abscess), visceral leishmaniasis (kala-azar), trypanosomiasis – all of which are tropical infections; toxoplasmosis, world-wide in distribution, is usually acquired in this country.
- *Fungal diseases*: histoplasmosis, coccidioidomycosis, systemic candidiasis.
- *Filariasis*: a tropical helminth infection: during the first few years of infection with the microfilariae of *Wuchereria bancrofti*, *Brugia malayi* or *Onchocerca volvulus*, and before the development of localizing signs, episodes of fever are a common feature.

Imported diseases

The common causes of PUO in the UK are very different from those seen abroad. Air travel has allowed the importation of tropical diseases within their incubation period, so they may present in this country as undiagnosed fevers. It is essential to take an accurate 'geographical history' from all patients. Malaria is the most important disease in this category. Nowadays almost all cases of typhoid fever and a significant proportion of cases of brucellosis have been acquired abroad.

Lassa fever, Ebola fever and Marburg disease are viral diseases imported from Africa – all rare and very serious. Once suspected, patients need to be investigated and nursed in strict isolation because of the danger of infecting nursing and other staff in attendance.

Investigation

Often time-consuming; below are the main examinations carried out: emphasis has been placed on those that help to establish an infective cause for PUO.

Clinical history

To include patient's previous illnesses; family illnesses, e.g. tuberculosis; foreign travel; contact with pets or farm animals; occupation; currently prescribed drugs; abuse of drugs.

Physical examination

Especially to detect lymphadenopathy, enlargement of liver or spleen, or areas of tenderness.

Laboratory examinations

1. *Bacteriology*:

- *Blood culture*: serial cultures should be taken: isolation of viridans streptococci points to infective endocarditis; isolation of coliforms, enterococci, *Streptococcus milleri* or 'bacteroides' suggests intra-abdominal sepsis.
- *Urine microscopy and culture*: serial specimens may be necessary to detect intermittent bacteriuria in chronic pyelonephritis; microscopic haematuria is often present in infective endocarditis and hypernephroma.
- *Stool culture and microscopy*: indicated if there is a history of diarrhoea: again, several specimens should be examined.
- *Serology*: appropriate tests for enteric fever (Widal reaction), brucellosis, infectious mononucleosis, Q fever, leptospirosis, and some other infections listed above. *Note*: a single raised titre must be interpreted with caution, since many people have had previous exposure to these organisms; do not attribute a PUO to a rare cause unless there is other supporting evidence.

2. *Haematology*:

Full blood count: blood films, for differential white cell count and examination for malarial parasites (Fig. 48.2); erythrocyte sedimentation rate – a very high result (e.g. more than 100 mm/h) suggests tuberculosis, a connective tissue disease or malignancy.

3. *Biochemistry*:

Liver function tests, etc.

Radiological examination: straight radiographs of chest, abdomen, sinuses and teeth.

Further investigations: should be planned at this stage if the diagnosis has not been made. The order in which they are carried out depends on what is considered the most likely cause of the PUO. Examples are listed below:

- *Serological tests* for connective tissue diseases, e.g. antinuclear factor, rheumatoid factor, other autoantibody tests. Immunoglobulin studies in myeloma.
- *Specialised radiology and ultrasonography*: to identify the site of disease, e.g. cholecystogram, excretion urogram, barium studies (in inflammatory bowel disease), isotope and CT scanning.
- *Biopsy*: of lymph nodes, bone marrow, muscle, liver, kidney, and of any lesion localized by other investigations.
- *Laparotomy*: a last resort if there is evidence of intra-abdominal pathology.

37. Tuberculosis and leprosy

TUBERCULOSIS

A chronic debilitating disease, once the scourge of Victorian Britain ('consumption', 'phthisis') – which remains a major health problem in much of the world today. It is a particular problem in HIV-infected patients.

Causal organisms: *Mycobacterium tuberculosis* and *M. africanum* – both human tubercle bacilli; less often, *M. bovis*, the bovine tubercle bacillus.

CLINICAL FEATURES

Tuberculosis is a slowly progressive, chronic, granulomatous infection which most often affects the lungs; other organs and tissues may also be involved. Clinically, tuberculosis is seen in two forms:

- *primary*: generally the more invasive, with marked lymph node involvement
- *post-primary*: in which the development of delayed-type hypersensitivity modifies the infection, with limitation of spread and considerable fibrotic reaction.

Primary infection

Primary tuberculosis usually involves the lung.

Symptoms: clinically, many cases are symptomless. Symptoms, if present, are vague and nonspecific – malaise, anorexia, weight loss, fever, sweats, tachycardia; cough may not be prominent.

Site of primary complex: the commonest form is a local lesion (Ghon focus), with marked enlargement of the regional hilar lymph nodes. The Ghon focus develops at the lung periphery, usually just below the pleura in the midzone, and is a small lesion. In most cases it heals with fibrosis.

A primary focus with enlargement of the draining lymph nodes can alternatively involve other sites, e.g. the tonsils with cervical adenitis, the intestine with mesenteric adenitis, peritonitis.

Progressive primary infection

Primary infection may progress:

- *Tuberculous bronchopneumonia*: an acute diffuse extension of the infection throughout the lung, due to discharge into the bronchial tree of caseous material from an expanding Ghon focus or, more often, from caseous hilar lymph nodes (Fig. 37.1). A serious and often fatal complication if untreated. *Caseation* – the production of thick cheesy material consisting of pus cells and necrotic tissue – is characteristic of tuberculous inflammatory lesions.
- *Miliary tuberculosis*: small tuberculous foci (tubercles) disseminated widely throughout the body, as a result of haematogenous (blood-borne) spread of infection.
- *Tuberculous meningitis*: blood-borne spread of infection to penetrate the blood-brain barrier and involve the meninges: uniformly fatal before the antibiotic era and still a serious disease, with considerable mortality and disabling sequelae in some survivors.
- *Bone and joint tuberculosis*: affects different sites: a common form is spinal tuberculosis, in which there may be collapse of the vertebrae, causing kyphosis and formation of a 'cold' *psoas abscess* in the groin, due to tracking of pus down the psoas muscle from the infective process in the spine.
- *Genitourinary tuberculosis*:
  a. *Renal tuberculosis* presents with frequency and painless haematuria: the urine shows a 'sterile' pyuria – numerous pus cells on microscopy, but no growth of pathogens when cultured on standard media.
  b. *Endometrial tuberculosis* in females.
  c. *Tuberculous epididymitis* in males.

Cold abscess: tuberculosis also causes 'cold' abscesses, i.e. without an acute inflammatory reaction. Neck abscesses, now rare and formerly associated with *M. bovis* infection, originate in an enlarged cervical lymph gland, with discharge of caseous pus and the formation of draining sinuses. Psoas abscess is another example.

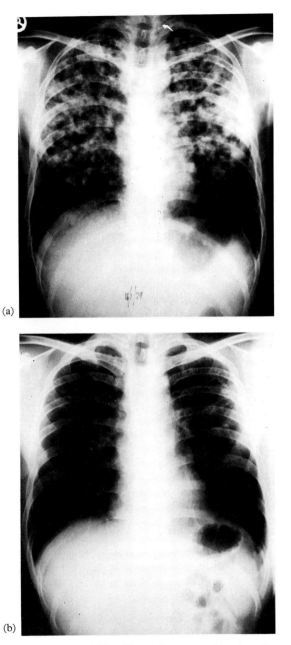

Fig. 37.1   Tuberculosis: (a) Chest X-ray of a patient with tuberculous bronchopneumonia. (b) Chest X-ray of the same patient 10 months after antituberculous therapy. (Courtesy of Dr R. S. Kennedy.)

Clinical features of post-primary infection

The lesions of post-primary tuberculosis are characteristically localized and fibrotic, due to the development of hypersensitivity. There may be a *latent period*, during which the tubercle bacilli remain dormant before initiating active disease years after the primary infection.

Post-primary tuberculosis generally involves the lungs, with lesions in the apices: if untreated, progressive chronic disease develops, with areas of exudation and caseation surrounded by dense fibrosis. Caseous lesions enlarge to coalesce and cavitate: cavities, sometimes large and containing fluid, can then be seen on radiography. Lymph node enlargement is much less marked in this form of tuberculosis than in the primary form.

Presenting symptoms: non-specific ill health, with fever, night sweats, weight loss; respiratory symptoms include cough, haemoptysis and a pneumonic illness that fails to respond to conventional antibiotics.

Source of post-primary infection can be:

- *endogenous*: reactivation of latent foci formed at the time of primary infection
- exogenous: reinfection, by inhalation of infected respiratory secretions from a case of 'open' tuberculosis (i.e. with tubercle bacilli in the sputum).

Patients: today in Britain, patients with tuberculosis are often immigrants, the elderly or the immunocompromised. Tuberculosis is a particular problem in AIDS, often causing a rapidly fatal infection. In the USA, multi-resistant bacteria are common, often making the treatment of HIV-positive patients difficult.

Dissemination: post-primary infection may disseminate, and cause the manifestations listed above as progressive primary infections.

Delayed hypersensitivity in tuberculosis

Tubercle bacilli are readily phagocytosed, but can then multiply within mononuclear cells and resist digestion. This *intracellular parasitism* is associated with the development of *delayed hypersensitivity* (cell-mediated immunity), and of activated macrophages with increased ability to kill ingested bacilli.

Delayed hypersensitivity modifies the host response to a second challenge from tubercle bacilli, and differentiates primary from post-primary lesions. *Koch* recognized the phenomenon a century ago. He demonstrated that inoculation of tubercle bacilli into a guinea-pig already suffering from a primary lesion, with caseating lymph nodes and disseminated infection, resulted in only a small superficial lesion at the site of the second inoculation – which healed rapidly without lymph node enlargement. (The guinea-pig nevertheless died, from the disseminated primary infection.)

Skin tests in human infection: delayed hypersensitivity can be demonstrated by the *tuberculin test*. This is the intradermal inoculation of Purified Protein Derivative (a purified filtrate from cultures of *M. tuberculosis*), either by multiple puncture (*Heaf* test) or by intradermal injection by syringe (*Mantoux* test). Result:

- Positive test (indicating delayed hypersensitivity) produces induration, followed by papule formation after 24–28 h.
- Negative test: no reaction.

Diagnosis

Specimens:
- *Respiratory: sputum* – if none available, laryngeal swab, bronchial washings or from gastric lavage.
- *Meningitis*: CSF.
- *Bone and joint*: samples removed at operation or by aspiration.
- *Renal*: early morning urine (i.e. the 'overnight' urine voided on waking).
- *Repeated specimens*: three are usually necessary – especially with suspected respiratory and renal tuberculosis.

Direct microscopy: detection of typical bacilli in a smear stained with Ziehl–Neelsen (see Fig. 14.1) or auramine confirms a diagnosis of tuberculosis in most cases. Care is necessary with urinary deposits, however, as these may contain other types of acid-fast bacilli (smegma bacilli).

Culture: all specimens must be cultured on Löwenstein–Jensen or other suitable medium, e.g. containing pyruvic acid. Culture is a more sensitive method of detecting *M. tuberculosis* than direct demonstration which, even if positive, should be followed by culture for antibiotic sensitivity test. Cultures are examined weekly: *M. tuberculosis* and *M. bovis* can be distinguished by cultural characteristics:

- *Human* strains grow as dry, crumbly yellowish colonies – often described as 'rough, tough and buff' (see Fig. 14.2).
- *Bovine* strains grow as smoother colonies; glycerol does not enhance their growth, in contrast to human strains.

Cultures should not be discarded as negative until they have been incubated for 8 weeks.

Treatment

The discovery of streptomycin in 1944 revolutionized the treatment of tuberculosis. However, resistant strains emerge readily and combinations of two or more drugs are used to minimize this risk.

Streptomycin has to be given by injection: it is toxic and side-effects include deafness and vertigo (due to damage to the eighth nerve) and nephrotoxicity.

Present recommended therapy

This is a combination of:

- Isoniazid
- Rifampicin
- Pyrazinamide
- Ethambutol

for 2 months

Followed by:

- Isoniazid
- Rifampicin

for a further 4 months

Ethambutol may be omitted if there is a low risk of isoniazid resistance. In non-respiratory tuberculosis, treatment may have to be continued for longer than 6 months.

Alternative or second-line antituberculous drugs, now used mainly abroad as they are both effective and cheap: streptomycin, thiacetazone but also in the case of resistance to first line drugs: capreomycin, cycloserine, ethionamide.

The choice of drugs should be reviewed when the sensitivity of the infecting strain has been reported. In patients successfully treated, cultures from the site of infection soon become negative for tubercle bacilli. If they remain positive, the sensitivity of the isolated organism must be tested again to determine whether resistance has emerged.

Tuberculosis is emerging as a major problem in AIDS patients – especially in Africa, but also in the USA. A particular difficulty is that the infecting strains in these cases are often multiply drug-resistant.

Epidemiology

Route of infection: inhalation of infected respiratory secretions.

Reservoirs of infection: patients with 'open phthisis': tubercle bacilli are coughed up in the sputum.

Bovine tuberculosis: formerly common in cattle in Britain, and transmissible to humans through drinking infected milk. The compulsory tuberculin testing of all cattle, and the slaughter of positive reactors, has eradicated the disease in cows: combined with *pasteurization* of milk, this has resulted in human cases acquired from cattle becoming very rare – although still a problem in some developing countries.

Occupation: some occupations used to be associated with a high mortality rate from tuberculosis, e.g. workers exposed to inhalation of stone or metal dust such as quarrymen, blasters and tin miners, especially if there is contamination with silica. Doctors and nurses also have an increased risk of tuberculosis.

Age incidence: formerly largely a disease of childhood, tuberculosis is now not uncommon in the elderly.

Race: Black people and American Indians are more susceptible to tuberculosis than Caucasian (white) Americans; in the UK, the disease is especially common in Asian immigrants.

Immunocompromised patients, especially those infected with HIV (see Chapter 42), are extremely susceptible to tuberculosis: in them, the infection can be rapid and overwhelming.

Prevention and control

BCG vaccine

Consists of live attenuated *M. bovis* grown in bile-containing medium: known by the names of the workers who developed it, i.e. bacille Calmette–Guérin.

Administration: intradermally, into the site of the insertion of the deltoid muscle.

Mode of action: confers hypersensitivity and therefore partial immunity to infection; prevents the invasive disease characteristic of primary infection.

Indications: give to children between 10 and 13 years of age, but only if they react negatively in a Heaf (tuberculin) test. Give also to tuberculin-negative health care staff in contact with patients or specimens likely to be infected.

Contraindications: Must *not* be given to immunocompromised patients, pregnant women, people with fever or generalized skin sepsis, or people with a positive tuberculin skin test.

Immigrants

Immigrants from areas (especially South East Asia) with a high prevalence of tuberculosis should be screened on entry to the UK. The infants and children (wherever born) of such immigrants should be offered BCG vaccination.

Contacts

Contacts of carriers need to be traced, screened and considered for chemoprophylaxis with isoniazid, with or without rifampicin; if they react negatively in a Heaf test, give BCG vaccine.

LEPROSY (HANSEN'S DISEASE)

The scourge of the ancient world, and still afflicting millions of patients, mainly in Asia and Africa. Now, the outlook has been revolutionized by the introduction of effective treatment.

Clinical features

Leprosy is a slow, chronic and progressive infection affecting mainly the skin, where lesions present as nodules or thickened patches, sometimes with loss of pigmentation. Thickening of the peripheral nerves, with anaesthesia, is common: this leads to trophic changes in the tissues of the extremities (due to repeated trauma as a result of loss of sensation) and so to the distressing mutilation characteristic of the disease. Lesions affect mainly the skin and exposed, cooler extremities such as nose and ears.

Causal organism: M. *leprae*.

Incubation period: long, usually 3–5 years.

Two forms of leprosy, depending on the patient's immunity, are recognized:

1. **Lepromatous (multibacillary)** leprosy: numerous bacilli are present in the lesions; sensory skin nerves are affected, causing 'glove and stocking' anaesthesia, with skin lesions causing nodules and diffuse thickening, and the characteristic 'leonine facies'. This

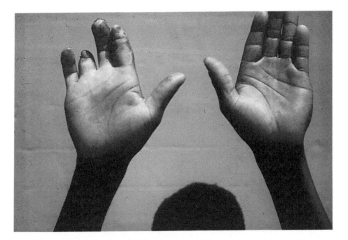

Fig. 37.2   Leprosy. Mutilation of fingers due to trophic changes associated with anaesthesia caused by infection of peripheral nerves.

form of leprosy is a systemic disease, with *M. leprae* spreading via the bloodstream: amyloidosis is a common complication.

2. **Tuberculoid (paucibacillary)** leprosy: the lesions are localized to the skin and peripheral nerves, with anaesthesia. There are only scanty *M. leprae* in the lesions, which tend to be benign, and the disease is often self-healing.

Delayed hypersensitivity mainly determines the clinical type of disease produced: patients with a high degree of hypersensitivity develop the tuberculoid form; in those with no, or only a low degree of, cell-mediated immunity, the disease tends to be lepromatous.

Demonstration of delayed hypersensitivity: by the lepromin skin test: heat-killed bacilli are inoculated intradermally: in the *Mitsuda reaction*, induration up to 28 days after inoculation indicates a positive reaction in tuberculoid leprosy – usually negative in lepromatous leprosy.

Diagnosis

Specimens: skin biopsy or scrapings from lesions in the nasal mucosa.

Direct demonstration of acid-fast bacilli in smears or sections from lesions.

Propagation in the laboratory: *M. leprae* does not grow on artificial media in the laboratory; it can be cultivated in vivo by inoculation of armadillos and into the foot-pads of mice. Culture is not used for diagnosis.

Treatment

- Dapsone
- Rifampicin
- Clofazimine

Triple therapy is required for lepromatous (multibacillary leprosy): duration at least 2 years

Tuberculoid (paucibacillary) leprosy: give rifampicin and dapsone, for 6 months.

Epidemiology

Spread in the community is slow.

Leprosy is often subclinical, and although patients with lepromatous leprosy shed numerous organisms from the nose, the incidence of disease in contacts is low. Leprosy is potentially quite infectious, but has a low expression of disease in infected people: the route of infection is probably mainly inhalation. The incubation period is long – often years.

Geographic distribution is widespread (10 million cases worldwide), especially in tropical climates. The disease is also found in the southern United States and in mediterranean Europe.

Control

The traditional horror of the disease may prevent early cases getting treatment. Hospitalization may be indicated at the start of treatment, but thereafter patients regarded as non-infectious can resume their normal activities.

Vaccine

BCG vaccine may offer a degree of protection, especially in children.

DISEASES DUE TO ATYPICAL MYCOBACTERIA

Atypical mycobacteria, or MOTT (mycobacteria other than tubercle bacilli), form an ill-defined group of mycobacteria usually found as saprophytes in soil or water. Their laboratory characteristics differ from those of *M. tuberculosis*: for example, many produce pigment on culture and grow at lower or sometimes higher temperatures. Also, their pathogenicity and infectivity are much lower. In lung infections they are often present as 'fellow travellers' along with *M. tuberculosis*, but do not play a significant pathogenic role.

Diseases

- *Pulmonary*: mainly seen in immunocompromized patients, e.g. those with AIDS: most often due to the *M. avium* complex, i.e. *M. avium*, *M. intracellulare*, *M. scrofulaceum*. Also associated with *M. malmoense* and *M. kansasii*, and occasionally *M. fortuitum*.
- *Cervical adenitis*: usually seen in children; can be due to *M. tuberculosis*, but also to MOTT such as *M. scrofulaceum*.
- *Skin ulcers*: e.g. 'fish-tank granuloma' and 'swimming-pool granuloma': due to *M. marinum*; occur in tropical countries. Progressive ulcers may be due to *M. ulcerens*.

Treatment

Initial therapy: standard antituberculous drugs, but resistance is common. Clarithromycin is effective against *M. avium* complex: rifabutin-a. Rifamycin is used for prophylaxis in AIDS patients.

The choice of drug combinations depends on the results of laboratory sensitivity tests. The identity of the isolate may indicate appropriate treatment, because some species have a predictable sensitivity pattern.

Epidemiology

Little is known.

38. Infections of bone and joint

Predominantly infections of childhood. Delay in diagnosis and inadequate treatment can result in protracted illness, with permanent disability.

The two main diseases are

- Osteomyelitis
- Septic arthritis.

ACUTE OSTEOMYELITIS

Clinical features

Most common in children under 10 years old. The classical sites are the distal femur, proximal tibia and proximal humerus (Fig. 38.1) and, in adults, the vertebrae.

Presentation: bone pain with fever, and local tenderness: the child is reluctant to move the affected limb. There may be a history of preceding mild trauma to the involved bone.

Causal organisms: *Staphylococcus aureus* (75% or more of cases); other organisms include *Haemophilus influenzae* (in pre-school children); *Streptococcus pyogenes*; coliforms or group B streptococci in neonates. Rarer organisms include salmonellae, *Pseudomonas aeruginosa* (especially in drug addicts) and non-sporing anaerobes such as 'bacteroides'.

Source: not always apparent; sometimes a septic focus elsewhere, e.g. a pustule or boil.

Spread to bone is *haematogenous*. Infection at any age may also follow *direct contamination* of exposed bone, after major trauma (compound fracture) or orthopaedic operation – obviously, the features of this type of osteomyelitis are different.

309

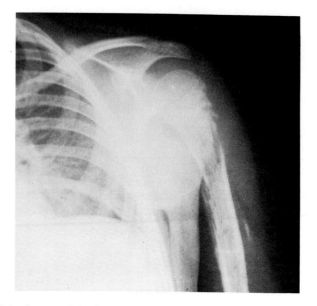

Fig. 38.1   Osteomyelitis of the upper humerus, showing bone destruction. (Reproduced with permission from Abbott Laboratories *Slide Atlas of Infectious Diseases*, 1982, Gower Medical Publishing, London. Photograph by Professor H. Lambert.)

Laboratory diagnosis

Isolation of the causal organism, with antibiotic sensitivity tests, confirms the clinical diagnosis and directs treatment: but not always possible.

Culture:

Blood: positive in many cases; several cultures may be necessary.

Pus: collected from the diseased bone, either by needle aspiration or at open operation.

Haematology: will show a polymorphonuclear leucocytosis and raised ESR.

Treatment

Antibiotics are usually effective, especially if started early. Surgery is necessary if there is evidence of bone destruction or accumulation of pus.

Antibiotic treatment: initially parenteral: later, the oral route is adequate.

In the absence of positive cultures, give flucloxacillin on the assumption that the pathogen is *S. aureus*. Other drugs include cephalosporins, erythromycin, fusidic acid and clindamycin (the latter two are particularly effective at penetrating bone). Sometimes a combination of antistaphylococcal drugs is preferred.

For other pathogens:

- Group B streptococci: penicillin
- *S. pyogenes*: penicillin
- *H. influenzae*: ampicillin
- Coliform organisms: ciprofloxacin or a cephalosporin.

Note: Treatment must be continued for several weeks.

CHRONIC OSTEOMYELITIS

Sometimes due to progression from acute osteomyelitis: may complicate a penetrating wound which directly contaminates bone: predisposing conditions include peripheral vascular disease, diabetes.

Clinical features

Pain; bone destruction with the formation of sequestra and discharging sinuses. If the vertebral column is involved there may be vertebral collapse, resulting in paraplegia. Small bones of the feet may be affected.

Causal organisms: *Staphylococcus aureus* – the most common pathogen; less often, *Mycobacterium tuberculosis*, coliform organisms, *Pseudomonas aeruginosa*, *Salmonella species*, *Brucella species*, 'bacteroides'.

Laboratory diagnosis

Isolation of the causal agent from blood culture; a discharging sinus or material obtained at operation; or possibly from an infective focus elsewhere (e.g. from culture of cold abscess pus in tuberculosis).

Treatment

Surgery is usually necessary for the drainage of pus and for the removal of sequestra. A variety of orthopaedic procedures, such as bone grafting, have an important role in management.

Antibiotics:

- *Chronic staphylococcal osteomyelitis*: long-term flucloxacillin, fusidic acid or clindamycin: often given in combination
- *Tuberculous osteomyelitis*: isoniazid, pyrazinamide and rifampicin
- *Salmonella or coliform osteomyelitis*: ciprofloxacin, a cephalosporin or co-trimoxazole
- *Brucella osteomyelitis*: doxycycline, with either rifampicin or streptomycin.

SEPTIC ARTHRITIS

Usually seen as:

- a complication of septicaemia, especially if there is pre-existing joint disease – particularly rheumatoid arthritis.
- an extension of osteomyelitis, or other infection near to the joint
- infection following intra-articular injection, arthroscopy, or orthopaedic surgery – especially insertion of joint prostheses.

Clinical features

The most striking feature is severe pain, which limits movement of the affected joint: in general, only one joint is involved. The onset may be sudden with fever, swelling and redness over the joint. Crippling sequelae are common, despite antibiotic therapy.

Causal organisms: similar to those responsible for osteomyelitis, but in addition *Neisseria gonorrhoeae* (an important cause in sexually active adults, especially women), *Neisseria meningitidis* and *Streptococcus pneumoniae*.

Laboratory diagnosis

- *Examination of fluid aspirated from the joint*:
  Direct film: observe for polymorphs and bacteria; the appearance may allow a presumptive diagnosis and advice regarding immediate chemotherapy.
  Culture: on a variety of media to isolate the causal pathogen.
- *Blood culture*.
- *Culture of specimens from any other infected site*, e.g. throat, genital tract, meninges. If tuberculosis is suspected, examine sputum and urine.
- *Serological tests* for salmonellosis and brucellosis.

Treatment

Antibiotic therapy on a 'best-guess' basis should be started as soon as diagnostic specimens have been taken. When a causal organism has been isolated, the drug of choice is the same as for osteomyelitis. Treat arthritis due to *N. gonorrhoeae* with penicillin: for resistant strains, use a cephalosporin or ciprofloxacin.

INFECTION IN PROSTHETIC JOINTS

The insertion of artificial joints, usually hip or knee, has a high long-term success rate (over 90%): failure is due to either mechanical loosening or infection. The introduction of inert material predisposes to infection, often with organisms of low pathogenicity.

Clinical features

Pain in the new joint with limited movement, as a rule soon after operation – but infection may be delayed for several months or longer.

Causal organisms: *Staphylococcus aureus*; skin commensals, e.g. *Staphylococcus epidemidis*; coliform organisms.

Source of infection: contamination of the site at the time of operation, with bacteria from the patient's skin or from the surgical team, by contact or via the theatre air. *Late infection* may be due to organisms settling in the implant from a transient asymptomatic bacteraemia.

Laboratory diagnosis

Diagnosis of infection may be impossible because of difficulty in accessing the joint. Try blood culture, or examine tissue if secondary operation is carried out. Bacteria in the exudate of the superficial surgical wound are not necessarily the same as those in the infected joint.

Treatment

Often must be blind, with flucloxacillin, cephalosporins or fusidic acid; gentamicin may be given in addition.

Prevention

Careful preparation of the skin site and scrupulous surgical technique: surgeons may wear special gowns and masks and operate in a laminar-flow ventilated theatre, which provides ultra-clean air.

Antibiotic prophylaxis: peri-operative, usually with a cephalosporin, often cefuroxime.

Infection rate with adequate precautions should be 1% or less.

REACTIVE ARTHRITIS

Acute arthritis of varying severity, affecting one or more joints, which develops 1–4 weeks after infection of either the genital or gastrointestinal tracts.

Due to an immunological mechanism: it is not the result of infection in the joint: culture of joint exudate is sterile.

Two forms of reactive arthritis are recognized:

1. **Post-sexual reactive arthritis** in which the arthritis, usually accompanied by ocular inflammation (conjunctivitis, sometimes also iritis), presents after non-gonococcal urethritis – often caused by *Chlamydia trachomatis*. Almost all patients are males: the condition is common in the UK.

2. **Post-dysenteric reactive arthritis** in which the arthritis presents after gastrointestinal infection with Gram-negative bacilli, such as shigella, salmonella, campylobacter or yersinia. Affects both men and women; patients may also develop urethritis or conjunctivitis. The condition is common in continental Europe, and is now being diagnosed more often in the UK.

Reiter's syndrome is a term used to describe patients who develop the triad of symptoms of arthritis, urethritis and conjunctivitis: much more common in post-sexual reactive arthritis.

Predisposing factor may be the antigen HLA-B 27, present in 7% of the population but found in more than half of patients with reactive arthritis. Numerous hypotheses have been proposed to explain this apparent genetic predisposition, but the pathogenic mechanisms that link it with infection and arthritis remain speculative.

39. Sexually transmitted diseases

Some infectious diseases are transmitted by sexual intercourse. The causal organisms are generally delicate, and do not remain viable for long outside the body: their survival as pathogens therefore depends on transmission by direct contact between mucosal surfaces.

Sexually transmitted diseases often (but not always) produce genital lesions – however, several give rise to systemic, severe, disease. After an increase in incidence during the 1970s and early 1980s, possibly due to changing social attitudes, increased travel amongst the young, urbanization, etc., there has been a decline during the late 1980s and 1990s – particularly in gonorrhoea. Fear of AIDS and promotion through the media of 'safe sex' may have played a part in this.

Sexually transmitted diseases affect male homosexual partners as well as heterosexual relationships. AIDS – or rather, HIV infection – is predominantly transmitted through homosexual (anal) intercourse – at least in the USA and the UK. Variations in sexual behaviour can result in sexually transmitted diseases producing lesions in the rectum or oropharynx.

The main sexually transmitted diseases are listed in Table 39.1.

GONORRHOEA

A world-wide disease, although now declining in incidence in the UK. Considerably less common than non-specific urethritis.

Causal organism: Neisseria gonorrhoeae.

Clinical features

Acute onset of purulent urethral or vaginal discharge: often with dysuria and frequency in males. Asymptomatic infection is

315

Table 39.1   Sexually transmitted diseases

Disease	Cause
Gonorrhoea	*Neisseria gonorrhoeae* (the gonococcus)
Nonspecific urethritis	*Chlamydia trachomatis* types D – K
Trichomoniasis	*Trichomonas vaginalis*
Vaginal thrush*	*Candida albicans*
Syphilis	*Treponema pallidum*
Vaginitis	*Gardnerella vaginalis*, anaerobes
Genital herpes	Herpes simplex virus type 2 (less often, type 1)
Genital warts	Papilloma virus
Hepatitis B*	Hepatitis B virus
AIDS*	Human immunodeficiency virus (HIV)
Chancroid	*Haemophilus ducreyi*
Lymphogranuloma venereum	*Chlamydia trachomatis* types L1, 2, 3
Granuloma inguinale (donovanosis)	*Calymmatobacterium granulomatis*
Pubic lice (crabs)	*Phthirus pubis*
Genital scabies	*Sarcoptes scabei*

*Not always sexually transmitted.
Note: This chapter deals only with gonorrhoea, nonspecific urethritis, trichomoniasis, thrush, syphilis, and *Gardnerella vaginalis*. AIDS is considered in chapter 42.

common in females. The disease may involve the rectum or the oropharynx.

Complications

Due to local spread.

Males: prostatis, epididymitis; rarely, urethral stricture in untreated cases.

Females: salpingitis, sometimes leading to infertility.

Occasionally: septicaemia, arthritis, meningitis, due to haematogenous spread.

Neonates: ophthalmia neonatorum or gonococcal conjunctivitis, due to infection during birth from maternal disease.

Gonococcal vulvovaginitis: a rare form of gonorrhoea in young girls, either following a sexual offence or sometimes acquired non-sexually by contact with infected exudates or fomites.

Diagnosis

Specimens: urethral, cervical, rectal or throat smears and swabs – swabs directly plated or transported to the laboratory in Amies' transport medium.

Direct Gram film: examine for typical intracellular Gram-negative diplococci in smears: often convincingly positive in males (see Fig. 16.1) but less useful in females due to difficulty in interpreting the microscopic appearances in the mixed normal flora.

Isolation

Culture: on gonococcal selective media (e.g. Thayer–Martin or modified MNYC media), because of contamination of sites such as vagina or rectum with other organisms: incubate in CO_2 for 48 h.

Observe: typical translucent colonies, turning purple on addition of oxidase reagent.

Identification: by rapid carbohydrate utilization test for enzyme; alternatively, or in addition, by co-agglutination with monoclonal antibody in Phadebact test kit.

Treatment

Patients tend to default, and whenever possible, antibiotics should be given in one curative dose. Numerous different regimens have been proposed.

Standard treatments include a large single oral dose of:

1. *Amoxycillin*, with oral *probenecid* to delay renal excretion
2. *Ceftriaxone*
3. *Spectinomycin*: if gonorrhoea due to penicillin-resistant *N. gonorrhoeae*, or if patient is allergic to penicillin; do *not* use for pharyngeal gonorrhoea (use ceftriaxone or ciprofloxacin)
4. *Ciprofloxacin*: for infection complicated with *Chlamydia*
5. *Erythromycin*: for children or pregnant women.

Penicillin resistance

Normally *N. gonorrhoeae* is extremely sensitive to penicillin, but two types of resistance are now seen:

- *Low-level*: strains remain sensitive to high concentrations of penicillin: relatively common and not due to β-lactamase production.
- *High-level*: due to a plasmid-coded β-lactamase: strains are totally resistant to penicillin; still seen in only a minority of strains in the UK.

Penicillin-resistant gonorrhoea should be treated with spectinomycin, ciprofloxacin, erythromycin or tetracycline.

NONSPECIFIC URETHRITIS OR CERVICITIS

Nonspecific genital infection is now the commonest sexually transmitted disease in Britain. Predominantly seen in males – presumably because infection in females is often symptomless.

Causal organism(s): almost certainly due to more than one infectious agent, but *Chlamydia trachomatis* is the most common identified cause. *Ureaplasma urealyticum,* a mycoplasma, may be responsible for a small proportion of cases.

Clinical features

Acute purulent urethral discharge, indistinguishable clinically from gonorrhoea; sometimes cervicitis in females (but this is usually symptomless).

Reiter's disease or *syndrome* is a triad of urethritis, arthritis and conjunctivitis (with or without iritis), often seen as a complication of nonspecific urethritis; sometimes only two of the three symptoms are present (see p. 314).

Diagnosis

Isolation

Specimens: smears and swabs of urethral or cervical discharge.

Culture: now rarely done, but necessary for forensic cases: in tissue cultures.

Observe: intracytoplasmic inclusions, by immunofluorescence.

Serology

Examine for chlamydial antigen by indirect immunofluorescence with monoclonal antibody, or by ELISA.

Treatment

Tetracycline (doxycycline) for 7–10 days – but relapses are common. *Alternatively,* ciprofloxacin or azithromycin.

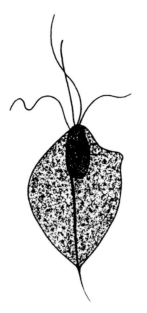

Fig. 39.1   *Trichomonas vaginalis.* This common protozoon is pear-shaped, with four flagella.

TRICHOMONIASIS

A common disease in women: mainly, if not entirely, transmitted as a result of sexual intercourse with males who have a symptomless infection. See also Chapter 48.

Causal organism: a pear-shaped protozoon, *Trichomonas vaginalis*: motile by means of four flagella (Fig. 39.1).

Clinical features

Vaginal discharge – typically frothy, offensive and greenish-yellow. There may also be urethral discharge and excoriation of vulva and perineum; the mucosa of vagina and cervix is reddened and inflamed. The bladder may be involved, with dysuria and frequency. Infection is usually symptomatic, but varies from an acute severe vaginitis to a mild, low-grade or even symptomless infection.

Diagnosis

Specimen: swab of vaginal discharge in Amies' transport medium.

Direct: observe wet film for motile protozoa, or stain for typical protozoal forms with acridine orange.

Culture: in special medium for trichomonas, for 5 days: examine for motile protozoa at 2 and 5 days.

Treatment

Metronidazole: orally for 7 days, or a large single dose. Whenever possible, the male partner should be identified, examined and treated.

THRUSH (CANDIDIASIS)

Vaginal thrush is seen in females; genital candidiasis is rare in men.

Causal organism: *Candida albicans*, a normal commensal of mucous membranes, including those of the vagina and bowel. Infection may be endogenous and precipitated by systemic disease (e.g. diabetes) or drug treatment (e.g. broad-spectrum antibiotics), but some cases are sexually transmitted.

Clinical features

White, membranous patches with itching and irritation of vulva or vagina; white, thick or sometimes watery discharge may be present; many cases are virtually symptomless.

Diagnosis

Can usually be made clinically – but best with laboratory confirmation.

Specimen: swab.

Direct Gram film: look for characteristic Gram-positive yeast cells, with budding pseudohyphae (see Fig. 27.1).

Culture: on Sabouraud's medium.

Observe: typical waxy-surfaced colonies.

Identification: by observation of germ tubes when grown in serum.

Treatment

Imidazole, e.g. clotrimazole, econazole, miconazole, applied locally for 3–14 days. Nystatin, applied locally, is also useful.

SYPHILIS

Now a relatively rare disease, at least in the UK, but important because of its severity and long-term effects if inadequately treated or missed: may be associated with concomitant HIV infection.

Causal organism: the spirochaete *Treponema pallidum*.

Clinical features

Incubation period: 2–4 weeks.

There are four clinical stages: primary, secondary, tertiary and late or quaternary.

Primary syphilis

A papule, usually on the genital area, which ulcerates to form the classical *chancre* of primary syphilis: a flat, dull, red indurated ulcer which exudes serous fluid (Fig. 39.2). This heals spontaneously in 3–8 weeks. There is painless enlargement of local lymph nodes.

Secondary syphilis

6–8 weeks after the primary lesion has healed, the infection becomes generalized with a rash, most often papular, of mucous membranes as well as of the skin. The lesions are highly infectious and contain many treponemes; they may coalesce in intertriginous

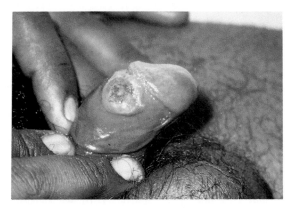

Fig. 39.2   Primary chancre, showing indurated ulcer on penis. (Reproduced with permission from Abbott Laboratories *Slide Atlas of Infectious Diseases*, 1982, Gower Medical Publishing, London. Photograph by Dr. R. D. Caterall.)

areas (especially perianal region) to form wart-like *condylomata lata*. There is generalized lymphadenopathy in half the patients at this stage, and there are snail-track mucosal ulcers in the mouth in about a third of patients. Rarer manifestations include periostitis, arthritis, hepatitis, glomerulonephritis and occasionally iridocyclitis and choroidoretinitis.

Tertiary syphilis

3–10 years after the primary lesion: *gumma* or granulomatous nodules in skin, mucous membrane or bones: gummata commonly break down to form shallow punched-out ulcers.

Late or quaternary syphilis

10–20 years after primary syphilis: there are two main clinical forms:

1. *Cardiovascular*: aortitis, aneurysm (classically of the aorta), aortic incompetence, coronary ostial stenosis (i.e. narrowing of the origins of the coronary arteries in the aortic sinus).
2. *Neurosyphilis*: may take the following forms:
   - *Tabes dorsalis*, with characteristic ataxic gait and trophic changes in joints (Charcot's joints): often associated with optic atrophy
   - *General paralysis of the insane*, with dementia, tremor, spastic paralysis
   - *Meningovascular syphilis*, with headache, cranial nerve palsies, pupillary loss of reaction to light (Argyll-Robertson pupil).

Latent syphilis

The disease can lie dormant for many years with no clinical symptoms (but with positive serology). Latent syphilis can eventually develop into cardiovascular syphilis or neurosyphilis.

Congenital syphilis

Syphilis is one of the infections – rare amongst bacteria – capable of crossing the placental barrier to infect the fetus.

Transmission can take place early (10th week) until late in pregnancy; fetal infection is usually seen only with primary or secondary syphilis in the mother.

Congenital syphilis is clinically seen as:

1. *Latent infection*: more than half the infected infants have no symptoms – but they are serologically positive.

2. *Early*: up to the end of the second year of age. Most infants appear healthy at birth; symptoms develop in the first few weeks of life, starting with failure to thrive, then generalized infection with skin rash, snuffles, nasal deformity (saddle nose), hepatitis, bone lesions, meningitis, anaemia.

3. *Late*: manifestations appear after the second year of life: interstitial keratitis, bone sclerosis, joint effusions and arthritis, juvenile general paralysis of the insane and tabes, notching of incisor teeth (Hutchinson's incisors), deafness.

Diagnosis

Direct demonstration

Rarely done: demonstration of spirochaetes in fluid or scrapings from chancre or ulcerated secondary lesions, by dark-ground microscopy.

Serology

The most effective laboratory diagnostic methods are serological. Two types of antigen are used:

1. *Cardiolipin or lipoidal antigen*: not derived from spirochaetes, but sensitive in detecting syphilitic antibody, probably directed against cross-reacting cardiolipin in the infecting treponemes. The antibody disappears with treatment. Biological false-positive reactions are common.

Test

- *VDRL* (Venereal Disease Reference Laboratory): uses a non-specific antigen consisting of a mixture of cardiolipin, cholesterol and lecithin. Syphilitic antibody (IgM or IgG), probably directed against cross-reacting cardiolipin in infecting treponemes, causes suspension of this antigen to flocculate.

2. *Specific treponemal antigen*: using *T. pallidum* as antigen. Tests using specific antigen involve fewer false-positive reactions than those using non-specific antigens, and they remain positive after treatment.

Tests

- *TPHA* (*T. pallidum* haemagglutination test)
- *FTA-ABS* (fluorescent treponemal antibody-absorption test): this test can be used to detect IgM as well as IgG antibody
- *ELISA*, using *T. pallidum* antigen: now being used increasingly as a screening test: detects IgG antibody, but with some false positives.

The earliest serological test to become positive is usually the FTA-ABS.

Screening for syphilis on a large scale (e.g. antenatal specimens) is best done by VDRL and TPHA.

Other treponemal diseases, such as yaws, also give positive reactions in all serological tests for syphilis. Table 39.2 lists the typical serological reactions in the different stages of syphilis.

Note: always test a patient with positive syphilis tests for HIV infection.

Treatment

Penicillin: large doses continued for 10–21 days.

Late or latent syphilis: large doses of penicillin for 21 days, usually followed by 10 injections at weekly intervals.

Erythromycin or tetracycline (doxycycline) can be used if patient is hypersensitive to penicillin.

Table 39.2 Serological tests for syphilis

Stage of disease	VD Reference Laboratory (VDRL)	*Treponema pallidum* Haemagglutination (TPHA)	Fluorescent Treponema Antibody-absorption (FTA-ABS)
Primary	+ or −	−	+
Late primary	+	+ or −	+
Secondary and tertiary	+	+	+
Late (quaternary)	+	+	+
Latent	+ or −	+	+
Treated syphilis	−	+	+
Congenital syphilis	+	+	+*

*IgM and IgG positive: detection of IgG only might represent passively transferred maternal antibody.

Note: The success of treatment can be monitored by the VDRL test, which becomes negative on successful treatment. The other two tests remain positive.

BACTERIAL VAGINOSIS

Many episodes of vaginosis remain unexplained. *Gardnerella vaginalis* has been implicated in some cases, apparently in conjunction with anaerobes such as 'bacteroides'. Infection is probably transmitted sexually, but infectivity appears to be low.

Causal organisms: G. *vaginalis* a Gram-variable microaerophilic bacillus of uncertain classification; various anaerobes.

Clinical features

Thin, grey-white watery offensive discharge with pH > 4.5. The odour is due to amines, and can be intensified by mixing secretions with a drop of potassium hydroxide – the *amine test*.

Diagnosis

Microscopy: demonstration of '*clue cells*', i.e. squamous epithelial cells with many Gram-variable adherent bacilli in wet or stained films. Few polymorphs are present.

Isolation: of little value in diagnosis: although numbers increase by a hundredfold in bacterial vaginitis, the organism can be isolated from the secretions of 60% of symptomless females.

Treatment

Metronidazole.

CONTROL OF SEXUALLY TRANSMITTED DISEASES

'Sexually transmitted diseases are now second only to respiratory tract infections as a cause of morbidity due to communicable diseases in Europe' (WHO, 1992): prompt diagnosis and treatment are essential.

Whatever the disease, determined attempts should be made to persuade patients to name consorts, and for the consorts to submit themselves to examination and treatment. The tracing of partners' contacts, although difficult and time-consuming, is of great importance in the control of sexually transmitted diseases.

40. Infections of the eye

EYELID INFECTIONS

Blepharitis

Acute or chronic infection of the hair follicles and glandular structures often with an associated conjunctivitis, and sometimes corneal ulceration in chronic infection.

Clinical features: red eyelids with fine crusts at the roots of the lashes.

Stye

An abscess or small boil in one of the glands of the lash follicles: external styes point to the outer side of the lid margin, internal styes to the inner surface of the eyelid.

Causal organism: Usually *Staphylococcus aureus*.
Source: endogenous, e.g. from the anterior nares or implantation via the fingers from a septic lesion elsewhere.
Diagnosis:
- Culture of a swab from lid margin or of pus
- Antibiotic sensitivity tests to topical drugs.

Antibiotic treatment: often unnecessary.

CONJUNCTIVITIS

The conjunctival sac is often colonized by Gram-positive bacteria (see p. 154). Tears act as a defence mechanism by flushing away foreign material; in addition, they contain lysozyme, lactoferrin and immunoglobulins.

Conjunctivitis is the result of microbial invasion of the conjunctival sac by pathogens; children and the elderly are most often affected.

Clinical features: inflammation of conjunctiva, unilateral or bilateral, with gritty and sticky sensation; excessive lacrimation with a mucoid or purulent discharge.

Causal organisms: *Staphylococcus aureus*, *Haemophilus influenzae*, *Streptococcus pneumoniae*, *Maraxella lacunata*; often, viruses – especially adenoviruses.

Source and spread: exogenous: often via contaminated fingers or fomites; endogenous: from infections of eyelids or respiratory tract.

Ophthalmia neonatorum

Conjunctival infection of the neonate, acquired either during birth, from the maternal genital tract, or from some external source after delivery.

Causal organisms:

1. *From the genital tract*:
   - *Neisseria gonorrhoeae*: gonococcal ophthalmia: now rare, but formerly an important cause of blindness in children. Clinically, severe purulent conjunctivitis with a tendency to involve the cornea, causing ulceration and even perforation. Usually develops within 36–48 h of birth. Can be prevented by instillation of 1% silver nitrate solution into the eyes at birth.
   - *Chlamydia trachomatis*: inclusion conjunctivitis. Clinically, an acute conjunctivitis with mucopurulent exudate: less severe than gonococcal ophthalmia and with a longer incubation period (5–12 days). There is often an associated infection of the respiratory tract.
   - *Streptococci* of Lancefield group B.
2. From an external source:
   - *Staphylococcus aureus*: 'sticky eye': the commonest eye infection, probably spread via medical and nursing staff. Outbreaks of staphylococcal sticky eye in maternity-hospital nurseries are well recognized.

Diagnosis

Bacterial infections

Specimens:
- Exudate collected directly from the patient's eye with a platinum bacteriological loop: films and cultures should if possible be made at the bedside
- Swab of exudate paced in Stuart's transport medium
  Direct film: examine by Gram's stain for characteristic bacteria.
  Culture: on blood and chocolate agar plates, incubated for 48 h at 37°C in the presence of 5–10% carbon dioxide.
  Observe: growth.
  Identification: by usual methods.

Chlamydial infections

Specimen: conjunctival scrapings.
  Direct film: examine by immunofluorescence.
  Culture: in irradiated or cycloheximide-treated McCoy cells for 2–3 days.
  Observe: intracytoplasmic inclusions when stained by Giemsa method or fluorescent-labelled monoclonal antibody.

MICROBIAL KERATITIS

Keratitis is infection of the cornea, often with ulceration: always potentially sight-threatening.

Clinical features: pain, photophobia, lacrimation and lid spasm. Ulceration, with grey-white areas and loss of corneal reflex: severe ulceration is accompanied by iritis and collection of pus at the lower recess of the anterior chamber, and may be complicated by corneal perforation, leading to endophthalmitis.

Causes: abrasion or trauma, e.g. due to a foreign body, with secondary infection – wearing contact lenses is a common predisposing factor. Infecting microorganisms include:
- bacteria (pyogenic cocci, pseudomonas)
- *Chlamydia trachomatis*
- viruses (notably herpes simplex)

- filamentous fungi and yeasts
- parasites (notably onchocera, acanthamoeba).

Diagnosis: take multiple corneal scrapings for microscopy and culture on a wide range of appropriate media.

Treatment: aggressive topical antimicrobial therapy: choice of drug based on laboratory results. Severe infections, with impending perforation, treated as for endophthalmitis (see below).

ORBITAL CELLULITIS

A serious infection of the cellular tissues of the orbit, which may follow penetrating injury or spread of infection from the nasal sinuses: sometimes 'spontaneous' without any recognized cause.

Clinical features: painful swelling and protrusion of the eyeball are accompanied by general systemic upset. Surgical incision may yield pus – an essential specimen for accurate bacteriological diagnosis. *Complications* include endophthalmitis, meningitis, brain abscess and cavernous sinus thrombosis – rare nowadays unless treatment inadequate.

Causal bacteria: *Staphylococcus aureus*, *Streptococcus pyogenes*, *Streptococcus pneumoniae*, *Haemophilus influenzae* (in children).

ENDOPHTHALMITIS

Inflammation of the inner eye (iris, vitreous, retina and choroid), which often results in total destruction: may be acute, subacute or chronic. Early diagnosis and treatment are necessary to save vision. Usually due to:

- penetrating wounds – traumatic or surgical (especially after cataract surgery with implant)
- spread of infection from a perforated corneal ulcer or orbital cellulitis
- haematogenous spread from septic focus, e.g. in endocarditis
- injection of infected material by intravenous drug abusers.

Causal microorganisms: wide range of infecting agents (see causes of keratitis). Bacteria are most commonly responsible: infections with *Staphylococcus aureus* and pseudomonas are fulminating; those caused by *Staphylococcus epidermidis* and other less virulent bacteria are often chronic.

Diagnosis: culture of a conjunctival swab gives misleading results. As soon as possible, the vitreous should be aspirated: examine the pus microscopically and culture on appropriate media.

TREATMENT OF BACTERIAL INFECTIONS OF THE EYE

Superficial infections

Bacterial infections usually respond readily to topical treatment:

- *General measures*: removal of exudate, irrigation with simple solutions, e.g. saline
- *Antibiotics*: either as drops or ointments: many agents are available, including chloramphenicol, aminoglycosides (framycetin, gentamicin, neomycin), cephalosporins, tetracycline, fusidic acid, polymyxin.

Chlamydial infections should also be treated orally, with tetracycline or erythromycin.

Endophthalmitis

More aggressive antibiotic treatment is necessary: systemic antibiotics penetrate the eye poorly, and in addition to intravenous therapy, drugs have to be given by the intravitreal and subconjunctival routes. A recommended initial regimen is gentamicin and cephazolin.

CHOROIDITIS AND CHORIORETINITIS

Granulomatous reaction in the choroid or retina is usually the result of invasion by microorganisms or parasites: clinically, grey-white choroidoretinal lesions, which heal to form scars.
Causal organisms:

- *Bacteria*: *Mycobacterium tuberculosis*, *Brucella abortus*, *Treponema pallidum* – all now very rare.
- *Viruses*: rubella and cytomegalovirus infection – usually congenital; varicella-zoster virus (ophthalmic zoster involves the choroid and ciliary body); herpes simplex virus can cause necrotizing retinal vasculitis
- *Fungi*: e.g. *Candida albicans*: a cause of retinitis in intravenous drug abusers
- *Protozoa*: *Toxoplasma gondii* (in congenital and acquired toxoplasmosis)
- *Helminths*: *Toxocara canis* (mainly retinitis).

Chorioretinitis may develop in patients with AIDS: causes include *Pneumocystis carinii* and cytomegalovirus.

41. Zoonoses

Zoonoses are infections between vertebrate animals and humans. Not surprisingly, many of those acquired by humans affect agricultural workers and veterinary surgeons, but the general public are also at risk, for example through contaminated meat and milk.

Table 41.1 lists the main bacterial zoonoses. Other zoonoses are caused by rickettsiae, chlamydiae, viruses, protozoa and fungi; animal ringworm is perhaps the commonest infection world-wide.

Domestic animals are more likely to be sources of infection than wild animals, due to their closer contact with people. Table 41.2 shows the principal sources and routes of infection acquired from domestic animals.

Bacterial food poisoning caused by salmonella, campylobacter or *Escherichia coli* is by far the most common zoonosis in Britain. These infections, and tuberculosis due to *Mycobacterium bovis*, are described in Chapters 28 and 37 respectively.

BRUCELLOSIS

Although brucellosis in Britain is now a rare disease, it remains world-wide in distribution. The causal *Brucella species* are named after David Bruce, who discovered the cause of one form of the disease while serving as an army doctor in Malta.

Causal organisms – brucellae – are small Gram-negative coccobacilli: the main species are listed in Table 41.3. Infection with *B. suis* is less common than that due to *B. abortus* or *B. melitensis*.

Clinical features

Incubation period: 1–3 weeks, occasionally several months.

Signs and symptoms: undulant fever, a prolonged debilitating febrile illness with remissions and relapses – often becoming chronic

Table 41.1 Bacterial zoonoses

Disease	Causal organism	Main animal host
Food poisoning	*Salmonella species*	Cattle, poultry
Food poisoning	*Campylobacter species*	Poultry, other domestic animals
Food poisoning	*Escherichia coli* (VTEC)	Cattle
Tuberculosis	*Mycobacterium bovis*	Cattle
Brucellosis	*Brucella abortus* *Brucella melitensis* *Brucella suis*	Cattle Goats, sheep Pigs
Anthrax	*Bacillus anthracis*	Cattle
Plague	*Yersinia pestis*	Rats
Mesenteric adenitis, enteritis	{ *Yersinia pseudotuberculosis* *Yersinia enterocolitica*	Various animals
Septic animal bite	*Pasteurella multocida*	Dogs, cats
Tularaemia	*Francisella tularensis*	Squirrels, other rodents
Leptospirosis	*Leptospira interrogans*	Rats, pigs, dogs, cattle
Lyme disease	*Borrelia burgdorferi*	Small mammals, deer
Listeriosis	*Listeria monocytogenes*	Various domestic and wild animals
Erysipeloid	*Erysipelothrix rhusiopathiae*	Pigs, fish, other animals
Rat-bite fever	*Streptobacillus moniliformis* *Spirillum minus*	Rats, mice
Cat-scratch disease	*Bartonella henselae*	Cats

when it persists for months or even years. The main symptoms are sweating, anorexia, constipation, rigors, weakness and lassitude; the spleen and lymph nodes are often enlarged, and there may be arthritis, orchitis and neuralgia. Acute brucellosis is a *septicaemic* illness: abortion is not a feature of human brucellosis. In chronic brucellosis the symptoms are of vague ill-health: 'psychiatric morbidity' (usually depression) may overshadow physical symptoms.

Duration: on average, 3 months: even without therapy, symptoms of acute brucellosis usually disappear within 1 year.

Table 41.2 Domestic animals: sources and routes of infection

Source	Route	At risk
Infected animals	Contact	Farm workers, veterinary surgeons, slaughtermen: may be associated with injury
Contaminated pastures, straw, dust, soil	Inhalation, contact	Farm workers, veterinary surgeons
Milk	Ingestion	People drinking unpasteurized milk*
Meat	Ingestion	Anyone eating meat
Hides, bones, other animal products	Contact Inhalation	Industrial workers handling animal products; occasionally, general public

*Almost all milk retailed in the UK is heat-treated. The sale of raw milk is no longer permitted in Scotland but, although discouraged, is not yet prohibited in England and Wales.

Severity: brucellosis due to *B. melitensis* tends to be a more severe disease than that due to *B. abortus*. Even before antibiotics, brucellosis had a low case fatality rate – around 2%.

Pathogenesis

Route of infection: usually by drinking unpasteurized *contaminated* milk, or eating cheese made from it. Farm workers, slaughtermen and veterinary surgeons are not uncommonly infected by direct contact with infected animals or their products – especially the placenta or uterine discharges from parturient animals.

Spread in the body is via lymph channels to lymph nodes and the bloodstream: the organism then becomes widely distributed in organs and tissues, to produce the symptoms of acute brucellosis.

Intracellular parasitism: brucellae have a particular tendency to persist intracellularly, notably in spleen, liver and lymph nodes: this is the reason for the well-known difficulty in eradicating the infection by antibiotic therapy. Antigen release from these sites may

Table 41.3 *Brucella species*

Species	Usual animal host	Geographical distribution
B. abortus	Cattle	World-wide
B. melitensis	Goats and sheep	Mediterranean area
B. suis	Pigs	USA, Denmark

lead to an immune-complex syndrome, and cause the symptoms of chronic brucellosis.

Diagnosis

Isolation

Specimen: blood culture in glucose serum broth, incubated in CO_2.
   Observe: growth: retain cultures for 8 weeks.
   Identification: by testing tolerance to dyes; H_2S production; CO_2 requirement for growth; agglutination with monospecific antisera; and lysis by specific bacteriophage.
   Positive blood cultures make certain the diagnosis of acute brucellosis, but numerous sets should be taken because the organism is difficult to isolate: *B. melitensis* is much more readily cultured than *B. abortus*.

Serology

Detect antibody levels against both *B. abortus* and *B. melitensis*. Confusingly, some biotypes of *B. abortus* have a preponderance of melitensis antigen, with a minor content of abortus antigen: infection with *B. abortus* may therefore result in higher titres of antibody to *B. melitensis* than to *B. abortus*. The most widely used tests are:

   1. *Direct (standard) agglutination test*: dilutions of the patient's serum are tested against a brucella suspension and examined for agglutination: *prozones* (i.e. absence of agglutination in low dilutions of serum which contain high levels of antibody) are common – excess antibody binds to bacteria, but fails to link them together in clumps. Agglutination is mainly due to IgM antibody: a titre of 80 or more is significant.
   2. *Complement fixation test*: useful in detecting incomplete antibody, which combines with organisms in the brucella suspension but is unable to agglutinate them. This antibody is mainly IgG: a titre of 16 or more is significant.

Acute brucellosis: at the time of presentation, antibody levels are almost always high – direct agglutination titres of perhaps 1000 or more: IgM and IgG are raised, and titres decline slowly to low levels or zero with clinical recovery.
Chronic brucellosis: levels of IgG (but not IgM) are elevated: the complement fixation test may be positive and the direct aggluti-

nation test negative. Similar findings to those in chronic brucellosis are encountered in healthy individuals whose immunity is being repeatedly stimulated by contact with brucella organisms: 'positive' serological tests are common in those at occupational risk. It is impossible by serological tests to distinguish chronic active brucellosis from seropositive but inactive infection – especially in rural areas where exposure to infection is common.

The administration of tetracycline or co-trimoxazole (a 'therapeutic test') may result in clinical improvement and a fall in antibody levels.

Delayed hypersensitivity: the *brucellin* skin test is similar to the tuberculin test and indicates present or past infection with brucellae: often positive in healthy people from agricultural areas. Of little diagnostic value – in fact, the test may stimulate antibody production and make assessment of serological tests even more difficult.

Treatment

Acute brucellosis should be cured if appropriate treatment is given promptly and continued for an adequate period. Monotherapy is ineffective. Give *doxycycline*, a tetracycline, for 6 weeks, with either *rifampicin* for the duration of treatment or *streptomycin* for the first 3 weeks of the course.

BRUCELLOSIS IN ANIMALS

Animal brucellosis is also a chronic debilitating, septicaemic disease: animals are particularly infectious at parturition because of the heavy contamination of placenta and products of conception. *Erythritol*, which is contained in bovine placental tissue, is a growth factor for brucellae.

Abortion is a common sequel of brucellosis in cattle and can result in serious economic losses in herds.

Milk: mammary gland involvement results in the excretion of brucellae in the milk of infected animals.

Control

Eradication

Brucellosis was eradicated in cattle in Britain in 1981 by a policy of identifying affected herds and slaughtering infected animals.

Vaccination

Vaccination of calves with a live attenuated vaccine (S19) results in significant protection from, but not the elimination of, infection and abortion. Some countries follow this policy, but in Britain, vaccination was abandoned in favour of eradication.

Human brucellosis in britain today

Eradication in animals and the pasteurization of milk supplies has led to a dramatic decline in the disease in the UK. In the early 1970s, some 300 cases of brucellosis were reported each year. In the 1990s, this number had decreased to between 10 and 20: many of these cases and infections due to *B. melitensis* and are either contracted abroad or acquired from imported dairy products, e.g. cheese made from unpasteurized milk.

ANTHRAX

Anthrax is a disease of animals which occasionally infects humans. Although a wide variety of animals is susceptible, anthrax is mainly a disease of herbivores, especially cattle and sheep.

   Causal organism: *Bacillus anthracis*: a large, sporing, capsulated, Gram-positive bacillus.

Clinical features

Cutaneous anthrax

Cutaneous anthrax, or *malignant pustule*, is due to direct inoculation of the skin from infected animals or animal products: an inflamed but painless lesion with surrounding oedema and a characteristic black eschar. Local lymph nodes are usually enlarged. If untreated, it may progress to septicaemia, with death from overwhelming infection. In the UK almost all cases are of this type: about 11 per year were reported in the 1960s, but this has dwindled to an average of less than one annually.

   Acquired in two ways:

- *Occupational*: the majority of cases: most often in those associated with the meat trade, but also in workers handling leather or wool, tanners, workers in bone-meal factories and in agriculture. Malignant pustule of the neck and shoulders was an occupational hazard of hide porters, due to rubbing of infected hides carried on their backs.

- *Non-occupational*: occasionally affects the general public: formerly due to contact with infected shaving brushes, leather goods and clothes: now sometimes seen in amateur gardeners who use bone-meal.

Pulmonary anthrax

Also called *woolsorter's disease* – a name indicating its mode of spread, by inhalation of spores by workers handling contaminated wool: now a rarity – a disease of the 19th century. A severe disease with high mortality.

Gastrointestinal anthrax

Also a lethal disease: due to ingestion of *B. anthracis* or its spores: fortunately, very rare.

Pathogenesis

Long regarded as a classic example of a disease purely due to the invasive properties of the causal organism – however, *B. anthracis* is now known to produce three important toxins:

- Oedema factor
- Protective factor (antibody to this is responsible for immunity to the disease)
- Lethal factor.

Diagnosis

Specimens: swab or sample of exudate from malignant pustule; sputum from suspected pulmonary anthrax.

Direct film: Gram-stained: observe typical large Gram-positive bacilli.

Culture: on ordinary media: observe growth of typical 'curled hair lock' colonies.

Confirm identity of isolated bacilli by subcutaneous inoculation of guinea pigs: observe local lesion with typical gelatinous oedema, and death from septicaemic infection.

Treatment

Penicillin, erythromycin in patients hypersensitive to penicillin.

Animal anthrax

Animal anthrax is a rapidly fatal, septicaemic infection in which huge numbers of organisms are present in the blood and are shed in discharges from the body orifices. *Pastures* used by infected animals become contaminated with anthrax spores, and may remain infective for many years.

Diagnosis

Specimens: blood from a sick animal; an ear cut off post-mortem and sent to the laboratory (packed with due precautions).

Direct demonstration for large Gram-positive bacilli – usually very numerous – in a blood smear: *B. anthracis* does not form spores in the animal body; *McFadyean's reaction*: the demonstration of pink-stained capsular deposits lying between the bacilli in a blood film stained by methylene blue (see Fig. 17.1).

Culture: on ordinary media, for typical colonies.

Control

The decline in incidence of anthrax in occupational 'at risk' groups is probably due to the introduction in 1965 of vaccination with an alum-precipitated toxoid, prepared from the protective factor – and to the wearing of protective clothing.

Animals suspected of being infected must be notified to the authorities. Dead animals must be disposed of by burning or, if this is not possible, by burying in quicklime: a careful check must be kept on the rest of the herd.

Animal products imported from countries where anthrax is a problem are subject to inspection and disinfection.

PLAGUE

Plague is a natural disease of rats, which occasionally spreads to humans via the bite of infected fleas: one of the great epidemic diseases, it was the Black Death (which killed millions in the 14th century) and the Great Plague of London and elsewhere in Britain during the mid-17th century. Plague still exists in endemic foci in the Western USA, South America, Africa and the Far East.

Causal organism: *Yersinia pestis*, a small Gram-negative bacillus.

Clinical Features

There are three forms of plague: bubonic, pneumonic and septicaemic.

- *Bubonic plague*: the most common form: characterized by fever, prostration, mental confusion and enlargement, with profuse pus formation, of the inguinal glands to produce *buboes*. High mortality rate: about 50% in untreated cases. Not contagious – acquired by the bite of fleas.
- *Pneumonic plague*: a rare but highly infectious form of plague, affecting the lungs. The route of infection is by inhalation of infected respiratory secretions: virtually always fatal.
- *Septicaemic plague*: either bubonic or pneumonic plague may progress to an invariably-fatal septicaemia characterized by haemorrhages: the Black Death was septicaemic plague.

Diagnosis

Isolation

Specimens: needle aspirate of lymph node (bubo pus); sputum; blood culture.

Gram film: examine for Gram-negative bacilli, stained darker at the ends than in the middle (bipolar staining).

Culture: ordinary media.

Identification: biochemical and serological reactions.

Treatment

Streptomycin: tetracycline or chloramphenicol are other effective drugs.

Epidemiology

Reservoir is mainly rural or sylvatic rats: most human epidemics have been due to spread of the disease to urban rats.

Vector: the rat flea *Xenopsylla cheopis*: plague spreads amongst rats via infected fleas. Infected fleas transmit the disease during biting: the bacilli multiply in the flea, and are injected from its proventriculus when it bites and sucks blood again.

Spread: the disease may become epidemic in the rat population, causing heavy mortality. Rat fleas do not usually infest humans, but if there are insufficient rats, the fleas turn to humans and spread the disease through human populations.

Control

The prevention of rats coming ashore from ships: although there seems little danger of epidemic plague nowadays, precautions and sampling regulations remain in force.

INFECTIONS WITH OTHER *YERSINIA* SPECIES

Gastrointestinal infection with *Yersinia enterocolitica* and *Yersinia pseudotuberculosis* is considered on page 219.

PASTEURELLA INFECTIONS

Pasteurella multocida, also known as *P. septica*, is a commensal of the mouths of dogs and cats: it is a not uncommon cause of sepsis, which is sometimes severe, after bites by domestic animals.

TULARAEMIA

A plague-like disease spread from rodents, e.g. squirrels, in the USA and elsewhere – but not yet in the UK; due to *Francisella tularensis*, a small Gram-negative bacillus.

LEPTOSPIROSIS

Leptospires infect many different wild and domestic animals, which usually remain well. Leptospires are transmitted to humans by direct or indirect contact with animal urine. Human disease, often due to occupational contact, predominantly affects males and is most common in late summer and autumn. In an average year about 50 cases are diagnosed in the UK, with three deaths.

Causal organism: *Leptospira interrogans*. This species is divided into more than 200 serovars, but three of them: hardjo, ictero-haemorrhagiae and canicola, are responsible for almost all human cases in Britain.

Clinical features

Incubation period: about 10 days.

An initial *septicaemic phase*, lasting 3–7 days, presents as an influenzal illness: the diagnosis is rarely made at this stage. There follows an *immune phase*, when leptospires have disappeared from the blood and antibodies begin to appear: characterized by signs of meningeal irritation (headache, vomiting), conjunctival suffusion and evidence of renal involvement (proteinuria). Leptospirosis is a recognized cause of *aseptic (lymphocytic) meningitis*.

Severe leptospirosis *(Weil's disease)*, associated with jaundice, haemorrhages and serious renal damage, is uncommon and usually due to icterohaemorrhagiae infections. It is likely that many mild cases of leptospirosis are never diagnosed.

Sources of infection

Hardjo infections

Natural host: cattle.

At risk: farmers, often infected from cow urine during milking, and others in close contact with cattle, e.g. veterinary surgeons, abattoir workers, meat inspectors. The hardjo serovar is responsible for about half of the diagnosed cases of leptospirosis, and many infections must pass unnoticed: in a serological survey, 10% of dairymen showed evidence of previous contact with this organism.

Icterohaemorrhagiae infections

Natural host: brown rat.

At risk: agricultural workers, fish handlers, miners, sewage workers and others working in a moist environment contaminated with rat urine: also water-sport enthusiasts.

Farm workers are now the occupational group most commonly affected by icterohaemorrhagiae infections in the UK: formerly it was a disease primarily of sewage workers and miners, but in recent years they have been protected by pest-control measures and protective clothing.

Entry of the pathogen is through skin cuts and abrasions, or sometimes via the nasopharynx or conjunctiva following bathing or accidental immersion in infected water – usually stagnant ponds or canals.

Canicola infections

Natural hosts: pigs and dogs.

At risk: those who tend pigs and dogs. The infection, formerly responsible for some 10% of human cases, is now rare because the disease in dogs has been controlled by immunization.

Diagnosis

Isolation

Difficult, and rarely accomplished.

Specimens: blood, during the first week of illness; urine (the sample *must* be fresh) during the second and third weeks of illness.

Inoculate and observe:

- A suitable serum-enriched liquid medium: growth of leptospires
- Guinea-pigs, intraperitoneally: jaundice and death.

Serology

The usual method of diagnosis: antibodies are not present in the first week of illness, but as a rule can be detected in the second and third weeks: initially of the IgM class, but IgG is developed later and may persist for years. Detection of IgG antibody can be taken as evidence of previous exposure.

1. *Screening tests using a genus-specific antigen,* usually the saprophytic patoc strain of *L. biflexa*:
   - ELISA test, which can be used to detect IgM or IgG
   - Complement fixation test
   - Macroscopic slide agglutination test.
2. *Confirmation tests using serovar-specific antigens* – suspensions, either live or formalin-killed, of leptospires representative of those serovars prevalent in the area – in a *microscopic agglutination test.*

Demonstrate a rising titre to the infecting serovar in serial samples. Cross-reactions may be found in early tests; results from later samples are more specific and diagnostic.

Treatment

Penicillin, erythromycin or doxycycline; antibiotics are of value in leptospirosis, but it is essential to start therapy early in the disease.

LYME DISEASE

A bacterial non-occupational zoonosis with widespread clinical manifestations, which usually follows an initial skin eruption, erythema chronicum migrans (ECM). Although ECM was attributed to a tick bite in 1910, the bacterial cause was only established in the early 1980s.

Causal organism: a spirochaete, *Borrelia burgdorferi*.

Clinical features

ECM starts as a red macule at the site of the tick bite: often associated with fever and malaise. It spreads to become an annular erythema with central clearing. Weeks or months later, in a proportion of patients there is involvement of:

- *Nervous system* – chronic meningoencephalitis, peripheral neuritis.
- *Joints* – arthritis of large joints, often recurrent: common in USA, less so in UK.
- *Heart* – myocarditis, pericarditis, conduction defects.

Diagnosis

Detection of antibody in serum and CSF, by indirect immunofluorescence or ELISA. Rising IgM antibody titres may be demonstrable in acute early infection, but the results of serological tests are often difficult to interpret.

Treatment

For ECM: doxycycline or amoxycillin.

For later stages: cefotaxime or ceftriaxone are more effective.

Epidemiology

Reservoir of infection: field mice, voles and larger mammals such as sheep and horses: importance of deer uncertain.

Route of infection: transmission by the bite of a hard tick, in Europe usually *Ixodes ricinus*.

Geographical distribution: ticks especially numerous in wooded or long-grassed areas: in UK, disease most common in the New Forest, Exmoor, East Anglia and the Scottish highlands.

At risk: farmers, forestry workers, walkers.

LISTERIOSIS

Formerly a rare disease: a tenfold increase in incidence in 10 years resulted in over 300 cases being recorded in the UK in 1988, but the incidence has declined sharply, by almost two-thirds, since then. The increase was thought to be real and not due to better diagnosis.

Causal organism: *Listeria monocytogenes*, a diphtheroid-like Gram-positive bacillus.

Clinical features

Mild or inapparent infection – as a nonspecific febrile illness – is probably not uncommon in the general population.

Non-pregnancy-associated listeriosis is rare in the healthy: usually found in the immunocompromised or elderly who develop either a septicaemia or a meningoencephalitis.

Pregnancy-associated listeriosis affects the fetus: in early pregnancy results in abortion, later causes still birth or neonatal septicaemia/meningitis. Maternal infection often asymptomatic.

Mortality of fully developed disease at any age is high – about 30%.

Diagnosis

Isolation

Specimens: blood cultures, CSF, swabs from genital tract.

Culture: onto blood agar.

Observe: small colonies surrounded by a narrow zone of β-haemolysis.

Identification: small Gram-positive bacilli, like corynebacteria but actively motile when grown in broth at 25°C. Use biochemical tests to distinguish from other listeria.

Treatment

Ampicillin, or ampicillin and gentamicin.

Epidemiology

Source: *L. monocytogenes* is widely distributed in nature: in soil, silage, water and a wide range of animal hosts (cattle, pigs, rodents, birds, fish); asymptomatic human faecal carriage is not uncommon.

Infection is probably food-borne: often sporadic, but food-associated outbreaks incriminating coleslaw, milk, pâté and several types of soft cheese have been reported. Listeria can multiply slowly at 6°C and is therefore able to grow in refrigerated foods.

Reduction in incidence since 1988 is probably due to 'at risk' groups following advice to avoid pâtés, soft cheeses and cook-chill foods; also to increased vigilance by the food industry.

ERYSIPELOID

An inflammatory lesion of the skin, usually of the fingers, hand and forearm, resembling erysipelas but due to a Gram-positive bacillus, *Erysipelothrix rhusiopathiae* – the cause of swine erysipelas, but also found in other animals, birds and fish.

Occupational hazard of meat and fish handlers, veterinary surgeons.

Treatment: penicillin or tetracycline.

RAT-BITE FEVER

Includes two separate, rare diseases transmitted to humans through rat bites: sometimes seen in laboratory workers handling experimental rats.

Causal organism: either *Streptobacillus moniliformis*, or *Spirillum minus*, a spiral organism.

BARTONELLA INFECTIONS

Cat-scratch disease

Clinically, a benign granulomatous disease of skin and sometimes internal organs, with regional lymph node involvement. Lesions may progress to abscess formation. Children and adolescents are usually affected. The condition is well recognized in USA, but rarely diagnosed in UK.

Cause: *Bartonella henselae*, a rickettsia-like organism. Acquired after close contact with apparently healthy cats, often kittens: normally, history of scratch or bite.

Diagnosis

Serology: by immunofluorescence test for antibodies to *B. henselae*.

Culture: on enriched blood agar or in Vero cell cultures.

Histology: still often diagnosed by histological examination of biopsied lymph node.

Bacillary angiomatosis

A rare complication of AIDS and some other immunosuppressed states is usually due to infection with *B. henselae*. The purplish lesions can be confused clinically with those due to Kaposi's sarcoma.

Bacillary angiomatosis can also be caused by *B. quintana*, which was responsible for trench fever in both World Wars. This epidemic infection, transmitted by the body louse, was characterized by relapsing fever and crops of erythematous maculopapules on the trunk.

42. Infection in immunocompromised patients

Increased susceptibility to infection in certain clinical conditions has been recognized for a very long time: for example, tuberculosis and staphylococcal skin sepsis are unduly common in diabetics, and when there is an obstructive element in the pathological process, such as a kidney stone or a bronchial carcinoma, infection is common.

Modern medicine has resulted in many more patients with increased susceptibility to infection whose immune system is defective because of disease or therapy. These patients present special problems to both clinicians and microbiologists.

The microorganisms responsible include recognized pathogens, but also some considered non-pathogenic in the normal host.

The infections, sometimes called *opportunistic,* are often unusually severe and may present with unusual signs and symptoms.

Source of infection: is either *endogenous* or *exogenous* – the latter often due to organisms acquired from the hospital environment.

IMMUNOCOMPROMISED PATIENTS

Deficiencies of the immune response may affect antibody production, cell-mediated immunity, neutrophil function or combinations of all these defence mechanisms. The most important risk factor for infection, especially due to bacteria, is neutropenia.

Table 42.1 shows the principal causes and results of infection in immunocompromised patients.

The immune response may be compromised by:
- Disease
- Therapy
- Congenital deficiency
- Special care

349

Table 42.1 Causes and results of infection in immunocompromised patients

Type of infectious agent	Main microorganisms involved	Clinical manifestations of infection
Bacteria	*Escherichia coli* *Klebsiella* species *Pseudomonas aeruginosa* Other coliforms	Urinary infections; sepsis of colonic origin (e.g. ischiorectal abscess); pneumonia; septicaemia; meningitis
	Legionella pneumophila	Pneumonia
	Mycobacterium tuberculosis	Pulmonary; miliary tuberculosis
	Mycobacterium avium complex	Pulmonary; disseminated disease
	Staphylococcus aureus	Soft tissue sepsis; pneumonia; septicaemia
	Streptococcus pneumoniae	Pneumonia; septicaemia; meningitis
	Listeria monocytogenes	Septicaemia; meningitis; arthritis
	Nocardia asteroides	Pneumonia; metastatic abscesses, especially brain
Fungi	*Candida albicans*	Local thrush; systemic candidiasis
	Cryptococcus neoformans Aspergillus: especially *A. fumigatus* *Mucor* species	Meningoencephalitis Pulmonary; occasionally disseminated infections
Viruses	Herpes simplex virus	Severe cold sores
	Varicella-zoster virus	Zoster, sometimes generalized zoster
	Cytomegalovirus	Pneumonitis; retinitis
	JC (human polyoma) virus	Progressive multifocal leucoencephalopathy
	Papilloma virus	Warts (may be florid)
Protozoa	*Toxoplasma gondii*	Severe toxoplasmosis with involvement of retina and brain
	*Pneumocystis carinii**	Interstitial pneumonia
	Cryptosporidium	Chronic diarrhoea; malabsorption

*see Chapter 48

DISEASE

Many diseases depress the immune response:

1. *AIDS* (see below): in which a virus (HIV) specifically attacks the T-cells of the cellular immune system.

2. *Neoplasms of the lymphoid system*, e.g. leukaemia, where there is suppression of all the defence mechanisms mentioned above. In *Hodgkin's disease*, the major deficiency is in cell-mediated immunity, with an increased susceptibility to viral infections; in *non-Hodgkin's lymphoma*, humoral immunity is depressed. A decrease

in normal immunoglobulin levels, with an increase in the characteristic monoclonal antibody, is seen in *multiple myeloma*.

3. *Solid tumours*: but these have much less effect.

4. *Other diseases*: diminish immunity in a variety of ways: the exact mechanisms involved are complex and often incompletely understood. These diseases include *renal failure, diabetes* and *autoimmune* diseases such as systemic lupus erythematosus and rheumatoid arthritis.

ACQUIRED IMMUNE DEFICIENCY SYNDROME (AIDS)

First recognized in the USA in 1981, although cases probably date from much earlier. There is now a world-wide AIDS epidemic. AIDS is characterized by an extreme degree of immune deficiency – largely due to depletion of CD4 (helper) T-lymphocytes.

Causal organism: human retrovirus: human immune deficiency virus type 1 (HIV-1). A similar but antigenically-distinct virus, HIV-2, is endemic in areas in West Africa and has appeared in patients in Europe and elsewhere: usually in patients with a history of travel to, or residence in, West Africa. HIV-2 causes a milder form of immune deficiency syndrome than HIV-1. HIV-2 infection is very rare in the UK.

Pathogenesis

HIV has a predilection for CD4 T-lymphocytes, in which it replicates – causing a widespread defect of immunity in the host, who then becomes susceptible to a variety of infections and some tumours. Virus replication also takes place in macrophages, neurones, and probably many other cell types throughout the body.

Clinical features

Incubation period: long: on average, about 8–10 years elapse after infection before full-blown AIDS symptoms develop: other opportunistic infections appear earlier.

Seroconversion: antibody appears 1–2 months after exposure.

Initial disease: an infectious mononucleosis-like syndrome, some 6 weeks after exposure: seen in some patients, but many are symptomless at this stage.

Symptomless period: lasts 5–15 years.

Progression of infection: can be measured by the number of CD4 T-lymphocytes in the peripheral blood. CD4 counts of less than 200 cells/µl represent a severe degree of deficiency of immunity.

Indicator diseases: are those which are most important in heralding the onset of AIDS:

- Pneumocystis pneumonia
- Kaposi's sarcoma
- Lymphoma, especially cerebral
- Oesophageal candidiasis
- Tuberculosis
- Cytomegalovirus infections
- Encephalopathy
- Wasting disease.

Symptoms: are of opportunistic infections and tumours. The most important are listed in Table 42.2.

AIDS patients

Still largely a disease of homosexual males, (especially in the age range 25–39 years old) in western Europe and the USA; women can acquire infection from an infected partner, and babies can be infected from their mothers (probably mostly perinatally).

Africa and Asia: AIDS is spread mostly heterosexually: an African partner, or residence in Africa, is also associated with increased risk. Ulcerative sexually transmitted disease increases the risk of acquiring HIV infection.

Haemophiliacs: in the early 1980s, about a third of haemophiliacs in the UK became infected due to contaminated factor VIII: this source of infection is now prevented by screening blood donations.

Drug abusers: another high-risk group: infection is spread through sharing contaminated syringes.

Routes of infection with HIV

These are shown in Table 42.3.

There is considerable public concern over the risk of infection being transmitted from surgeons, dentists, nurses and other health care workers during invasive procedures. The risk is extremely small. To date there have been only two documented incidents –

Table 42.2   AIDS: some of the opportunistic infections and other diseases associated with AIDS

Disease	Cause
Parasitic	*Pneumocystis carinii* pneumonia* Cryptosporidiosis Isosporidiosis Toxoplasmosis (cerebral)
Tumour	Kaposi's sarcoma Lymphoma (usually cerebral) Cervical cancer (invasive)
Fungal	Candidiasis (oesophagus, lower respiratory tract) Cryptococcosis
Bacterial	Tuberculosis Anonymous mycobacterial infection Salmonellosis Pneumonia (recurrent)
Viral	Herpes simplex Cytomegalovirus pneumonitis, retinitis Progressive multifocal leucoencephalopathy HIV: encephalopathy and dementia; wasting syndrome (weight loss, fever, diarrhoea)

*see Chapter 48

a dentist in the USA infected a small number of patients, and a surgeon in France apparently infected a patient during operation.

Health care workers have a very low risk of acquiring infection from infected patients, via needle-stick or other injuries.

Prognosis

A small proportion of patients remain symptom-free apparently indefinitely, but the risk of AIDS after HIV infection is high.

Once full-blown AIDS has developed, the disease seems uniformly fatal. Treatment with two, or preferably three, anti-retroviral drugs prolongs survival, and prophylaxis and treatment of the infections associated with AIDS can control some of the manifestations. Tuberculosis is a particularly difficult complication: often multi-resistant and rapidly fatal in AIDS patients. The rate of progression of AIDS depends on age, and is lower in younger patients.

Table 42.3   Modes of HIV transmission in AIDS cases, UK*

Transmission	Males		Females
		Percentage	
Sexual intercourse			
– Between men	80		–
– Between men and women	9		67
Intravenous drug abuse	5		18
Blood or blood products	6		15

*Based on 1996 cumulative totals.

Therapy which depresses the immune function and induces neutropenia is now widely used. This includes:

- Drugs
  - Immunosuppressive drugs
  - Steroids
  - Cytotoxic drugs
- Radiotherapy
- Splenectomy: results in increased susceptibility to infection with *Streptococcus pneumoniae*.

Drugs in the categories listed, often in combination, are used to treat malignant disease and to prevent graft rejection after organ transplantation. Thus both the disease itself and the treatment administered predispose to infection.

Patients with acute leukaemia, receiving chemotherapy to achieve remission, often develop neutropenia (neutrophil count less than 0.5×10^9/L): they are at special risk of infection, including bacteraemia.

Patients after organ transplantation are maintained on an immunosuppressive regimen designed to reduce the cell-mediated immune response which causes graft rejection: infection in these patients is a common cause of death.

CONGENITAL DEFICIENCY OF THE IMMUNE SYSTEM

Rarely, children are born with congenital deficiency of the immune system. This may involve:

1. **Immunoglobulin synthesis**, e.g. B-cell deficiency with depressed production of immunoglobulins. All immunoglobulins

may be affected, as in Bruton's agammaglobulinaemia, or only some, as in hereditary telangiectasia with deficient IgA and IgE.

2. **Cell-mediated immunity**: T-cell deficiency, e.g. thymic hypoplasia (DiGeorge's syndrome).

3. **Combined immunodeficiency**: lack of differentiation of the common lymphoid stem cell, resulting in both B- and T-cell deficiency, e.g. Swiss-type agammaglobulinaemia, in which there are no lymphocytes or plasma cells in lymphoid organs, and the thymus is very small.

4. **Neutrophil function**: several syndromes affect different aspects of phagocytosis, e.g. chronic granulomatous disease; Chediak–Higashi syndrome.

SPECIAL CARE

PATIENTS IN SPECIAL CARE UNITS

The management of these patients often involves risk factors for infection, such as indwelling catheters (see below). In modern intensive care, patients have prolonged intubation of the respiratory trait: their tracheal secretions often contain coliforms, e.g. *Escherichia coli*, *Klebsiella* species, *Pseudomonas aeruginosa*, *Acinetobacter* species – although the significance of these organisms in the respiratory tract is doubtful.

Indwelling catheters

Catheters in veins, arteries or the urinary tract are associated with a high risk of infection: usually extending from the site of insertion in veins and arteries. Infection associated with venous or arterial catheters is most often due to Gram-positive cocci. The longer the catheter remains in situ, the greater the risk of infection.

Prostheses

In recent years the use of metal and plastic prostheses (i.e. foreign bodies) at sites deep within the patient has enormously increased: unfortunately these devices sometimes fail – often because of infection.

Orthopaedic prostheses (e.g. hip and knee joints): the bacteria responsible for the infection are usually skin commensal flora.

Artificial heart valves: often infected with *S. epidermidis*, a micro-organism not traditionally associated with natural valve endocarditis.

SOURCE OF INFECTION IN THE IMMUNOCOMPROMISED

Endogenous infection: caused by microorganisms that are part of the normal flora, e.g. septicaemia from colonic bacteria, thrush from candida in the mouth.

Exogenous infection: acquired from the environment, e.g. MRSAs, *C. difficile*, *P. aeruginosa*.

Note: An exogenous potential pathogen, often an antibiotic-resistant hospital strain, can colonise the patient and become part of the normal flora before causing infection.

Infections may be either newly acquired or the result of reactivation of asymptomatic latent infection, e.g. tuberculosis, toxoplasmosis, pneumocystis pneumonia, infections due to herpes viruses.

Transplanted tissue can be the source of a variety of infections, e.g. primary cytomegalovirus infection acquired by a sero-negative recipient from a sero-positive donor.

PREVENTION OF INFECTION

1. *Surveillance*:
   - Careful clinical examination to detect infection early: institute treatment without delay
   - Screening for colonization by potential pathogens: take repeated cultures from a variety of body sites – of debatable value.
2. *Antibiotics*: avoid indiscriminate use of 'prophylactic' broad-spectrum antibiotics: this promotes an abnormal flora of resistant bacteria. During periods of neutropenia prescribe ciprofloxacin (antibacterial), acyclovir (antiviral) and fluconazole (antifungal). Co-trimoxazole may be given in addition, to protect against pneumocystis pneumonia.
3. *Isolation*: indicated to protect the patient from infection if severely neutropenic: the measures can be either simple (reverse barrier nursing to protect the patient from infection in a single room) or elaborate (nursing in a laminar-airflow bed or room and the preparation of sterilized food).

43. Infection in hospital

Incidence: 20% of hospital patients suffer from infection: half of them are admitted with, and often because of, their infection, i.e. it is *community-acquired*; the other half develop their infection during their hospital stay, i.e. it is *hospital-acquired*.

COMMUNITY-ACQUIRED INFECTIONS

The commonest infections are of:

- lower respiratory tract (about one-third of the total)
- skin and soft tissues
- urinary tract.

Patients with these infections are most often found in paediatric, general medical and geriatric wards.

HOSPITAL-ACQUIRED INFECTIONS

Sometimes called *nosocomial* infections. Commonest are:

- urinary tract infection (about one-third of the total)
- wound infection
- lower respiratory tract infection
- skin and soft tissue infection
- gastrointestinal infection
- septicaemia (often associated with intravascular lines).

Patients are most likely to be in special intensive care units or in wards for genitourinary surgery, orthopaedics, general surgery, gynaecology or geriatrics.

Hospital infection is probably as great a problem today as it was in the pre-antibiotic era. Although antibiotics have reduced mortality, they have failed to alter the incidence of infection. Present-day

Table 43.1   Some treatments and associated infections

Treatment	Infection	Common cause
Surgery	Wound infection	*Staphylococcus aureus*
Urinary catheterization	Urinary tract infection	Coliforms
Intravenous infusion line	Septicaemia	*Staphylococcus epidermidis*
Antibiotic therapy	Antibiotic-associated colitis	*Clostridium difficile*

pathogens are often antibiotic-resistant, especially strains of coliforms, *Staphylococcus aureus* and enterococci. British hospitals are presently suffering from outbreaks of infection due to strains of *S. aureus* multi-resistant to many antibiotics including flucloxacillin (MRSA) and to enterococci resistant to vancomycin (VRE). The widespread use of antibiotics in hospitals creates an environment conducive to the survival of these organisms and their spread from patient to patient. Multi-resistant coliforms pose special problems in intensive care units; MRSA are encountered in both surgical and medical wards; VRE infect immunocompromised patients particularly.

Treatments often predispose to infection: surgery, use of invasive devices and drug therapy all carry risks (Table 43.1). When the use of catheters, intravenous lines, etc. is unavoidable, they should be removed as soon as possible.

Age: infection is commonest at extremes of age. Neonates and the elderly are more likely to spend a longer time as in-patients, and therefore run a greater risk of infection. Neonates and the elderly are also less able to resist infection, possibly because of less efficient immunity.

Susceptible patients: advances in medical care have resulted in new 'at risk' groups, e.g. the immunocompromised, patients in special care units or with prosthetic implants. Some infections in these patients are unusual, e.g. due to organisms normally regarded as virtually non-pathogenic, or with an atypical, and usually more severe, clinical presentation.

The majority of hospital-acquired infections are due to common organisms, e.g. urinary infections due to coliforms, wound infections due to *Staphylococcus aureus*, pneumonia due to *Streptococcus pneumoniae*. Septicaemia is the most serious infection and is associated with significant mortality: it is most often due to coliforms, *S. aureus* or *Staphylococcus epidermidis*. The commonest cause is now *S. epidermidis*, as a result of the increasing use of intravascular devices.

Sporadic (endemic) infections are daily occurrences in hospital: only of concern if they threaten the recovery of an individual patient.

Outbreaks of cross-infection are, however, not uncommon. Sometimes they have been traced to a common source, e.g. staphylococcal wound sepsis due to a surgeon operating with a boil on his wrist; postoperative endophthalmitis due to antibiotic eyedrops in which pseudomonads were growing. Whenever cross-infection is suspected, the Infection Control Team should be alerted so that appropriate investigations can be carried out without delay.

Classical contagious diseases (e.g. measles, chickenpox, infantile gastroenteritis) sometimes cause outbreaks in children's wards: these can be life-threatening if the ward contains leukaemic children. Influenza can be a problem in geriatric institutions, where outbreaks give rise to considerable mortality.

Community epidemics of respiratory syncytial virus infection occur every year, and cause bronchiolitis and pneumonia in infants. A sick child who requires in-patient treatment may be the source of a hospital outbreak.

Sources

Infection may be acquired either:
- *Endogenously*: with microorganisms from the patient's own normal flora, or
- *Exogenously*: with microorganisms from other people, or inanimate objects (fomites) in the environment.

Endogenous infection

Many hospital infections are *autogenous*: caused by bacteria from the patient's own normal flora. Although steps can be taken to reduce their incidence, they cannot be eliminated: they are not due to cross-infection. Examples are:

- *Chest infection*, following tracheal and nasogastric intubation associated with anaesthesia – which results in the aspiration of bacteria from the naso-pharynx and stomach into the lower respiratory tract. Most patients who develop pneumonia in hospital are surgical patients.
- *Urinary infection*, after catheterization – which inevitably transmits bacteria normally present in the distal urethra, into the bladder. Indwelling catheters create a permanent channel

between the outside of the catheter and the urethral mucosa, along which bacteria can ascend.

- *Wound infection*, after colonic surgery, caused by the extensive large bowel flora.

Exogenous infection

People are by far the most important source, e.g. members of the hospital staff (medical, nursing, ancillary) or other patients – either suffering from infection or asymptomatic carriers able to disperse infection.

Inanimate objects ('fomites') can also spread infection. These include:

- *Surgical instruments* (especially those which cannot be heat-sterilized, e.g. optical-fibre endoscopes)
- *Anaesthetic apparatus and ventilators*: formerly difficult to decontaminate between patients: risk of infection now much reduced by new equipment with disposable and autoclavable parts
- *Humidifiers*: should be either heat-sterilized or disposable: both types must be filled with sterile water and the circuits changed every 48 h
- *Parenteral fluids*, although sterile at source, are easily contaminated if drugs such as heparin are added.

The hospital environment contains other potential sources of exogenous infection, including floors, blankets, lockers, baths and wash-basins, commodes, bedpans, urinals and toilets, food and water, dust, air-conditioning systems. In a well-run hospital the risk should be low.

Note: Potentially pathogenic bacteria on inanimate objects may be spread without increase in numbers – but in the presence of moisture, certain organisms (e.g. pseudomonads) multiply and so enhance the risk of infection. Fomites which remain moist pose a greater risk than those which can be kept dry.

Operating theatres

Organisms which cause wound infections gain entry during surgery either *endogenously* or *exogenously* – often from skin scales shed by staff. Avoid overcrowding, which increases the number of bacteria in the environment, and unnecessary door-opening, which interferes with effective ventilation.

Spread

The routes of infection are via contact, the air, or ingestion.

Contact

Probably the most important, it may be via:

- the hands or clothing of staff transmitting microorganisms, either from their own bodies or from other patients, i.e. acting as a vehicle for patient-to-patient spread
- inanimate objects (see above).

Airborne

This may be via:

- droplets of respiratory infection, spread by inhalation from person to person
- dust from floors and bedding; exudate dispersed from a wound during dressing; scales shed from skin to a susceptible site, usually a surgical wound – particularly important with *S. aureus*
- aerosols created by nebulizers, humidifiers, suction machines, air-conditioning systems – notably incriminated in the spread of Gram-negative bacilli (e.g. coliforms, legionella) to the respiratory tract. Patients with endotracheal tubes receiving artificial ventilation are especially at risk.

Ingestion

Outbreaks of food poisoning (e.g. due to salmonella, *Clostridium perfringens*) are not uncommon in hospitals, especially if it is difficult to maintain a high standard of hygiene, e.g. in over-crowded, long-stay psychiatric or geriatric wards. Institutional food often contains large numbers of coliforms and, although their ingestion does not cause gastroenteritis, they can become established in the faecal flora of patients. Reservoirs of antibiotic-resistant bacteria, e.g. klebsiella, pseudomonads, are thus created within the ward environment.

A particular and increasing problem in general hospitals, involving faecal–oral spread, is antibiotic-associated colitis due to *Clostridium difficile* (see p. 217).

Prevention

Prevention of hospital-acquired infections can be achieved by education, sterilization and disinfection, isolation, antibiotics, staff health, surveillance and organizational strategy. These are described below.

Education

Medical, nursing and ancillary staff must be educated in the basic concepts of infection control. *All* staff (and *medical staff must not default*) must follow good practice to minimize the risk to patients. For example:

- *Frequent hand washing*: this is the *single most important measure* for preventing cross-infection. Staff must be taught how to wash hands effectively.
- *Hygiene* in theatres, wards and kitchens: including special attention to the safe disposal of excreta, soiled dressings, etc.
- *Good nursing* in an open ward can limit the dissemination of exogenous infection by the contact and faecal–oral routes, but cannot contain airborne spread; can also reduce some endogenous infections, e.g. chest infection in postoperative and unconscious patients.
- *Safe patient environment*: adequately spaced beds; sufficient wash-basins, toilets etc; enclosed linen storage shelves.
- *Techniques* of theatre asepsis, wound dressing, bladder catheterization, care of intravenous lines, etc.
- *Good surgical technique* minimizes tissue destruction and haematoma formation: reduces soiling, especially during operations on the colon.

Sterilization and disinfection

There should be policies to ensure:

- *Provision of sterile instruments*, dressings, surgical drapes, etc.
- *Proper use of disinfectants* in the environment and antiseptics on the skin of patients and on the hands of staff.
- *Use of disposable items* such as syringes, catheters, tubing, etc.

Isolation

Single-bedded rooms (cubicles) are necessary to avoid infection by the airborne route; in addition, strict precautions (e.g. gowns, masks, gloves) for anyone coming into contact with the patient, i.e. barrier nursing.

Source isolation: aims to prevent the spread of infection from an infected patient. A 'risk assessment' is made and the appropriate isolation category imposed: precautions to be taken are set out in a series of nursing care plans, each matched to the isolation category (Table 43.2).

Protective isolation aims to prevent a susceptible (i.e. immuno-compromised) patient being exposed to infection: requires 'reverse' barrier nursing, ideally in a cubicle ventilated with sterile (i.e. filtered) air, delivered under positive pressure. Staff should wear plastic aprons to prevent dissemination of bacteria from clothing, wash hands before touching patient, and never tend patient if suffering from any infection.

Table 43.2   Two examples of source isolation

Infection	Mode of spread	Risk assessment considerations	Appropriate nursing care plan
1. Salmonella	Faecal–oral	Amount of diarrhoea	Private toilet facilities
		Personal hygiene	Educate patient to wash and dry hands effectively
		Ward facilities	Patient not to enter ward kitchen
			Check for possible outbreak
			Gloves and aprons for staff in direct contact
			Disinfection of spillages with a phenolic disinfectant
2. Methicillin-resistant *Staphylococcus aureus*	Direct or indirect contact (skin scales)	Amount of wound exudate	Cubicle with extract (negative pressure) ventilation
		Virulence of strain	Plastic aprons for staff in direct contact
		Vulnerability of other patients	Wash patient with chlorhexidine gluconate
			Swab nose, groin, axilla, to assess colonization

Antibiotics

A rational policy for the use of antibiotics must be followed: prophylaxis with carefully chosen drugs can reduce postoperative infections significantly (see p. 398). Prohibit topical application – which encourages the emergence of drug resistance – of antibiotics that can be life-saving when given systemically.

Staff health

Staff suffering from infection, e.g. viral respiratory infections, septic lesions, should be excluded from contact with patients. Staff should be protected by appropriate immunization, e.g. BCG vaccine, hepatitis B vaccine.

Surveillance

Surveillance of infection within a hospital is of prime importance. Vigilance by all members of staff is essential, and information from wards, theatres and laboratories should be collated daily by an Infection Control Team, whose key members are the Infection Control Nursing Officer (a specially trained nurse) and the Infection Control Officer (usually a microbiologist). Records should be kept with the aid of a computer to:

- follow the spread of potentially dangerous bacteria within the hospital: these 'alert organisms' include MRSA, *Streptococcus pyogenes*, *Clostridium difficile*, etc.
- Monitor infection rates in certain selected units (accurate assessment of infection rates in every ward of a hospital is an impossible task).

A source of trouble is often an infected patient transferred from another ward or hospital. The Infection Control Team should be contacted if two or more patients develop symptoms of infection, e.g. diarrhoea, for which there is no obvious cause.

Organization

Management and medical advisory committees must be made aware of the importance of infection in hospital, and its prevention. Policy making to prevent hospital infection should be the responsibility of a group, the Control of Infection Committee, composed of the

Infection Control Team, together with clinicians, community medicine specialist, pharmacist, administrator, etc.

Policies should ensure good accommodation (including kitchens, toilet facilities), avoidance of overcrowding, adequate provision of nurses, and so on.

Audit, with feedback, is essential so that problems can be identified and appropriate action taken without-delay.

44. Infection in general practice

Infections form a large part of the general practitioner's workload: they may be bacterial, viral or fungal.

Antibiotics have radically changed the management of bacterial illness, not least because their use means that fewer patients require hospital admission. However, problems with antibiotic therapy can arise from:

- choice of an inappropriate antibiotic
- poor clinical response – especially in severe infection
- lack of compliance
- inadequate absorption, e.g. due to vomiting
- hypersensitivity or allergy to the chosen drug (not uncommon with penicillin).

Best guess. Most antibiotic therapy in general practice is prescribed on this basis. Laboratory data on the organism and its antibiotic sensitivity are rarely available early in infection, and it is necessary to start treatment without delay.

EPIDEMIOLOGY OF INFECTIONS IN PRIMARY CARE

In the UK, the average general practitioner looks after approximately 2000 patients. Each year about 70% of patients consult their doctor – although not all the consultations are because of infection.

Frequency of consultations due to infection: the lists below show some common and less common infections – bacterial, viral and fungal – that are encountered in general practice. Note that sexually-transmitted diseases are increasing in importance.

Infections seen by the average general practitioner more than once per week

Note: The order of listing does not necessarily reflect the frequency with which each infection is encountered: this will vary with season, type of practice, etc.

- Upper respiratory infection
- Acute bronchitis; other lower respiratory tract infections
- Sore throat; tonsillitis
- Urinary tract infections
- Vaginal discharge
- Gastrointestinal infections
- Otitis media; otitis externa
- Warts
- Conjunctivitis
- Skin infections (e.g. impetigo).

Infections seen by the average general practitioner more than once per 3 months

Note: The frequency of virus infections in this list:

- Varicella and zoster
- Herpes simplex
- Other childhood fevers
- Infectious mononucleosis
- Sexually transmitted diseases.

COMMON INFECTIONS

Upper respiratory infection

Most often due to viruses: management depends on recognizing bacterial infections, such as acute sinusitis (which may also complicate a previous viral infection) or streptococcal sore throat, which require antibiotic therapy. Treatment of viral infection is supportive – although observe for onset of respiratory distress in infants, due to extension of upper respiratory infection with respiratory syncytial virus to lower tract, causing bronchiolitis or bronchopneumonia – this requires hospital admission and ribavirin therapy.

Acute bronchitis and lower respiratory infection

Sometimes related to complications of asthma (sometimes themselves infective), or a primary bacterial infection such as pneumonia. Bacterial pneumonia still carries a significant case fatality rate, although the causal organisms are usually sensitive to a variety of antibiotics. Bacterial pneumonia can complicate influenza, and contributes largely to influenza-related deaths.

Chronic bronchitis

Also known as chronic obstructive airways disease. Acute exacerbations common during winter, and most often associated with *Haemophilus influenzae*.

Treatment: tetracycline, amoxycillin: may require prolonged or maintenance antibiotic therapy.

Acute tonsillitis/sore throat

May be due to *Streptococcus pyogenes*, but only 30–40% of these are bacterial: most are viral in origin. A bacterial cause can be suspected clinically if there are tender tonsillar lymph nodes or pus visible on the tonsils.

Treatment: oral penicillin or amoxycillin.

Urinary tract infection

A common problem, which requires careful clinical assessment, with laboratory investigation of a urine sample.

Treatment: on a 'best-guess' basis, e.g. trimethoprin.

Further investigation is required in the following patients:

- Children under 15 years of age: males with one proven infection and females with at least two proven infections
- Adult males, 15 to 64 years of age
- Adult females of the same age range, with infections which are either frequent or slow to clear
- Elderly males with blood in the urine
- Elderly females who have had few if any urinary infections in earlier life.

Vaginal discharge

This is a very common symptom, and has several causes:

Candida: not usually sexually transmitted: a common infection which can be diagnosed clinically. Female patients quickly learn to recognize recurrences – a frequent complication. Exclude diabetes as an underlying precipitating factor.

Treatment: a single oral dose of fluconazole, local nystatin or clotrimazole.

Trichomonas vaginalis: also common: causes vaginal discharge, usually profuse and offensive. Laboratory confirmation is desirable.

Treatment: oral metronidazole for 7 days; if possible, treat the patient's partner also.

Gardnerella: cause of bacterial vaginosis and a frequent commensal, so isolation is not diagnostic: laboratory confirmation is best based on detection of 'clue cells' (see Ch. 39) or the amine test. The discharge in bacterial vaginosis is often profuse and offensive compared to that due to vaginal candidiasis.

Treatment: oral metronidazole for 7 days.

Chlamydia: infection with *C. trachomatis* is the commonest cause of nonspecific urethritis in males. In females, genital infection is often asymptomatic but the organism is important as a cause of pelvic inflammatory disease and salpingitis. Investigate with urethral swabs (males) and endocervical swabs (females), submitted to laboratory in specimen transport medium.

Treatment: tetracycline or erythromycin.

Virus genital infections: genital warts and genital herpes are notoriously difficult to eradicate, and genital warts often very difficult to treat. In most cases, refer to a specialist.

Gastrointestinal infection

Common at all ages, but in small children there is a risk of developing severe dehydration. Causal organisms are often unidentified and even when specimens are taken, often only around 20% yield positive cultures.

Treatment: maintain fluid balance with rehydration sachets.

If symptoms persist, consider antibiotic treatment – s*almonella:* ciprofloxacin; *campylobacter:* erythromycin or ciprofloxacin if there are persistent or generalized symptoms. Campylobacter infection may be accompanied by marked abdominal pain: relieve with codeine phosphate, to reduce gut motility.

Otitis media

Very common: the graph of its incidence follows that of acute respiratory infection in childhood, indicating it is often a complication of previous viral respiratory infection. Remember that catarrhal congestion of the middle ear may also complicate upper respiratory infection, and can mimic bacterial middle ear infection.

Treatment: antibiotics (e.g. amoxycillin – because *H. influenzae* is often responsible).

Otitis externa

Usually a complication of eczema; often involves fungal infection.

Warts

Due to human papilloma viruses: often disappear spontaneously, but this may take time.

Conjunctivitis

Usually seen in young children. In infants in first few days of life, take specimens to exclude gonorrhoea. *Note*: allergic conjunctivitis can be mistaken for conjunctivitis due to infection.

Skin infections

May be bacterial or fungal. Bacterial infection, e.g. impetigo, is usually purulent. Fungal infection is difficult to confirm because specimens are not easy to take.

Treatment: Bacterial: if possible, on the basis of a positive laboratory report: if not, 'best-guess' is oral flucloxacillin. Fungal: topical clotrimazole.

RARE INFECTIONS

Some infections, not seen very often, are nevertheless important in general practice. These are:

- tuberculosis
- erysipelas and erythema nodosum
- viral hepatitis
- meningitis and encephalitis
- malaria.

Tuberculosis

Largely controlled in the UK, tuberculosis has recently shown a slight but worrying upward trend. The disease remains endemic in developing countries in Africa and Asia, and *immigrants* to the UK are a high-risk group. *Immunosuppressed patients*, especially those suffering from HIV infection, are at particular risk. In the USA, tuberculosis is a major problem in AIDS patients, in whom the disease is often rapidly fatal. These patients show a high incidence of multi-resistant bacilli, making treatment difficult.

General practitioners need to maintain constant vigilance, and be aware of the possibility of tuberculosis in patients with nonspecific symptoms of vague ill health.

Erysipelas and erythema nodosum

Seen approximately once every 2 years in general practice.

Erysipelas: presents as an acutely inflamed area of skin, commonly on the face, accompanied by fever and signs of generalized infection.

Treatment: penicillin.

Erythema nodosum: not a true infection: an immunological reaction often due to sarcoidosis, presenting with painful, raised inflammatory lesions in the skin. Investigate with chest radiograph (to detect enlarged hilar lymph nodes) and biochemically (for raised blood calcium levels). There is no specific treatment, but steroids may be used if the lesions are particularly extensive or persistent.

Viral hepatitis

Seen by most general practitioners at least once a year: most often due to hepatitis A. Confirm serologically, to establish the diagnosis and to identify the less common hepatitis B (with its implication of risk of infecting others).

Meningitis and encephalitis

Uncommon: most practitioners see a case only once in every 4 or 5 years. Diagnosis early in the disease can be very difficult, but is also vital because of the need for immediate treatment – especially in meningococcal meningitis.

Watch for adults and older children who complain of headache or neck pain, photophobia or vomiting:

Classic sign is a stiff neck (see Ch. 33) but is often a relatively late manifestation.

Refer to hospital *urgently* if meningitis or encephalitis suspected on clinical grounds, and give penicillin intramuscularly straight away.

Treatment: intramuscular penicillin. In infants, meningitis may be due to *H. influenzae*: treat with chloramphenicol, ampicillin or cefotaxime.

Malaria

Seen in general practice from time to time in patients who have travelled to endemic areas. Travellers to infected areas are often not aware of the risk and do not take, or fail to take regularly, prophylactic drugs. The disease is easily misdiagnosed as 'flu. Malaria can be fatal unless appropriately and promptly treated.

LABORATORY INVESTIGATION OF INFECTION

Clearly, it is less easy to obtain laboratory tests in general practice than in hospital practice. Nevertheless, diagnostic laboratories are increasing their commitment to general practitioners and most offer specimen transport arrangements, with rapid transmission of results by telephone or by fax. Laboratory specialists are also available for advice or consultation.

PREVENTION

Preventive immunization is available for many infections, and forms a most important element of primary care. Immunization schedules are listed and discussed in detail in Chapter 46.

Treatment and prevention of bacterial disease

45. Antimicrobial therapy

Bacterial infections are among the few diseases in medicine for which specific therapy is available. Despite this, infections are still common and treatment may fail.

ANTIBIOTICS

More than a century ago, Pasteur observed that the growth of one microorganism could be inhibited by the products of another. However, most of these early products or 'antibiotics' were toxic to mammalian as well as to bacterial cells, and were therefore of no therapeutic use. Penicillin, discovered in 1929 but not available for clinical trials until 1940, is the product of a mould, *Penicillium notatum*, and was the first antibiotic drug: it is still the best. Other antibiotics are the products of soil streptomycetes and bacteria of the genus *Bacillus*. Many recently introduced antibiotics, e.g. the semi-synthetic penicillins and cephalosporins, have been prepared by the chemical manipulation of existing drugs.

Selective toxicity is the ability to kill or inhibit the growth of a microorganism without harming the cells of the host: an essential requirement for any successful antibiotic.

Chemotherapeutic agents, e.g. sulphonamides, trimethoprim and many of the antituberculous drugs, are synthetic drugs with this selective toxicity.

Antimicrobial therapy aims to treat infection with a drug to which the causal microorganism is sensitive. This can be achieved if a sound knowledge of microbiology indicates the most likely pathogen in a given patient and its usual antibiotic sensitivity, i.e. on a *'best-guess'* basis: it is better still if the infection is investigated bacteriologically by culture and in vitro sensitivity testing.

Antimicrobial drugs are often classified as *bactericidal* – when they kill the infecting bacteria – or *bacteriostatic* – when they prevent

Table 45.1   Antibiotics and other antimicrobial agents

Drug	Principal use
Penicillins	Wide variety of infections
Cephalosporins	Mainly second-line drugs
Co-trimoxazole	Urinary and chest infections
Trimethoprim	Urinary infections
Aminoglycosides	Severe infections with coliforms
Tetracyclines	Chest infections
Metronidazole	Anaerobic infections
Macrolides	Second-line drugs to the penicillins
Glycopeptides	Staphylococcal infections resistant to other drugs
Quinolones	Urinary and gastrointestinal infections; infections with *Pseudomonas aeruginosa*
Chloramphenicol	Typhoid fever, meningitis
Fusidic acid	Staphylococcal infection
Nalidixic acid	Urinary infection
Nitrofurantoin	Urinary infection
Isoniazid	Tuberculosis
Rifampicin	Tuberculosis
Pyrazinamide	Tuberculosis
Ethambutol	Tuberculosis

multiplication but do not kill the bacteria. This classification is not always clear-cut, and may depend on the local concentration of the drug. In all but a few conditions, notably infective endocarditis, appropriate bacteriostatic drugs give excellent therapeutic results.

This chapter deals with the main antibiotics and antimicrobial agents in current use, from the point of view of a clinical bacteriologist. Pharmacokinetics are not considered.

The principal drugs are listed in Table 45.1. Subsequent tables summarize information about particular antibiotics, including their clinical use: inevitably they are oversimplified, and should be used only as a guide to antibiotic therapy.

PENICILLINS (PENAMS)

Chemical structure:

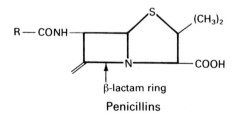

Penicillins

Mode of action: bactericidal: inhibit cell wall synthesis by combining with the transpeptidase responsible for cross-linking of the peptidoglycan; activity depends on an intact β-lactam ring.

Resistance: common: due to production by bacteria of an enzyme, *β-lactamase*, which inactivates penicillin by acting on the *β-lactam* ring: often, bacterial β-lactamases are plasmid-coded.

Antibacterial spectrum: varies with individual penicillins: activity determined by the side-chain of the penicillin nucleus. The principal penicillins and their antibacterial spectra are shown in Table 45.2.

Toxicity: virtually non-toxic: very large doses can be given if required. Hypersensitivity can occur in the form of rashes (especially with ampicillin) and, rarely, anaphylaxis (with any penicillin given by injection).

Co-amoxiclav

Contains: amoxycillin and potassium clavulanate.

Administration: oral; also intravenous.

Mode of action: clavulanic acid, a β-lactam compound without useful antibacterial activity, is an irreversible inhibitor of most plasmid-mediated and some chromosomal β-lactamases. Combined with a β-lactamase-susceptible penicillin (e.g. amoxycillin), it enables the penicillin to resist degradation by β-lactamases.

Antibacterial spectrum: broad: active against β-lactamase-producing coliforms, staphylococci and 'bacteroides'.

Clinical use: relatively expensive: reserve for infections of urinary and respiratory tracts, skin and soft tissues due to amoxycillin-resistant, co-amoxiclav-sensitive bacteria.

Ticarcillin with clavulanic acid

Combination of ticarcillin and potassium clavulanate analogous to co-amoxiclav.

Administration: intravenous.

Clinical use: alternative to carbenicillin or acylureidopenicillins.

PENEMS AND CARBAPENEMS

Semisynthetic β-lactam compounds: a double bond has been introduced into the penam structure.

Table 45.2 The penicillins

Penicillin	Administration	Antibacterial spectrum	Clinical use
Penicillins			
Benzylpenicillin (Penicillin G)	i.m., i.v.	Gram-positive bacteria; *Neisseria species*	Streptococcal, pneumococcal, clostridial infection; sensitive Staphylococcal infection; meningitis, gonorrhoea, syphilis, anthrax, actinomycosis
Phenoxymethyl penicillin (Penicillin V)	Oral		
Aminopenicillins			
Ampicillin Amoxycillin	Oral, i.m., i.v.	Similar to penicillin but in addition enterococci, almost all *Haemophilus influenzae* and many coliforms	Urinary and respiratory infections, enteric fever; in combination with other drugs in severe systemic infections
Isoxazolyl penicillins			
Cloxacillin Flucloxacillin	Oral, i.m., i.v.	Similar to penicillin, but less active drugs. Stable to staphylococcal β-lactamase	Staphylococcal infections
Carboxypenicillins			
Carbenicillin Ticarcillin	i.m., i.v.	Similar to aminopenicillins but in addition *Pseudomonas aeruginosa* and most *Proteus* species. Some activity against 'bacteroides'	Urinary, respiratory, burns and other infections due to sensitive bacteria, especially *Pseudomonas aeruginosa*; severe sepsis, usually in combination with other drugs
Acylureidopenicillins			
Mezlocillin	i.m., i.v.	Similar to carboxypenicillins but in addition, *Klebsiella species* and greater activity against pseudomonads	As for carboxypenicillins
Azlocillin	i.v.		
Piperacillin	i.m., i.v.		
Amidinopenicillins			
Mecillinam	Oral, i.m., i.v.	Coliforms; low activity against Gram-positive bacteria	Urinary infections; salmonellosis, including enteric fever

i.m.: intramuscular; i.v.: intravenous.
Note: In this book, reference to penicillin is taken to mean Penicillin G or Penicillin V.

Chemical structure:

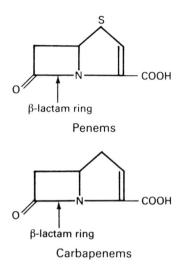

β-lactam ring

Penems

β-lactam ring

Carbapenems

Imipenem with cilastatin

Imipenem is the first carbapenem available for clinical use. Rapidly metabolized in the kidney by a dipeptidase: therefore administered with an enzyme inhibitor, cilastatin, which increases urinary and serum concentrations of the antibiotic and also reduces the potential for nephrotoxicity observed in experimental animals.

Administration: intravenous.

Mode of action: bactericidal: potent inhibitor of bacterial cell wall synthesis. Extremely stable to degradation by β-lactamases: imipenem, like clavulanic acid, is itself a β-lactamase inhibitor.

Resistance: uncommon; resistance may develop in *Pseudomonas aeruginosa* during treatment.

Antibacterial spectrum: extremely broad; active against Gram-positive and Gram-negative aerobes and anaerobes.

Clinical use: initial empirical therapy of serious undiagnosed infection, especially if a polymicrobial cause is likely.

Toxicity: similar to other β-lactam antibiotics.

CEPHALOSPORINS

Chemically similar to the penicillins: antibacterial activity can be altered by variation in the side-chains of the cephalosporin nucleus. Cephalosporins are arbitrarily assigned to three generations: 'first generation' drugs were introduced in the 1960s. Progressive development has culminated in the availability of a large number of new 'third generation' cephalosporins.

Table 45.3 lists the main cephalosporins and some of their properties: it is not exhaustive and some drugs not available in the UK. Numerous other compounds are under development.

Administration: mostly parenteral, but a few oral drugs have been developed, e.g. oral cefuroxime.

Table 45.3 The cephalosporins

Cephalosporin	Administration	Antibacterial spectrum	Clinical use
First generation			
Cephaloridine	i.m., i.v.	Wide range of Gram-positive and Gram-negative bacteria: enterococci *Pseudomonas aeruginosa*, *Haemophilus influenzae* and 'bacteroides' are resistant; *Staphylococcus aureus* is sensitive, unless methicillin-resistant	Second-line drugs: formerly used in severe sepsis; oral drugs may be of value in 'difficult' urinary infections
Cephalothin	i.m., i.v.		
Cephalexin	Oral		
Cephradine	Oral, i.m., i.v.		
Cephazolin	i.m., i.v.		
Second generation			
Cefuroxime	i.m., i.v., oral	Wide: with marked stability to β-lactamases of Gram-negative as well as Gram-positive bacteria; active against *Haemophilus influenzae* and (especially cefoxitin) 'bacteroides'; inferior antistaphylococcal activity	Have largely replaced the first generation drugs in severe systemic infections; widely used in prophylaxis
Cefamandole	i.m., i.v.		
Cefoxitin	i.m., i.v.		
Third generation			
Cefotaxime	i.m., i.v.	Similar to second generation drugs, but in addition activity against *Pseudomonas aeruginosa* (especially ceftazidime)	Similar to second generation drugs, particularly in serious sepsis due to susceptible aerobic Gram-negative bacilli
Ceftazidime	i.m., i.v.		
Cefsulodin	i.m., i.v.	*Pseudomonas aeruginosa* only	

i.m.: intramuscular; i.v.: intravenous.

Chemical structure:

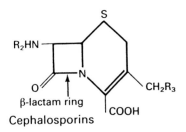

β-lactam ring
Cephalosporins

Mode of action: bactericidal: similar to penicillin. Stable to many bacterial β-lactamases, and this stability has been increased with the later generations: the inferior antistaphylococcal activity of the newer drugs is due to their less avid binding to the target site.

Clinical use: most cephalosporins are given parenterally, so are restricted to hospital patients: most useful in seriously ill patients infected with more than one susceptible organism. Valuable second-line drugs. Increasingly used as an alternative to an aminoglycoside, especially in patients with renal impairment. A major use is in short-term peri-operative prophylaxis.

Toxicity: low: rashes, fever, sometimes pain at site of injection. *Nephrotoxicity*: apparently limited to older drugs, especially cephaloridine. *Hypersensitivity*: about 10% of people hypersensitive to penicillin are also hypersensitive to cephalosporins.

MONOBACTAMS

Monocyclic β-lactam antibiotics, derived from 3-aminomonobactamic acid.

Chemical structure:

β-lactam ring
Monobactams

Aztreonam

First monobactam available for clinical use.

Administration: intramuscular, intravenous.

Mode of action: bactericidal: inhibits cell wall synthesis; β-lactamase-stable.

Resistance: uncommon.

Antibacterial spectrum: narrow: active against aerobic Gram-negative bacteria but *Pseudomonas aeruginosa* less sensitive; Gram-positive bacteria and anaerobes resistant.

Clinical use: infections with aerobic Gram-negative bacteria, e.g. urinary tract infections, septicaemia, gonorrhoea; mixed bacterial infections if given with another antibiotic.

Toxicity: as for other β-lactam antibiotics, but less likely to induce hypersensitivity: may be given *with caution* to patients known to be allergic to penicillins, cephalosporins or both.

SULPHONAMIDES AND TRIMETHOPRIM

Both drugs act sequentially in the synthesis of tetrahydrofolate: widely used in combination because of in vitro evidence of synergism. Trimethoprim and sulphonamides are also available separately.

Co-trimoxazole

Contains: sulphamethoxazole and trimethoprim in 5:1 ratio.

Administration: oral, intramuscular, intravenous.

Mode of action: bacteriostatic: sulphonamide and trimethoprim block sequential steps in DNA synthesis.

Resistance: not uncommon: mainly due to production of resistant enzymes; gene for trimethoprim resistance often present on a transposon.

Antibacterial spectrum: broad: active against both Gram-positive and Gram-negative bacteria; *Pseudomonas aeruginosa* is resistant.

Clinical use: widely used for urinary and respiratory tract infections: invasive salmonellosis, pneumocystis pneumonia.

Toxicity: nausea and vomiting; rashes; occasionally, thrombocytopenia, leucopenia; mouth ulceration; folate deficiency has been reported.

Sulphonamides

Rarely used on their own; occasionally, in combination with penicillin in meningitis because of their excellent penetration into the CSF.

The most widely used preparation is sulphadimidine.

Trimethoprim

Mainly used for urinary tract infections, but also respiratory infections: main advantage is reduced incidence of side-effects compared with co-trimoxazole.

AMINOGLYCOSIDES

Family of extremely useful antibiotics. Main aminoglycoside antibiotics are listed in Table 45.4.

Administration: intramuscular; intravenous for systemic infections.

Mode of action: bactericidal: inhibition of protein synthesis due to action on bacterial ribosomes; all aminoglycosides misread messenger RNA to produce amino acid substitution in proteins.

Resistance: due to acquisition of plasmid-coded inactivating enzymes, which cause acetylation, adenylation or phosphorylation of the drugs: amikacin is least affected. Resistance is also due to decreased transport of aminoglycoside into the bacterial cell and, in the case of streptomycin, may be the result of a mutation which renders the ribosome insusceptible.

Table 45.4   The aminoglycosides

Aminoglycoside	Main clinical use
Gentamicin Tobramycin Netilmicin Amikacin	Severe infections in hospital due to coliforms; gentamicin most widely used: in certain infections, given in combination with a β-lactam antibiotic
Streptomycin	Little used: most active aminoglycoside against mycobacteria
Kanamycin Neomycin	Given orally in 'gut sterilization' regimens prior to surgery; in leukaemia; in chronic liver disease; neomycin also as topical cream

Antibacterial spectrum: coliforms, *Pseudomonas aeruginosa*, staphylococci; streptococci and strict anaerobes intrinsically resistant.

Toxicity: ototoxicity (vertigo or deafness) and nephrotoxicity are major problems, because toxic levels are close to therapeutic levels necessary for treatment. Netilmicin *may* be safer than other aminoglycosides. In patients with renal impairment or on long-term therapy, serum levels must be monitored: ensure trough level not excessive (2 mg/L for gentamicin) and peak level therapeutic (5–10 mg/L for gentamicin).

TETRACYCLINES

Few specific indications for use, but have broad spectrum and are remarkably free of serious side-effects – particularly successful in the management of chronic bronchitis. The following are available:

Tetracycline
Chlortetracycline
Oxytetracycline
Doxycycline ⎱ more effective: can be given in
Minocycline ⎰ smaller dosage

Administration: almost always oral.

Mode of action: bacteriostatic: inhibit protein synthesis by preventing the attachment of amino acids to ribosomes.

Resistance: fairly common: generally plasmid-mediated.

Antibacterial spectrum: broad: both Gram-positive and Gram-negative bacteria: some strains of *Streptococcus pyogenes*, pneumococci and *Haemophilus influenzae* are now resistant; *Pseudomonas aeruginosa* and *Proteus species* are intrinsically resistant. Active against brucellae, *Mycoplasma pneumoniae*, rickettsiae, *Coxiella burneti* (the cause of Q fever), chlamydiae.

Main clinical use: acute exacerbations of chronic bronchitis, and long-term prophylaxis; treatment of nonspecific urethritis, brucellosis, atypical pneumonia, Q fever, psittacosis.

Toxicity: diarrhoea, due to disturbance of alimentary flora – common, but mild and self-limiting. Avoid in renal and hepatic failure; contraindicated in pregnancy, and in children because the drug may be deposited in the developing teeth, with permanent yellow staining, and also interfere with bone development.

METRONIDAZOLE

Exceedingly effective against anaerobic bacteria.

Administration: oral, rectal (suppositories), intravenous.

Mode of action: bactericidal: converted by anaerobic bacteria to active (reduced) metabolite with inhibitory action on DNA synthesis.

Resistance: almost unknown.

Antibacterial spectrum: strictly anaerobic bacteria, e.g. 'bacteroides', anaerobic cocci, clostridia. No effect on aerobic organisms; actinomyces are resistant. Active against anaerobic protozoa (e.g. *Trichomonas vaginalis*, *Entamoeba histolytica*, *Giardia lamblia*).

Clinical use: any anaerobic infection, e.g. abdominal and gynaecological wound sepsis, deep abscesses, peritoneal sepsis, Vincent's angina; peri-operative prophylaxis in abdominal and gynaecological surgery.

Toxicity: low; side-effects: nausea, metallic taste in mouth.

LINCOMYCINS

Clindamycin (7-chloro-7-deoxylincomycin) is active against Gram-positive bacteria and some anaerobes: penetrates tissue well and acts on *Staphylococcus aureus* and 'bacteroides'. Excellent agent for staphylococcal bone and joint infections, but because of a warning notice from the Committee on Safety of Medicines that it is associated with pseudomembranous colitis, it is now rarely used in the UK.

MACROLIDES

Erythromycin

Most widely used member of the macrolide group of antibiotics.

Administration: oral, intravenous.

Mode of action: bacteriostatic by inhibition of protein synthesis; may be bactericidal at higher concentrations.

Resistance: occurs in *Staphylococcus aureus*, pneumococci and *Streptococcus pyogenes*.

Antibacterial spectrum: penicillin-like, but includes in addition *Haemophilus influenzae*, *Bordetella pertussis*, 'bacteroides' *Campylobacter species*, *Legionella pneumophila*, *Mycoplasma pneumoniae* and chlamydiae.

Clinical use: staphylococcal infections; variety of respiratory infections (tonsillitis, sinusitis, bronchitis and pneumonia, diphtheria, whooping cough, atypical pneumonia, psittacosis, Legionnaires' disease); non-specific urethritis; campylobacter enteritis. Useful second-line drug in patients hypersensitive to penicillin.

Toxicity: safe antibiotic except for erythromycin estolate, which may be hepatotoxic.

Azithromycin and clarithromycin

New drugs with similar spectra to that of erythromycin. Have enhanced activity and achieve higher tissue concentrations.

GLYCOPEPTIDES

Vancomycin

Available for over 30 years but little used: nowadays, indications for its use are common.

Administration: intravenous, oral.

Mode of action: bactericidal: by inhibition of cell wall synthesis: mechanism different from that of β-lactams.

Resistance: occurs in coagulase-negative staphylococci (but not *S. aureus*) and enterococci.

Antibacterial spectrum: staphylococci (including strains resistant to methicillin and other drugs), streptococci (but less active against enterococci), clostridia.

Clinical use: *intravenous*: serious infections, e.g. endocarditis, septicaemia due to streptococci, coagulase-positive and coagulase-negative staphylococci, especially if multi-resistant or if the patient is hypersensitive to penicillins; *oral*: antibiotic-associated colitis; *intraperitoneal*: CAPD peritonitis.

Toxicity: phlebitis, ototoxicity, nephrotoxicity if given intravenously: monitor serum levels to control dosage.

Teicoplanin

Chemically related to vancomycin, with similar activity and toxicity. Once-daily dosage.

Note: Glycopeptides have no advantage over the penicillins in treating penicillin-sensitive infections.

CIPROFLOXACIN

First of the fluoroquinolones – antibacterial agents developed from nalidixic acid – available in the UK.

Administration: oral, also intravenous.

Mode of action: inhibits DNA-gyrase activity by binding to chromosomal DNA strands. Interferes with DNA replication and prevents supercoiling within the chromosome.

Resistance: uncommon: result of chromosomal mutation: most likely to develop during prolonged treatment of chronic infections. Plasmid-mediated resistance not reported.

Antibacterial spectrum: broad: active against aerobic Gram-negative bacteria, including *Pseudomonas aeruginosa* and staphylococci (including MRSA), but streptococci less sensitive. Anaerobes are resistant.

Clinical use: respiratory infections due to *Pseudomonas aeruginosa*, e.g. cystic fibrosis, Legionnaires' disease (combined with erythromycin or rifampicin); chronic urinary infections, often catheter-associated; gonorrhoea; prostatitis; wide range of gastrointestinal infections, including enteric fever; useful in travellers' diarrhoea; skin and soft tissue infections due to *P. aeruginosa*.

Toxicity: severe systemic adverse reactions rare: most important is CNS stimulation to produce anxiety, nervousness, insomnia, even convulsions. Avoid administration to children, because of potential to damage juvenile cartilage. Decreases metabolism of theophylline, caffeine and warfarin – so toxic effects of these drugs encountered if administered with ciprofloxacin.

OTHER ANTIBIOTICS AND ANTIMICROBIAL DRUGS

Some other less commonly used antibiotics and antimicrobial drugs are listed in Table 45.5.

ANTITUBERCULOUS CHEMOTHERAPY

Tuberculosis was successfully treated with a combination of streptomycin, para-aminosalicylic acid (PAS) and isoniazid for 30 years. Problems with streptomycin toxicity and the unpalatability of PAS have resulted in this regimen being replaced. A *combination of antimicrobial drugs* is essential in tuberculosis, to prevent emergence of resistant bacteria.

Antituberculous drugs in current use

Isoniazid

Isonicotinyl hydrazide.

Administration: oral; parenteral preparations available for intramuscular, intravenous, intrapleural and intrathecal use.

Table 45.5 Some other antimicrobial drugs

Drug	Admini-stration	Mode of action	Antibacterial spectrum	Clinical use	Other features
Fusidic acid	Oral, i.v.	Bacteriostatic	*Staphylococcus aureus*	Abscesses, osteo-myelitis, septicaemia	Good tissue penetration; resistance may emerge rapidly – give in combination
Chloram-phenicol	Oral, i.m., i.v., topical	Bacteriostatic: inhibits protein synthesis	Broad spectrum	Typhoid fever, meningitis; eyedrops for con-junctivitis	Rarely causes fatal aplastic anaemia: this has restricted its use
Nalidixic acid*	Oral	Inhibits DNA replication	Coliforms; not *Pseudomonas aeruginosa*	Lower urinary infections	Side-effects include nausea; rarely, visual disturbances
Nitro-furantoin*	Oral	Inhibits DNA replication	Enterococci but not proteus or *Pseudomonas aeruginosa*	Lower urinary infections	Nausea; peripheral neuropathy is sometimes seen
Spectino-mycin	i.m.	Bactericidal	*Neisseria gonorrhoeae* and other Gram-negative bacteria	Penicillin-resistant gonorrhoea	
Mupirocin (pseudo-monic acid)	Topical	Bactericidal: arrests protein synthesis	Staphylococci and streptococci	Skin infections; elimination of nasal carriage of *Staphylococcus aureus* (including MRSA)	

i.m.: intramuscular; i.v.: intravenous.
*Serum levels inadequate for treatment of systemic infections, including pyelonephritis.

Mode of action: bacteriostatic: penetrates well into tissues and fluids, and acts on intracellular organisms.
Resistance: develops readily.

Toxicity: uncommon: peripheral neuritis, psychotic and epileptic episodes.

Rifampicin

Administration: oral.

Mode of action: inhibits by combining with bacterial DNA-dependent RNA polymerase.

Resistance: develops rapidly unless other drugs used in combination.

Antibacterial spectrum: mycobacteria. Also active in vitro against a wide range of Gram-positive and Gram-negative bacteria.

Clinical use: tuberculosis; prophylaxis of meningococcal meningitis; in combination with another drug, to treat severe staphylococcal infections.

Toxicity: low: liver function may be affected; often transient hypersensitivity; rarely, thrombocytopenia. Contraindicated in first trimester of pregnancy. Patients should be warned that urine, sputum and tears become coloured red with rifampicin therapy.

Pyrazinamide

Administration: oral.

Mode of action: bactericidal: acts on intracellular organisms; good meningeal penetration. Not active against *Mycobacterium bovis*.

Resistance: develops rapidly unless other drugs used in combination.

Clinical use: main effect in early phase of combination therapy: especially useful in tuberculous meningitis.

Toxicity: low: may be hepatotoxic.

Ethambutol

Administration: oral.

Resistance: uncommon.

Toxicity: optic neuritis may develop: reversible, and uncommon with low dosages.

Other (second-line) drugs

- Streptomycin
- Thiacetazone
- Capreomycin

- Cycloserine
- Ethionamide.

Recommended schedule for tuberculosis

6 months' course of isoniazid, rifampicin, ethambutol, pyrazinamide: latter two stopped after 8 weeks.

Longer treatment may be necessary for bone and joint infections, for meningitis or for resistant organisms.

ANTIBIOTIC RESISTANCE IN BACTERIA

A major problem in antibiotic therapy is the emergence of drug-resistant bacteria. The frequency depends on the organism and the antibiotic concerned: some organisms rapidly acquire resistance, e.g. certain coliforms, *Staphylococcus aureus*; others rarely do so, e.g. *Streptococcus pyogenes*. Resistance to some antibiotics virtually never develops, e.g., metronidazole, whereas with others resistant strains readily emerge, e.g. penicillin, tetracycline, streptomycin.

Drug resistance in clinical practice is associated with antibiotic use: when a small number of resistant bacteria have emerged, they will be at a selective advantage in the presence of the antibiotic and will multiply at the expense of sensitive bacteria. Widespread often indiscriminate prescribing of antibiotics in hospitals has therefore favoured the survival and increase of drug-resistant bacteria.

Drug resistance is of two types:

- **Primary resistance**: an innate property of the bacterium unrelated to contact with the drug, e.g. resistance of *Escherichia coli* to penicillin.
- **Acquired resistance**: due to mutation or gene transfer.

Spontaneous mutation may be relatively infrequent or, as in the case of *Mycobacterium tuberculosis* and streptomycin, common.

Gene transfer is a major cause of resistance in bacteria: it enables resistance to spread from bacterium to bacterium, within and between species. (See Chapter 4).

Cross-resistance occurs when resistance to one antimicrobial drug confers resistance to other (usually chemically related) drugs, e.g. bacteria resistant to one tetracycline or one sulphonamide are resistant to all tetracyclines or all sulphonamides respectively. Conversely, *dissociated resistance* occurs when resistance to one drug is not accompanied by resistance to closely related drugs, e.g. resistance to gentamicin is not always associated with resistance to tobramycin.

Mechanisms of antibiotic resistance

There are three main mechanisms: modification of the permeability of the cell wall or of the site of action of the drug, or inactivation of the drug.

Permeability

The cell wall may become altered – by modification of proteins in the outer membrane – so that antibiotics or other antimicrobial drugs cannot enter and be taken up by the bacterial cell. This is often associated with low-level resistance to several drugs, but occasionally with high-level resistance to a single drug (e.g. tetra-cycline): a common type of antibiotic resistance in *Pseudomonas aeruginosa*.

Modification of site of action

Modification of the enzyme or substrate with which the anti-microbial drug reacts enables the bacterium to function normally in the presence of the drug, e.g. trimethoprim, sulphonamide. In the case of trimethoprim resistance, the bacterium acquires a plasmid or transposon coding for a resistant dihydrofolate reductase – while retaining its own chromosomal-coded trimethoprim-sensitive enzyme.

Inactivation of antibiotic

A common mechanism of resistance. The antibiotic is inactivated by enzymes produced by the bacterium, e.g. β-lactamase destruc-tion of the β-lactam ring responsible for the antibacterial action of penicillins and cephalosporins. Some of these enzymes are plasmid-coded, others chromosomal-coded. Acetylating, adenylating and phosphorylating enzymes in the case of resistance to the amino-glycosides are plasmid-coded.

PRINCIPLES OF ANTIMICROBIAL THERAPY

- *Administration*

Antimicrobial therapy is indicated for an established infection that makes a patient sufficiently ill to require specific treatment: trivial, self-limiting infections in healthy individuals should not be treated with antibiotics.

- *Choice of drug*

Successful chemotherapy depends on the infecting organism being sensitive to the drug chosen. Attempts to treat *viral* respiratory infections – a common practice – are doomed to failure unless there is secondary *bacterial* infection.

The choice of drug is based on:

Clinical diagnosis: implies prescribing on an informed 'best-guess' basis: most infections requiring antibiotics have to be treated before laboratory results are available: they vary in severity from exacerbations of chronic bronchitis to septicaemia. Sometimes the clinical diagnosis indicates a specific bacterial cause, e.g. boil, typhoid fever, but often the cause cannot be deduced from the clinical picture – e.g. peritonitis, urinary infection. All medical students must therefore have a working knowledge of the bacteriology of infection so that, when qualified, they can prescribe effectively.

Laboratory diagnosis: specimens adequate for diagnosis should, whenever possible, be taken before chemotherapy begins. Isolation of the pathogen and sensitivity tests take time – at least 24 h, and usually longer – and as soon as results are available, treatment should be reviewed: laboratory monitoring can make the difference between success and failure of therapy.

- *Route of administration*

Drugs must be given parenterally to seriously ill patients. Oral antibiotics for the treatment of systemic infections must be both acid-stable (e.g. penicillin V is acid-stable but penicillin G is not) and absorbed from the gastrointestinal tract.

- *Dosage*

Dosage must be adequate to produce a concentration of antibiotic at the site of infection greater than that required to inhibit the growth of the infecting organism. *In renal failure*, the dosage of drugs eliminated by the renal route may require either major adjustment (e.g. aminoglycosides, vancomycin) or more minor modification (e.g. β-lactams), whereas those eliminated by the hepatic route (e.g. erythromycin) can usually be given in normal dosage.

- *Duration*

Treatment of some severe infections, e.g. endocarditis, tuberculosis, needs to be prolonged and is aimed at eradication of the pathogen, but the majority of acute infections respond to a short course of antibiotics, leaving the body defence mechanisms to cope with any infection that remains.

- *Distribution*

The drug must penetrate to the site of the infection, e.g. in meningitis the antibiotic must pass into the CSF. Deep-seated sepsis is a particular problem, and an important cause of anti-biotic failure: antibiotics cannot penetrate 'walled-off' abscesses or internal collections of pus, and treatment will probably fail unless the pus is drained. Surgical intervention is also necessary if there are established pathological changes, e.g. urinary obstruction due to stones, chronic tuberculous cavities.

- *Excretion*

Agents used to treat urinary infections are excreted in the urine in high concentrations: some, e.g. nalidixic acid and nitrofurantoin, do not achieve useful serum levels: they are eliminated almost exclusively by the renal route, and are therefore indicated only for the management of lower urinary infections.

Urinary pH affects the activity of some drugs, e.g. the amino-glycosides are far more active in an alkaline medium. The reverse is true of nitrofurantoin, which therefore should not be used to treat infections caused by *Proteus species*, which raise the pH of the urine.

Erythromycin is excreted largely in the bile: only low con-centrations can be detected in urine.

- *Toxicity*

Although the antibiotics in general use are well-tested, safe drugs, patients should be warned of possible side-effects, e.g. the mild diarrhoea common with tetracycline therapy; red colouring of body fluids with rifampicin.

Serious toxicity can manifest itself in two ways:

- *Direct toxicity*, e.g. ototoxicity with the aminoglycosides; nephrotoxicity with vancomycin; (rare) bone marrow aplasia due to chloramphenicol.
- *Hypersensitivity*, most often due to the penicillins.

Other complications include *superinfection* with antibiotic-resistant microorganisms, e.g. coliforms and yeasts. This is surprisingly uncommon in immunologically normal patients, e.g. chronic bronchitics on repeated courses of tetracycline, but is a major problem in immunocompromised hosts. Antibiotic-associated pseudomembranous colitis is probably a special example: with the use of lincomycins restricted, broad-spectrum β-lactam antibiotics are often involved.

- *Use of drugs in combination*

This may be necessary to treat a mixed infection if no single agent is active against all the causal organisms, e.g. in peritonitis due to coliforms and non-sporing anaerobes it is usual to give an aminoglycoside or cephalosporin along with metronidazole. In addition to this indication, there are two possible advantages.

1 *Emergence of drug-resistant bacteria will be prevented*: this applies in the treatment of tuberculosis, and may apply in infections due to *Staphylococcus aureus* – an organism with a marked propensity to become resistant, especially during clinical therapy involving some antibiotics, e.g. fusidic acid.

2 *Enhanced antibacterial effect (synergism) will be achieved*: this is governed to some extent by the '*Jawetz Law*' (see below) on combined action, although there are exceptions. The combined effect of two antibiotics depends on whether each is bacteriostatic or bactericidal in action, and the law predicts that the effect of a combination will be as follows:

Bactericidal + bactericidal:	may be synergistic
Bactericidal + bacteriostatic:	may be antagonistic
Bacteriostatic + bacteriostatic:	will be additive

This working rule has some value in clinical practice. For example, the combination of a penicillin and an aminoglycoside, both bactericidal, is often synergistic, with an increase in the efficacy of antibacterial action – and this may be essential, e.g. to treat septicaemia successfully in immunocompromised neutropenic patients, or to eradicate infection in endocarditis.

● *Antibiotic prophylaxis*

Early but indiscriminate attempts to prevent infection by giving antibiotics for several days or more failed. This was because the infection to be avoided, e.g. pneumonia in unconscious patients, wound infection after surgery, was due to a number of different bacteria – not all of which were sensitive to the drugs chosen. Prolonged antibiotic administration therefore resulted in the selection of resistant organisms, which subsequently caused infection.

Prophylaxis should be considered when there is a high risk of infection, and the agent chosen must be active against the likely pathogens.

Short-term prophylaxis: one dose, or at most a few doses, of carefully chosen antibiotics given to cover the time when the risk of an infection being established is greatest – usually the peri-operative period. This is a controversial issue. Some examples are listed in Table 45.6.

Short-term (2–3 day) prophylaxis should also be given to close contacts of a patient with *meningococcal meningitis*, especially young children: rifampicin is the drug of choice: minocycline and ciprofloxacin are also effective, as are the sulphonamides if the strain is sensitive.

Long-term prophylaxis: may be continued for months or years.

Rheumatic fever: recurrence of rheumatic fever invariably follows throat infection with *Streptococcus pyogenes*, which is always penicillin-sensitive. Incidence of further attacks is greatly reduced by giving penicillin.

Urinary tract infection: may be avoided in women who suffer repeated episodes, by administration of trimethoprim or nitro-furantoin: some 90% of urinary pathogens are sensitive to these drugs.

Tuberculosis: close contacts of a case of open tuberculosis should be given rifampicin and isoniazid for 6 months.

● *Antibiotic policies*

The large number of antimicrobial agents now available, many with similar properties and overlapping activity, may make the choice of drug difficult. Many hospitals have drawn up guidelines to improve the quality of antibiotic prescribing and enable clinicians to select the most effective therapy. These policies aim to prevent the indiscriminate use of antibiotics and inappropriate

Table 45.6   Antibiotic prophylaxis

Clinical situation	Bacteria most likely to cause infection	Appropriate prophylactic regimen
Colonic surgery	Coliforms: anaerobes ('bacteroides', anaerobic cocci, clostridia)	Metronidazole plus gentamicin or cephalosporin
Appendicectomy	Anaerobes (as above)	Metronidazole
Gynaecological surgery	Anaerobes (as above)	Metronidazole
Biliary tract surgery	Coliforms enterococci	Cephalosporin or piperacillin
Urological surgery (if urine infected)	Coliforms	As indicated by antibiotic sensitivity tests, or cephalosporin
Open heart surgery	*Staphylococcus aureus* *Staphylococcus epidermidis*	Cloxacillin plus gentamicin or cephalosporin
Insertion of prosthetic joints	*Staphylococcus aureus* *Staphylococcus epidermidis* corynebacteria	Cephalosporin
Amputation of ischaemic limb	*Clostridium perfringens*	Penicillin
Dental extraction in patients with heart valve disease	Oral streptococci	Amoxycillin or clindamycin
Prevention of tetanus after wounding*	*Clostridium tetani*	Penicillin

*In conjunction with immunoprophylaxis.

treatment: they restrict the prescription of some drugs, often those that are new and expensive and not necessarily superior to established agents. As a result, antibiotic costs, a major item in pharmacy expenditure, are decreased (sometimes substantially), and there is evidence that the emergence of resistant bacterial pathogens is reduced.

- *'Chemotherapy without bacteriology is guesswork'*

Collaboration between clinician and bacteriologist is crucial, especially in combating the severe infections increasingly encountered in hospitals today. Frequent discussions are to be encouraged.

46. Prophylactic immunization

The introduction of immunization against infectious disease has been one of the most successful developments in medicine.

Immunization aims to produce *immunity* to a disease, artificially and without ill effects. Immunity can be classified under two main headings:

1. Active
- *a. Natural*: follows clinical or subclinical infection
- *b. Artificial*: induced by vaccination

2. Passive
- *a. Natural*: due to transplacental maternal IgG antibody, which protects the child for first 6 months of life
- *b. Artificial*: by injection of preformed antibody derived from serum of humans or animals

Immunization can therefore be used to produce either active or passive immunity.

Active immunity

Follows either natural infection after some, but not all, infectious diseases, or vaccination. Associated with the production of antibody, and often cell-mediated immunity also. The onset of immunity is delayed, but when established lasts for years, sometimes for life.

Antibody: protects in different ways, depending on the type of disease: most effective in virus diseases because antibody neutralizes virus infectivity. In bacterial disease due to exotoxin, antibody neutralizes the toxin. In both bacterial and virus infections, antibody enhances phagocytosis.

Cell-mediated immunity (delayed hypersensitivity): stimulated independently of antibody: particularly important in resistance to chronic bacterial infections characterized by intracellular parasitism (e.g. tuberculosis, leprosy, brucellosis), and in some virus diseases, e.g. herpes simplex.

Passive immunity

Either naturally acquired by fetus from mother, or artificially induced by injection of preformed antibody present in human or animal serum. Immediate immunity is conferred but it is short-lasting – usually for only a matter of weeks. There is no associated induction of cell-mediated immunity.

Antibody production

Figure 46.1 shows antibody levels after vaccination by passive immunization and active immunization, with either live attenuated or killed organisms.

ACTIVE IMMUNIZATION

Objective: to produce immunity with adequate antibody levels and a population of cells with immunological memory.

Long-lasting once produced, the immunity persists and even after many years, infection may still stimulate an accelerated antibody response.

TYPES OF VACCINE

Vaccines for producing active immunity are of three types: live attenuated organisms; killed (inactivated) organisms or cell components; and toxoids.

Live attenuated organisms

These organisms have been cultivated under conditions in which they lose virulence but retain the ability to stimulate a protective immune response. They multiply in the body and mimic natural infection, with antibody production but without symptoms: reactions are mild and are similar to the natural disease. A single dose gives long-lasting immunity, which can be reinforced with subsequent booster doses.

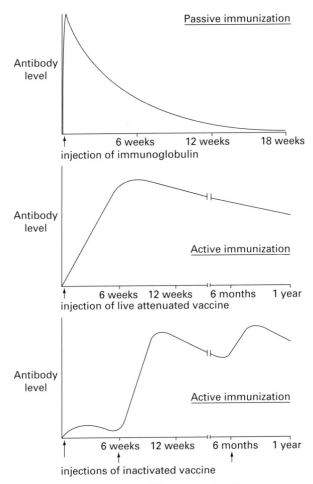

Fig. 46.1   Antibody levels following different methods of immunization.

Killed (inactivated) organisms or cell components

Several doses – usually three – are required, because there is no multiplication in the body. Generally the first and second doses are 4 or 6 weeks apart, and the second and third doses 6 months apart; subsequent booster doses are also necessary. Reactions do not resemble those of the natural disease, and usually follow soon after inoculation.

The older vaccines contain whole cells, but those recently introduced are often made from cell components such as purified proteins, e.g. obtained by genetic engineering (as in hepatitis B vaccine), or polysaccharides conjugated to proteins (as in *Haemophilus influenzae* vaccine).

Toxoids

Toxoids are very successful vaccines in diseases due to a single exotoxin, e.g. diphtheria, tetanus. Toxoids are toxins, rendered harmless – usually by formaldehyde – but retaining antigenicity. The antigenicity of toxoids can be increased by adsorption to a mineral carrier (such as aluminium salts) or by mixture with a suspension of other bacteria containing lipopolysaccharide endotoxin, e.g. the pertussis component of Triple Vaccine (pertussis, diphtheria, tetanus).

Future vaccines

Using molecular technology, research is being undertaken into novel vaccines, for example vaccinia virus whose DNA includes a gene coding for an immunogenic protein derived from a different organism. Synthetic peptides may also be used in the future, possibly in conjunction with carriers that present the antigen so as to enhance the immune response.

ASSESSING PROTECTION

Immunization should give a significant degree of protection against infection. Live attenuated organisms and toxoids are better vaccines than killed organisms.

Widespread vaccination of human populations – the aim is usually to achieve acceptance rates of at least 90% – has caused a dramatic fall in the incidence of many infectious diseases, e.g. diphtheria, poliomyelitis. However, in some instances the introduction of other measures (e.g. improved housing, sanitation, or nutrition, or chemotherapy which reduces the duration of infectivity) at the same time as a vaccine may have had more effect on the prevalence of the disease than vaccination, e.g. tuberculosis.

Field trials, studying the effect of a vaccine in a population which is 'at risk', are of crucial importance: *look for* a significant reduction in the attack rate or the severity of the disease in vaccinees. Extensive, carefully controlled field trials in human populations are essential for the final evaluation of most vaccines.

Vaccine trials involve the estimation after vaccination of antibody levels (*titres*), and occasionally of the appearance of cell-mediated immunity (e.g. tuberculin conversion after BCG vaccination). Detailed studies in human volunteers indicate the likelihood of the vaccine providing worthwhile protection. However, the ability to stimulate antibody production does not guarantee effective prophylaxis. The reasons for the failure of an apparently promising vaccine are often complex: in some instances it may be that inappropriate antibody is formed. For example, after parenteral administration of killed vaccine, IgM and IgG but not secretory IgA are formed, although the latter is the principal protective antibody at mucosal surfaces and therefore of great importance in respiratory virus infections (e.g. influenza), and also in poliomyelitis and cholera (where the gut is the site of primary multiplication).

CONTROL OF VACCINE PREPARATION

The manufacture of each batch of vaccine is subject to stringent legal control, to ensure safety and potency.

Safety

The following are the main problems – with modern control of vaccine production, they now represent more theoretical than actual risks:

- Contamination: by extraneous bacteria or viruses (derived from the cell cultures used in vaccine production)
- Inadequate inactivation of killed vaccine
- Reversion to virulence of attenuated vaccine: still an occasional problem, in vaccinees and in contacts who excrete vaccine virus which has undergone partial reversion to virulence on passage
- Residual toxicity of toxoids.

Potency

Ensured by the following measures:

- Live vaccines are prepared from organisms grown for only a few passages from the parent strain, to ensure that antigens essential for protection are not lost.

- Killed vaccines are prepared from organisms which have a full complement of the antigens involved in the protective immune response. The antigenic composition of the vaccine organisms sometimes has to be altered, if new variants of wild organisms appear in the population.
- Tests of potency: measure the antibodies produced on inoculation of the vaccine into experimental animals; other tests assess the survival of immunized animals after challenge with virulent organisms – but the method of the test may bear little relationship to the human disease, e.g. tests of pertussis vaccine measure the protection of mice against intracerebral injection with *Bordetella pertussis,* and this is said to correlate with the ability of the vaccine to prevent human disease.

ADMINISTRATION

Age

Immunization should be targeted at the age group at greatest risk. Some vaccines (e.g. typhoid, cholera) are indicated regardless of age for anyone entering an endemic area; others (e.g. influenza) are given primarily to the elderly or those with chronic cardiac or respiratory disease.

Childhood: most vaccines, however, are given to children because most of the diseases they prevent are encountered in childhood: e.g. more than two-thirds of deaths from pertussis are of infants under 1 year old.

There are two problems in starting immunization early in life.

- *The infant immune system is not fully developed* at birth, and the capacity to make antibody is therefore limited – nevertheless, it is probably adequate if the vaccine is potent.
- *Transplacental maternal antibody* may prevent a response to live virus vaccines, and reduce that to some killed vaccines.

Official policy in Britain is to start immunization at 2 months of age. This is a compromise: delay until the child is 6–9 months old would produce better responses, but the chance of establishing immunity when it is most needed would be lost.

Combined vaccines

Giving more than one vaccine at a time is attractive because it reduces the number of injections required, and therefore increases acceptability by the parent and child.

Combined vaccines may enhance antibody production (e.g. the presence of the pertussis component acts as an adjuvant for the toxoids in Triple Vaccine): there were fears in the past that the response to one organism might diminish that to others, but this has not been a problem in practice.

Complications of immunization

Side-effects are not uncommon after administration of some vaccines, e.g. many killed bacterial vaccines cause mild reactions, local (pain and redness at the injection site) and general (fever and constitutional upset). Although unpleasant, these are usually trivial.

Serious complications, although rare, are associated with some vaccines and include anaphylaxis, bronchospasm and laryngeal oedema. Other dangerous adverse reactions affect the CNS (e.g. convulsions), and can result in permanent brain damage.

The small but definite risk of serious reactions in a tiny proportion of vaccinees must be balanced against the benefits: the controversy some years ago over pertussis vaccine illustrates the difficulty that this may present.

Contraindications to vaccination

- Previous severe local or generalized reaction to that vaccine, or a history of hypersensitivity to some of its components, e.g. egg allergy in the case of virus vaccines grown in chick cells, antibiotic hypersensitivity with many virus vaccines.
- Live vaccines should never be given to:
  - *Immunocompromised* patients: because of the risk of severe generalized infection
  - *Pregnant women*: because of the danger of transplacental spread to the fetus.

VACCINES IN CURRENT USE

Table 46.1 lists the main vaccines in current use in the UK.

LIVE VACCINES

BCG vaccine

Contains: live attenuated *Mycobacterium bovis* (Bacille Calmette–Guérin). Killed vaccines are of no value as immunizing agents against tuberculosis: they do not produce a cell-mediated response.

Indications: policy in the UK is to vaccinate all children between their 10th and 14th birthdays, *after* a tuberculin test has shown that they are non-reactors. Infants should be immunized at birth if there is high risk of contact with tuberculosis, e.g. a close relative with the disease. Others at high risk of exposure to tuberculosis should be immunized if not already protected (e.g. health care staff, contacts of known cases, immigrants from countries with high prevalence of the disease).

Administration: one dose *intradermally* at the insertion of the deltoid muscle, near to the middle of the upper arm. Normally a red papule develops at the site of injection after some weeks, and soon subsides.

Adverse reactions: the papule may progress to an indolent ulcer and discharge pus: associated axillary lymphadenopathy is not uncommon. Keloid formation at injection site.

Protection: MRC field trials in the UK (1950–71) and studies in North America both showed durable (10–15 year) protection.

Table 46.1　Vaccines in current use in the UK

	Bacterial vaccines	Viral vaccines
Live	BCG (tuberculosis) Typhoid	Poliomyelitis (Sabin) Measles–mumps–rubella (MMR) Rubella
Killed or cell components	Typhoid Cholera Pertussis *Haemophilus influenzae* b (Hib) Pneumococcal Meningococcal	Influenza Hepatitis A Hepatitis B
Toxoids	Diphtheria Tetanus	

The incidence of clinical disease in vaccinees was reduced by 80%. However, other field trials have yielded less encouraging results.

Poliomyelitis vaccine

Contains: live attenuated strains of poliovirus types 1, 2 and 3 – Sabin vaccine. (Salk vaccine, which was developed earlier, contains inactivated strains of poliovirus types 1, 2 and 3: it is no longer in routine use in Britain, and can only be obtained on a named-patient basis.)

Indications: active immunization of all infants, starting when 2 months old.

Administration: orally: three spaced doses are needed to ensure multiplication in gut with both local (i.e. gut IgA) and serum antibody production to each of the three virus types. Booster doses are recommended at school entry and on leaving school. (Salk vaccine is given by injection and produces good protection, but serum antibodies only.)

Adverse reactions: minimal: rare cases of paralysis in adults due to Sabin type 3 virus.

Protection: excellent with both vaccines. Following a vigorous campaign with Salk vaccine in the UK, launched in 1956, there was a dramatic decrease in poliomyelitis notifications, with the vaccine giving an 80% protection against paralytic disease. Sabin vaccine, introduced in 1961, has been equally effective and has helped eliminate wild virus from circulation in the community.

Choice of vaccine type

Sabin vaccine is preferred to Salk vaccine because it produces gut immunity and is easier to administer, so can be given more quickly in the face of an epidemic.

However, in some circumstances Salk vaccine is preferred, e.g. in Third World countries where naturally occurring enterovirus infection of the gut is common, and may interfere with the multiplication of vaccine virus in the gut. Scandinavian countries traditionally prefer Salk vaccine – the newer preparations of which are considerably more potent than the earlier vaccine.

Current debate in the UK includes consideration of the reintroduction of Salk vaccine. This is because the risk of naturally-acquired paralytic poliomyelitis is now so low that the remote chance of vaccine-induced paralysis with Sabin live attenuated vaccine is almost as great.

Measles–mumps–rubella (MMR) vaccine

A new approach to virus vaccines in the UK was the introduction in 1988 of a combined live attenuated vaccine against measles, mumps and rubella.

Contains: live attenuated strains of all three viruses.

Indications: active immunization of all children in the second year of life, to prevent the complications associated with these three common childhood fevers, such as respiratory infections, encephalitis (measles), meningitis (mumps) and congenital infection (rubella).

Administration: two doses by intramuscular injection: the first in the 2nd year of life, the second at school entry. The second dose is to protect those who did not develop immunity after the first injection, and to prevent the development over years of sufficient susceptible children to sustain an epidemic.

Adverse reactions: few: the present vaccine is well tolerated; fever, malaise and transient rash may follow 6–12 days after vaccination, and occasionally, febrile convulsions. Around 1% of children have mild parotitis. Rarely, meningoencephalitis due to the mumps component.

Protection: good – of the order of 90% – and apparently long-lasting.

Note: In November 1994, with the prospect of a measles epidemic in schoolchildren, a programme of immunization of all children aged from 5 to 16 years with MR (i.e. measles and rubella) vaccine was successfully undertaken in the UK.

Rubella vaccine

Contains: live attenuated virus.

Indications: following the widespread acceptance of the MMR immunization scheme and the administration of MR vaccine in 1994, the schoolgirl rubella immunization programme was brought to an end. Previously in the UK, rubella vaccine had been admin-istered to all girls between 10 and 14 years of age. This policy was aimed at preventing congenital rubella, but did not affect the epidemiology of the disease and outbreaks of rubella continued to take place, in which some susceptible pregnant women contracted infection. The vaccine is still available and should be given to any susceptible (i.e. seronegative) women of child-bearing age.

Note: A past history of rubella not confirmed by laboratory tests is an unreliable guide to immune status: other virus diseases can mimic rubella clinically.

Administration: one dose by injection.

Adverse reactions: uncommon, but there may be mild rubella-like symptoms, including arthralgia, some 9 days after vaccination. Pregnancy must be avoided for 1 month after vaccination: the vaccine should never be given during pregnancy.

Protection: apparently good, with long-lasting immunity.

Typhoid vaccine (live)

A recently-introduced live attenuated vaccine.

Contains: the attenuated Ty 21a strain of *S. typhi*.

Indications: for those travelling to or living in areas where typhoid fever is endemic; health care staff at risk.

Administration: orally in enteric-coated capsules, in three doses on alternate days.

Adverse reactions: mild and transient nausea, vomiting, abdominal cramps and diarrhoea; occasionally urticaria.

Protection: efficacy similar to parenteral vaccines, but may be less durable: annual reimmunization with three doses is recommended if exposure is likely.

KILLED VACCINES

Typhoid vaccines

Classical vaccine

The classical vaccine is now being replaced by other preparations (see above and below), but is still the most widely used.

Contains: heat-killed, phenol-preserved suspension of *Salmonella typhi*.

Indications: for those travelling to or living in areas where typhoid fever is endemic, and health care staff at risk.

Administration: two doses 4–6 weeks apart, by injection; booster doses every 3 years.

Adverse reactions: local and general reactions are common: early in onset, they subside in 36 h.

412   NOTES ON MEDICAL BACTERIOLOGY

Protection: around 70–90%: extensive field trials in Yugoslavia, carried out by WHO in 1954–55, showed a good protection rate against typhoid. An alcohol-killed, alcohol-preserved vaccine evaluated at the same time was ineffective – although alcohol preserves the Vi ('virulence') antigen.

Capsular polysaccharide typhoid vaccine

This has been licensed in the UK recently.
Contains: the Vi capsular polysaccharide antigen of *S. typhi*.
Administration: one dose, by injection.
Adverse reactions: mild and transient: less than with whole cell vaccine.
Protection: 70–80%, lasting for 3 years or more.

Cholera vaccine

Contains: heat-killed *Vibrio cholerae* O1, serotypes Inaba and Ogawa.
Indications: for those travelling to areas where cholera is endemic. Evidence of vaccination is no longer a requirement for entry into any foreign country.
Administration: two spaced doses by injection; booster doses every 6 months.
Adverse reactions: local and general reactions are quite common; serious reactions are rare.
Protection: poor – estimated at 50%, and short-lasting – about 6 months.

Attempts have been made to produce better vaccines, e.g. live avirulent oral vaccines, to stimulate the production of secretory IgA antibodies in the gut (*coproantibodies*) as well as serum antibodies; also a toxoid prepared from cholera enterotoxin (exotoxin): none has so far gained acceptance.
Note: The vaccine does not protect against the non-O1 type 139 strain of cholera vibrios.

Pertussis vaccine

Contains: killed, freshly isolated, smooth strains of *Bordetella pertussis*. The vaccine should contain all the surface antigens of *B. pertussis* associated with epidemics: these antigens designate the three common serotypes – 1,3; 1,2,3; and 1,2.
Indications: official policy in Britain is the active immunization of all children, starting at 2 months old. The heated debate which

began in 1974 about the risk and efficacy of vaccination aroused much public concern. As a result, the acceptance rate declined and major outbreaks of pertussis resulted in 1977–79 and 1981–83.

Administration: three doses at 2, 3 and 4 months old: the vaccine is always given with diphtheria and tetanus toxoids, as Triple Vaccine. Booster doses are not recommended because pertussis is not a problem after 5 years of age.

Adverse reactions: usually local and trivial: a few infants develop excessive crying and irritability. Severe reactions attributed to the vaccine are convulsions and, rarely, permanent brain damage. Subsequent work has cast doubt on whether the severe reactions are, in fact, attributable to the vaccine.

Protection: mass vaccination was started in the UK in 1957. During the following years there have been conflicting claims about the efficacy of the vaccine. The protection is not solid, but is of the order of 80%. Whooping cough is a disease that has become less severe as living conditions have improved and children have become healthier – but it has not been eliminated. Nevertheless, the case fatality rate has fallen dramatically and there is good evidence that vaccination has prevented epidemics. Public confidence in immunization returned in the mid-1980s, and with it, control of whooping cough. Although the cyclical pattern remains, notifications reached an all-time low in 1995.

Note: Acellular vaccines which contain pertussis toxoid, sometimes combined with other pertussis antigens, are undergoing field trials in the UK at present, with promising results. An acellular vaccine is available on a named-patient basis.

Hib vaccine

Contains: capsular polysaccharide from *Haemophilus influenzae* type b, conjugated to protein carrier to enhance immunogenicity. *H. influenzae* is an important cause of invasive disease, especially meningitis and acute epiglottitis in infants.

Indications: introduced in October 1992 for routine immunization of babies. This has achieved a dramatic reduction in the incidence of invasive *H. influenzae* infection.

Administration: at 2, 3, 4 months old, at the same time as Triple Vaccine: a recent recommendation is for Hib vaccine to be mixed with Triple Vaccine, for simultaneous administration by a single injection.

Adverse reactions: minor – most common after the first dose.

Pneumococcal vaccine

Contains: a saline solution of 23 highly purified capsular polysaccharides, extracted from pneumococci of the most prevalent pathogenic types.

Indications: to prevent pneumococcal pneumonia, bacteraemia and meningitis in individuals at special risk, especially those who have had a splenectomy but also patients with chronic lung, heart, liver and kidney disease.

Administration: one dose, by injection.

Adverse reactions: local in about half, and fever in 10% of those vaccinated.

Protection: apparently good – but only against infections caused by the serotypes present in the vaccine. Efficacy in preventing pneumococcal pneumonia is about 60–70%, but the vaccine is less effective in young children and the immunosuppressed.

Meningococcal vaccine

Contains: outer capsular polysaccharide of groups A and C *Neisseria meningitidis*. (There is *no* effective group B vaccine available.)

Indications: selective use only: risk of infection is low, and in the UK group B strains are the major cause of disease. Recipients include: *close family contacts* of cases of group A or C meningitis (who should also receive chemoprophylaxis); *members of closed or semiclosed communities* (e.g. schools) affected by an epidemic (usually caused by group C organisms); *those travelling overseas* in areas where the disease is endemic, especially if living rough.

Administration: one dose, by intramuscular injection, to children and adults.

Adverse reactions: generally well tolerated.

Protection: antibody response detected in more than 90% of those immunized after 1 week: infants respond less well; lasts 3–5 years.

Influenza vaccine

Contains: inactivated virus, usually two of the currently circulating strains of influenza A virus plus the current influenza B strain. Vaccines contain either 'split' virus (i.e. partially purified, disrupted particles) or subunit antigens (highly purified haemagglutinin and neuraminidase).

Indications: elderly people with pre-existing cardiorespiratory or renal disease – especially useful for old people in residential homes or long-stay hospitals; if pandemic imminent, key personnel in essential services, e.g. hospital staff, the police force.

Administration: one dose by injection; vaccination needs to be repeated each winter.

Adverse reactions: few and mild, but a number of cases of polyneuritis (Guillain–Barré syndrome), some severe, were recorded in the USA following mass vaccination in 1976–77; there may be severe reactions in those hypersensitive to egg protein.

Protection: short-lived, i.e. about 1 year: the protection conferred is of the order of 70%.

Hepatitis A vaccine

Recently available.

Contains: formaldehyde-inactivated virus, grown in cell culture.

Indications: for non-immune frequent travellers to areas where hepatitis A is endemic, which include most tropical and semitropical regions.

Administration: two doses by intramuscular injection: the second 6–12 months after the first.

Protection: antibodies produced in response to a single injection persist for 1 year.

Hepatitis B vaccine

Contains: hepatitis B surface antigen (HBsAg), genetically-engineered and adsorbed onto aluminium salt.

Indications: those at special risk, e.g. parenteral drug misusers; homosexual and bisexual males; prostitutes; haemophiliacs; health care personnel and patients in hospitals for the mentally deficient and renal units; staff in casualty departments and laboratories; infants born to mothers who are HBsAg carriers.

Administration: in three doses intramuscularly, separated by 1 month and 6 months respectively.

Adverse reactions: local pain and redness.

TOXOIDS

Diphtheria toxoid

Contains: diphtheria formol toxoid (i.e. toxin treated with formaldehyde) – usually adsorbed onto aluminium phosphate or aluminium hydroxide, which act as adjuvants.

Indications: children and selected adults at risk, e.g. hospital or laboratory staff.

Administration: three spaced injections starting at 2 months old, as for pertussis vaccine, with which it is usually combined as part of the Triple Vaccine. Booster dose at school entry and on leaving school.

Older children (i.e. aged 10 years or more) and adults, use a low-dose vaccine: administer by deep subcutaneous or intramuscular injection.

Adverse reactions: mild and transient under 10 years of age; older children and adults may experience more severe side-effects.

Protection: excellent – the disappearance of diphtheria in the UK between 1941 and 1951 was due to immunization, and the disease is now extremely rare in this country. However, every few years a small outbreak – usually in the unvaccinated – is reported. (See page 237.)

Tetanus toxoid

Contains: tetanus formol toxoid adsorbed onto aluminium hydroxide or aluminium phosphate.

Indications: the aim is active immunization of the entire population: although tetanus is rare, it may develop after common, trivial wounds. Those at greatest risk are the non-immunized – now usually elderly people, and more often women.

Administration: three spaced injections, starting in infancy as part of the Triple Vaccine. In the unvaccinated, a course should begin when a situation of risk presents, e.g. after injury, at the casualty department. Booster doses are given at school entry, on leaving school and in the event of injury.

Adverse reactions: rare and minor; severe reactions may be seen in patients with hypersensitivity to a component, and occasionally in adults who have been hyperimmunized with too many booster injections.

Protection: excellent.

Triple Vaccine

Contains: killed *Bordetella pertussis*, diphtheria toxoid and tetanus toxoid.

Indications: active immunization of all infants.

Administration: three doses by injection, at 2, 3 and 4 months of age. At school entry: booster doses of diphtheria and tetanus toxoids only.

Adverse reactions: see sections on individual vaccines.

Protection: see sections on individual vaccines.

SCHEDULE OF IMMUNIZATION RECOMMENDED IN THE UK

This is shown in Table 46.2

TRAVEL ABROAD

Additional vaccination – and sometimes booster doses of previous vaccines – are often advisable for travel abroad. These are shown in Table 46.3.

PASSIVE IMMUNIZATION

Objective: to produce immunity immediately, by the injection of antibodies present in human or animal serum. The immunity that follows is *short lasting* and wanes in a matter of weeks or a few months. Antisera are also used in treatment.

Table 46.2 Schedule of vaccination and immunization recommended in the UK

Age	Vaccine	Notes
During the first year of life	Triple Vaccine, polio vaccine, Hib	Give in three doses at 2, 3 and 4 months
During the second year of life (at age 12–15 months)	Measles–mumps–rubella combined vaccine	Administer to both boys and girls
3–5 years (school entry)	Diphtheria and tetanus toxoids	Booster dose
	Polio vaccine	Booster dose
	Measles–mumps–rubella combined vaccine	Second dose
Between 10th and 14th birthdays	BCG vaccine	For tuberculin-negative children
13–18 years (on leaving school)	Polio vaccine	Booster dose
	Tetanus toxoid	Booster dose
	Diphtheria toxoid	Booster dose with low-dose vaccine

Table 46.3 Vaccines to be considered for travel

Vaccine	Indications; area of travel
Polio ⎫ Typhoid ⎭	Anywhere except Europe, North America, Australia, New Zealand
Cholera	Some countries in Asia, Africa, Middle East, South and Central America
Tetanus	If the traveller is unprotected and liable to be at risk
Yellow fever*	Some countries in South America and Africa
Rabies	Anywhere except Australia, New Zealand and various island communities (e.g. Cyprus) – if occupational exposure to animals
Meningococcal group A and group C	Endemic areas in north India, Nepal, Central Africa, Middle East
Tick-borne encephalitis	Endemic areas in Eastern Europe
Japanese encephalitis	Endemic areas in Nepal, Thailand, Korea, China
Plague	For workers in rat-infested, poor conditions, e.g. refugee camps
Hepatitis A	For travel to tropical or semitropical regions
Hepatitis B	For workers exposed to blood and its products in areas of Asia and Africa, with high carriage rate of HBsAg

*Vaccination certificate essential for travel to certain countries.

SPECIFIC IMMUNOGLOBULINS

Human

Prepared from plasma pools containing high levels of the appropriate antibody. Donations are taken from individuals after their plasma has been screened for antibody content: sometimes they are chosen because they are recovering from infection (convalescent serum) or have recently been actively immunized against the disease.

Human immunoglobulins have a half-life of 26 days after injection: significant protection may last up to 3 months, and sometimes longer.

Preparations

Some of the available preparations are:

- *Hepatitis B immunoglobulin*: indication: post-exposure prophylaxis after accidental inoculation with HBsAg-positive blood.
- *Tetanus immunoglobulin*: indication: prophylaxis and treatment of tetanus.
- *Varicella-zoster immunoglobulin*: indication: treatment of the disease in immunocompromised patients, who are susceptible to severe varicella or generalized zoster.
- *Rabies immunoglobulin*: indication: post-exposure prophylaxis in a non-immunized individual from a high-risk area.

Animal

Specific antibodies, raised in horses by active immunization, were used extensively in the past. Unfortunately, they contain foreign protein to which the recipient forms antibody, with the result that they are *rapidly eliminated* (much faster than human immunoglobulins) and can cause unpleasant and sometimes dangerous *hypersensitivity reactions*, including serum sickness (an Arthus reaction) and anaphylaxis. A few equine antisera are still available.

NONSPECIFIC IMMUNOGLOBULINS

Human immunoglobulin prepared from donations of pooled normal plasma: contains antibodies to the wide range of infective agents likely to have been encountered by most people.

Indications:

- *Prophylaxis of hepatitis A:* temporary protection for occasional travellers to areas where hepatitis A is endemic: now superseded by vaccine – which should be given to regular travellers or those staying for longer than 3 months.
- *Prophylaxis of measles:* given within 6 days of exposure, will prevent or modify the disease: use for immunocompromised children and adults.
- *To boost immunoglobulin levels* in children with hypogammaglobulinaemia.

Medical mycology

47. Fungal infections

Fungi, unlike bacteria, are *eukaryotic*: the cell nucleus contains multiple chromosomes enclosed by a membrane, and in the cytoplasm there are mitochondria and 80s ribosomes (see Ch. 2). Many fungi can reproduce sexually: this process involves meiosis. Most fungi grow as filaments (*hyphae*), which intertwine to form a mesh (the *mycelium*) – but most yeasts are exceptions: they are unicellular and reproduce by budding. Of the thousands of species of fungi, only a few are pathogenic for humans: some others cause disease in other animals or plants.

Habitat: fungi, like bacteria, are ubiquitous. In the soil they play an important role in the degradation of organic compounds, and they may produce antibiotics (e.g. penicillin) which inhibit the growth of competitive bacteria.

Culture: all fungi are aerobic, and most grow readily on simple media.

Classification: is complex and based on the method of spore production (sexual or asexual); the morphology of the colony; the vegetative hyphae which form the mycelium; and the specialized aerial hyphae which bear the spores. Fungi of medical importance can conveniently be divided into three groups:

- Yeasts
- Filamentous fungi
- Dimorphic fungi.

Diseases caused by fungi

Fungi cause three types of disease:

- Infections (mycoses)
- Mycotoxicoses
- Allergic reactions.

423

Infections (mycoses)

1. *Superficial infections* of the mucosa, with yeasts (causing thrush) and of the keratin of skin, nail and hair, with filamentous fungi called *dermatophytes* (causing ringworm). These infections are common in the UK. Although troublesome, they are usually trivial and do not involve deeper tissues.

2. *Subcutaneous infections*: the result of the traumatic implantation of environmental fungi, leading to progressive local disease with considerable tissue destruction and sinus formation. These infections are rare in the UK, but common in the tropics.

3. *Systemic infections*, with haematogenous spread throughout the body, are serious and often fatal. They are uncommon in the UK except in immunocompromised patients with impaired host defences (see Chapter 42), who may develop widespread disease due to yeasts or filamentous fungi such as *Aspergillus* species. In other parts of the world, certain forms of deep disseminated mycoses caused by dimorphic fungi are remarkably common in otherwise healthy individuals.

Mycotoxicoses

The result of eating mouldy food, in which the fungus has produced toxic metabolites. Examples are: poisoning following the consumption of food containing aflatoxins formed by the growth of *Aspergillus flavus*; ergotism after the ingestion of wheat infected with *Claviceps purpurea*.

Allergic reactions

Inhalation of fungal spores, notably those of *Aspergillus fumigatus*, may provoke a type I and/or a type III hypersensitivity reaction. Sometimes, the antigenic stimulus is prolonged because the fungal hyphae grow in the lumen of the bronchi: invasion of lung tissue does not take place.

YEASTS

Yeasts are round to oval unicellular fungi, which reproduce by budding. Some may develop *pseudohyphae* – chains of elongated budding cells – but only a few are able to form true hyphae.

CANDIDA

Several species are found in humans, but one species, *Candida albicans*, is responsible for 90% of infections. The other species capable of causing infection include *C. stellatoidea* (now regarded as a subtype of *C. albicans*), *C. tropicalis*, *C. krusei*, *C. guilliermondii* and *C. parapsilosis*.

CANDIDA ALBICANS

Habitat: the normal flora of the upper respiratory, gastrointestinal and femal genital tracts.

Laboratory characteristics

Morphology and staining: two forms, both Gram-positive, are recognized in clinical material and on culture:

- Spherical to oval budding cells (3–5 × 5–10 μm): the yeast or Y-form.
- Elongated filamentous cells, joined end to end (*pseudohyphae*) and producing buds (*blastospores*); also true hyphae. These constitute the mycelial or M-form. *C. albicans* is the only species to produce hyphae and pseudohyphae in vivo (see Fig. 27.1).

Culture: aerobic and easy to cultivate, but isolation from clinical material may be impeded by faster-growing bacteria:

1. *Sabouraud's medium*: a simple glucose–peptone agar, pH 5.6, often made more selective by the addition of antibiotics (e.g. chloramphenicol), is useful for primary isolation. Incubation at 37°C for 48 h may be necessary.

2. *Ordinary agar* and *blood agar*: colonies may be observed more easily around antibiotic discs which have inhibited bacterial growth.

Colonial morphology: colonies are cream to white, flat or hemispherical and have a waxy surface. The yeasts are predominantly Y-form, but M-forms develop in older cultures, and the pseudohyphae may project from the edge of the colonies.

Identification: *C. albicans* can be readily differentiated from other species by production of:

1. *Germ tubes*: method: grow in serum for 3 h at 37°C; make a wet film and examine for formation of filamentous outgrowths – *germ tubes*.
2. *Chlamydospores*: method: grow in a nutritionally poor medium (e.g. corn-meal agar) for 24 h at 28°C and examine for presence of round, thick-walled resting structures – *chlamydospores* – usually found at the ends of pseudohyphae, deep in the agar.

Biochemical activity: the results of fermentation (anaerobic metabolism) and assimilation (aerobic metabolism) of a range of carbohydrates are used in the identification of *Candida species*.

Antigenic structure: strains fall into two serotypes: A – antigenically similar to *C. tropicalis*; and B – antigenically similar to *C. stellatoidea*. Candida antibodies can be demonstrated in most human sera. Delayed-type hypersensitivity is common, and a positive candida skin test is almost universal in normal adults.

Pathogenicity

Source: usually endogenous, but cross-infection may occur, e.g. from mother to baby, from baby to baby in a nursery.

Host: infections are most common in babies who are premature and in adults debilitated by general ill health, notably diabetes. A special 'at risk' group is composed of patients immunocompromised by either the nature of their disease (e.g. AIDS; malignancy, in particular leukaemias or lymphomas) or the treatment they have received (e.g. long courses of broad-spectrum antibiotics, immuno-suppressive or cytotoxic drugs).

Clinical features

Infection is known as either *candidiasis* or *candidosis*. The lesions are usually superficial (mucous membranes and skin), but occasionally are deep and involve internal organs.

Superficial: *Mucous membranes*: thrush: white adherent patches on buccal mucosa or vagina.

Skin: red weeping areas, usually where skin is moist and traumatized, e.g. intertrigo in the obese.

Chronic mucocutaneous candidiasis: an intractable, disfiguring condition, especially affecting the face and scalp: onset generally in infancy. The condition is due to a defective immunological response, in which T-cell function is reduced, but antibody response to candida remains normal.

Deep: involvement of lower respiratory tract and urinary tract; septicaemia with localization in eye, endocardium, meninges, kidney, bone.

Diagnosis

- By demonstration of yeasts in a wet film or Gram-stained smear, followed by isolation of candida when the specimen is cultured.
- By detection of antigen, in serum or other body fluid.
- By detection of antibody in serum. A variety of methods is available, e.g. ELISA, but the tests are of limited value because antibody is present in more than half of the healthy adult population
- By detection of elevated levels of arabinitol (a metabolite of candida) in serum, using gas-liquid chromatography. A positive result may indicate systemic infection. Not a routine test in the UK.

Treatment

Candida are eukaryotic microorganisms, and are resistant to *all* antibacterial antibiotics.

Superficial infections can be treated topically with a polyene (nystatin, amphotericin B) or an imidazole (miconazole, clotrimazole). Systemic infections require intravenous amphotericin B, either given alone or with 5-fluorocytosine: the combination may be synergistic. Oral administration of fluconazole is effective in mucosal and systemic candida infections: it may also be used prophylactically in susceptible (e.g. neutropenic) patients.

CRYPTOCOCCUS

The one pathogenic species in the genus is *Cryptococcus neoformans*.

CRYPTOCOCCUS NEOFORMANS

Habitat: ubiquitous saprophyte: often found in soil, especially in ground contaminated with bird droppings; particularly associated with pigeons.

Laboratory characteristics

Morphology and staining: a capsulated, budding yeast with spherical cells 5–15 μm in diameter; does not usually form a pseudomycelium. Gram-positive, although the capsule may prevent staining.

Culture: aerobic: grows on a wide variety of common media at 37°C, but also at room temperature. Isolation from clinical material is best achieved by culture at 30°C: several days' incubation may be required before colonies develop.

Colonial morphology: on Sabouraud's medium, forms glistening mucoid cream colonies, which become duller and darker on extended incubation.

Identification: make a wet preparation of a portion of the colony in Indian ink to demonstrate the capsule. *Note*: the capsule, which is usually pronounced in clinical material, may be rudimentary in culture.

Biochemical activity: produces a urease; assimilates a number of compounds, including inositol but is unable to metabolize by fermentation; produces phenol oxidase, detected by the formation of brown colonies on birdseed agar.

Pathogenicity

Pathogenic for humans and a variety of animals.

Source: from the environment, usually by inhalation, especially of dust containing pigeon excreta.

Clinical features

A lung granuloma, usually symptomless, is the primary lesion. This resolves spontaneously in the vast majority of patients, without dissemination. Haematogenous spread results in subacute or chronic meningoencephalitis – the classic disease presentation – and sometimes involvement of skin, lungs, lymph nodes and other organs. Clinical disease is usually found in immunocompromised patients, especially those with AIDS.

Diagnosis

- By demonstration in CSF, exudate, urine or other appropriate specimen of an encapsulated yeast, confirmed by isolation on culture. *Note*: CSF changes resemble those in tuberculous meningitis, and the yeast may be confused with red blood cells or lymphocytes.
- By detection of antigen in CSF, blood or urine, using a latex agglutination test.
- By detection of antibody in serum: a variety of tests is available, including agglutination and immunofluorescence.

Treatment

Intravenous amphotericin B combined with 5-fluorocytosine. Fluconazole is an alternative, although perhaps less effective, treatment. After primary therapy, particularly in AIDS patients, fluconazole administration should be continued to prevent relapse.

MALASSEZIA

Malassezia furfur (formerly known as *Pityrosporum furfur, P. orbiculare* or *P. ovale*).
   Habitat: skin.

Laboratory characteristics

Morphology: oval yeast, reproducing by unipolar budding.
   Culture: dull, buff colonies on agar supplemented with lipids, e.g. olive oil.

Pathogenicity

Cause of tinea versicolor, in which large scaling patches develop on the skin of the trunk: brownish on light-skinned people, lighter on dark-skinned people; usually asymptomatic. This yeast is also associated with seborrhoeic dermatitis and dandruff.

Diagnosis

Although the yeast can be isolated on culture, diagnosis is usually made by the demonstration of short, curved, non-branching hyphae and yeasts in skin scales.

OTHER YEASTS

Torulopsis glabrata (Candida glabrata) is a skin commensal, and may be isolated from urine and blood as a contaminant. It can be a cause of infection in immunocompromised patients.

Rhodotorula species are yeasts which form pink colonies. They are skin commensals, and may be cultured from contaminated clinical specimens: grow at room temperature, but not at 37°C.

FILAMENTOUS FUNGI

DERMATOPHYTES

The dermatophytes comprise a group of fungi which cause infection – *tinea* or *ringworm* – of skin, nail and hair, without involvement of living tissue. They belong to three different genera: *Trichophyton*, *Microsporum* and *Epidermophyton*. The common species and the types of ringworm they cause are listed in Table 47.1.

Habitat: the keratin of humans and animals.

Source: by person-to-person spread, sometimes via fomites, or from contact with animals, as a zoonosis. A few species are present in the soil (Table 47.1).

Clinical features

These are summarized in Table 47.2.

Diagnosis

Specimen: scrapings of skin or nail; short lengths of plucked hair.

Preparation: make a wet preparation of the specimen in 20% potassium hydroxide: leave for 10–20 min to digest keratin.

Observe: filamentous branching hyphae: spores may also be seen. In tinea capitis, fungal elements may be seen either outside the hair – *ectothrix* infections, e.g. with *Microsporum canis* or, less commonly, inside the hair – *endothrix* infections, e.g. with *Trichophyton schoenleinii*.

Table 47.1 Dermatophytes and ringworm

Fungus	Source	Type of ringworm caused				
		Tinea capitis	Tinea corporis	Tinea cruris	Tinea pedis	Tinea unguium
Trichophyton rubrum	Human		+	++	+++	+++
Trichophyton mentagrophytes var. *interdigitale*	Human			+	++	+
Trichophyton mentagrophytes var. *mentagrophytes*	Animal: cattle, horses, rodents	+	++			
Trichophyton schoenleinii	Human	+ Usual cause of favus				
Microsporum audouinii	Human	+	+			
Microsporum canis	Animal: cats, dogs	+++	++			
Microsporum gypseum	Soil	+	+			
Epidermophyton floccosum	Human			++	+	+

+++: most commonly caused by; ++: commonly caused by; +: sometimes caused by.

Table 47.2   Clinical manifestations of ringworm

Site	Affects	Clinical features
Tinea capitis	Scalp and hair	Small scaling papules, which spread to leave areas of baldness: infected hairs break, to leave stumps. Skin may suppurate. *Favus* is a variety characterized by yellow lesions which later develop cup-shaped crusts that heal, leaving atrophic bald skin.
Tinea corporis	Skin, excluding scalp, bearded areas and feet	Circular spreading lesions: as the centre scales and heals, the periphery advances, with vesicles and pustules in inflamed skin.
Tinea cruris	Skin of groin and perineum	Spreading scaly dermatitis, with vesicopustular edge: little central healing.
Tinea pedis	Soles of feet and between toes	Inflamed skin with vesicles, leading to peeling and fissure formation (athlete's foot).
Tinea unguium	Nails of hands or feet	Affected nails appear opaque, thickened, brittle and distorted: they may separate from nailbed and be totally destroyed.

Culture: necessary to identify the causal fungus: *inoculate* the specimen onto a plate of Sabouraud's agar containing chloramphenicol: this antibiotic suppresses the growth of contaminating bacteria. *Incubate* aerobically at 25–30°C. *Examine* daily up to 21 days, for fungal colonies.

Colonial appearance: observe pigmentation and texture of the surface of the colony, and pigmentation of the reverse side, seen through the bottom of the plate. Colonial morphology can vary considerably (Table 47.3).

Microscopic features of colony: transfer growth to slide carefully: suspend in a drop of alcohol so that structural arrangement is preserved. Stain growth with a drop of lactophenol cotton blue, and place a cover slip over the preparation. Observe: hyphae and *conidia* – asexual spores. Two types of conidia are formed: small unicellular *microconidia* and larger septate *macroconidia*. Microscopic morphology aids identification: some characteristic features are listed in Table 47.3.

Treatment

Mild infections: topical imidazole (e.g. clotrimazole or miconazole), or topical terbinafine.

Severe infections: oral terbinafine and itraconazole are effective, as is oral griseofulvin: prolonged treatment is required if hair and especially nails are involved.

OTHER FILAMENTOUS FUNGI

ASPERGILLUS

Aspergillus fumigatus is the main pathogen: other species associated with infection include *A. niger* and *A. flavus*.

Habitat: soil and dust: spores are ubiquitous.

Laboratory characteristics

Culture: after 3–4 days' incubation on Sabouraud's agar at 25–37°C, the colonies have a velvety to powdery surface and are characteristically coloured: *A. fumigatus* dark green; *A. niger* black on white and *A. flavus* yellow-green.

Microscopic colonial appearance: a wet preparation stained with lactophenol cotton blue demonstrates septate hyphae and *conidiophores* – specialized aerial hyphae that bear conidia (i.e. spores). The conidiophores have swollen, rounded ends and the spores are formed in chains. The general morphology is characteristic of the genus, and there are also inter-species differences that are useful in identification (Fig. 47.1).

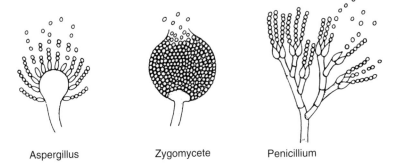

Aspergillus   Zygomycete   Penicillium

Fig. 47.1 Spore-bearing structures of some fungi.

Table 47.3   Identification of dermatophytes

Fungus	Colonial appearance*	Characteristic microscopic features of colony
Trichophyton rubrum	**Surface**: white, granular or fluffy **Reverse**: dark red to brown	**Microconidia**: tear-shaped 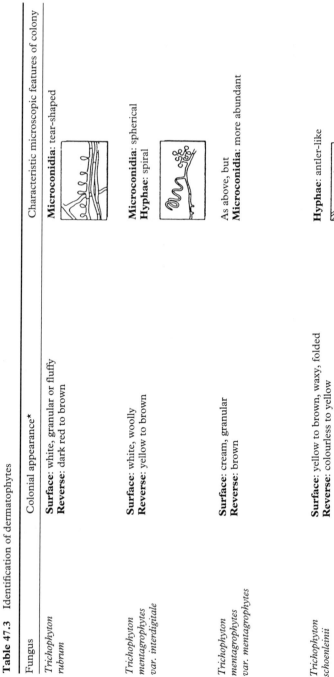
Trichophyton mentagrophytes var. interdigitale	**Surface**: white, woolly **Reverse**: yellow to brown	**Microconidia**: spherical **Hyphae**: spiral
Trichophyton mentagrophytes var. mentagrophytes	**Surface**: cream, granular **Reverse**: brown	As above, but **Microconidia**: more abundant
Trichophyton schoenleinii	**Surface**: yellow to brown, waxy, folded **Reverse**: colourless to yellow	**Hyphae**: antler-like

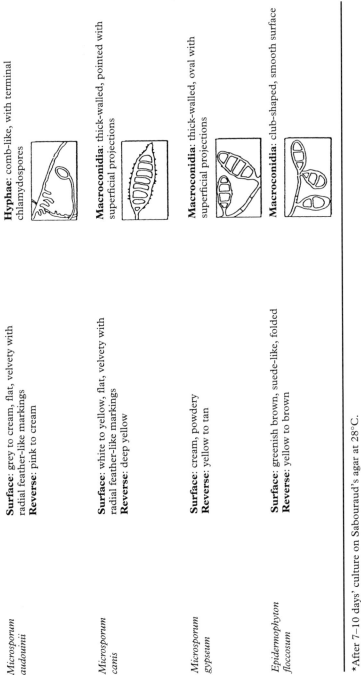

Microsporum audouinii	**Surface:** grey to cream, flat, velvety with radial feather-like markings **Reverse:** pink to cream	**Hyphae:** comb-like, with terminal chlamydospores
Microsporum canis	**Surface:** white to yellow, flat, velvety with radial feather-like markings **Reverse:** deep yellow	**Macroconidia:** thick-walled, pointed with superficial projections
Microsporum gypseum	**Surface:** cream, powdery **Reverse:** yellow to tan	**Macroconidia:** thick-walled, oval with superficial projections
Epidermophyton floccosum	**Surface:** greenish brown, suede-like, folded **Reverse:** yellow to brown	**Macroconidia:** club-shaped, smooth surface

*After 7–10 days' culture on Sabouraud's agar at 28°C.

Clinical features

Aspergillus species can cause a variety of clinical syndromes:

- *Allergic bronchopulmonary aspergillosis*: inhaled spores provoke a hypersensitivity reaction, which may be of:
  - Type I (asthma)
  - Type III (extrinsic alveolitis)
  - Types I and III combined.
- *Aspergilloma*, in which a fungal ball grows within, and is usually restricted to, an existing lung cavity, e.g. due to old tuberculosis, bronchiectasis.
- *Invasive aspergillosis*, in which the fungus establishes a pneumonia and later disseminates to involve other organs, e.g. brain, kidneys, heart: mortality is high. Patients who develop this type of disease are usually immunocompromised (see Ch. 42).
- *Superficial infections* of the external ear (*otomycosis*) and, less commonly, the eye (*mycotic keratitis*) and nasal sinuses.

Diagnosis

Direct microscopy to demonstrate septate hyphae: suggestive, but not diagnostic of, aspergillus infection.

Specimens:
Exudate, e.g. sputum: make wet preparation in 20% potassium hydroxide.
Tissue, e.g. biopsy or post-mortem material: stain sections by PAS (periodic acid–Schiff) method – hyphae are poorly stained by haematoxylin and eosin.
Isolation by culture: on Sabouraud's agar at 25–37°C. Colonies grow after 48 h, but longer incubation may be required before characteristic morphological features develop.
   Note: Since aspergillus spores are ubiquitous, colonies of the fungus are often found growing on cultures as the result of aerial contamination. Thus it may be difficult to interpret the significance of isolating a few colonies from a clinical specimen.
   Serology: precipitating antibodies to aspergillus antigens can be demonstrated by a number of laboratory methods, including counter-current immunoelectrophoresis, immunodiffusion and ELISA. Antibodies are usually absent from the sera of healthy individuals, but can be detected in the majority (70%) of patients

with allergic aspergillosis and approximately the same proportion of those with pneumonia or invasive disease.

Treatment

Invasive aspergillosis is treated with intravenous amphotericin B. Oral itraconazole may also be effective, especially for maintenance therapy following initial treatment, but mortality is high.

ZYGOMYCETES

The genera associated with human infection are *Mucor*, *Absidia* and *Rhizopus*.
  Habitat: ubiquitous in the soil: spores in air and dust.

Laboratory characteristics

All three genera are similar.
  Culture: after 3–4 days' incubation on Sabouraud's agar at 30–37°C, the colonies are grey-white with a thick cottony, fluffy surface.
  Microscopic colonial appearance: non-septate broad hyphae, with aerial *sporangiophores* which end in a *sporangium* – a sac containing spores (Fig. 47.1).

Clinical features

Zygomycosis (*mucormycosis*, *phycomycosis*) occurs as a systemic infection following dissemination from a primary focus, often in the lung: almost all patients are immunocompromised (see Ch. 42). The rhinocerebral form, in which the nose, nasal sinuses and orbit are involved, is a well recognized and usually fatal complication of diabetes: infection may penetrate to involve the frontal lobe of the brain.

Diagnosis

Direct microscopy: to demonstrate broad, non-septate hyphae.
Specimens:
Exudate: make wet preparation in 20% potassium hydroxide.
Tissue: hyphae stain readily with haematoxylin and eosin (unlike aspergillus).

Isolation by culture on Sabouraud's agar: may be difficult to achieve from necrotic material, even when abundant hyphae are seen.

Note: These common environmental moulds are frequent contaminants of culture plates.

Treatment

Intravenous amphotericin B combined, where appropriate, with surgical drainage. Good medical control of diabetes.

PENICILLIUM

A variety of species abound in the environment and grow on bread, jam, fruit, cheese, etc. In the laboratory penicillium is a common airborne contaminant of culture media. *Penicillium marneffei* has caused systemic infection in AIDS patients.

Colonies are blue-green with a white border, and have a powdery surface.

Microscopy demonstrates septate hyphae with branched conidiophores bearing chains of spores, the appearance likened to a 'brush or broom' (Fig. 47.1).

FUNGI CAUSING MYCETOMA

Mycetoma usually affects the foot (Madura foot), and can be caused by a variety of fungi and actinomycetes (usually *Nocardia species*: see page 115). Important filamentous fungi which cause mycetoma include *Madurella mycetomatis*, *Madurella grisea* and *Phialophora verrucosa*.

Habitat: soil.

Pathogenicity

Fungi implanted into subcutaneous tissue following trauma (e.g. by a splinter) produce destructive granulomatous lesions, with suppuration and abscess formation in soft tissue and bone, which drain through multiple sinus tracts. There is local spread, but no dissemination. A common condition in tropical and subtropical areas where people go barefoot.

Treatment

Surgical: chemotherapy is ineffective when mycetoma is due to filamentous fungi.

DIMORPHIC FUNGI

Dimorphic fungi grow as either yeasts or filaments. The *yeast form* (parasitic phase) is found in infected tissues and on artificial media at 37°C. The *filamentous form* (saprophytic phase) is present in the soil and on artificial media at 22–25°C.

Habitat: soil: some have a characteristic geographical distribution (Table 47.4).

Pathogenicity

Cause disease in humans (Table 47.4), and in wild and domestic animals.

Infection is usually acquired by inhalation, and the primary lesions are in the lungs. In most cases these heal, often without causing illness, and delayed hypersensitivity develops, with a positive skin-test reaction to the appropriate antigen. Progressive disease may affect the lungs, sometimes causing cavitation, and/or disseminate widely to involve the skin, mucous membranes and internal organs.

Table 47.4 Dimorphic fungi and disease

Fungus	Disease	Geographical distribution
Blastomyces dermatitidis	North American blastomycosis	North America, especially Mississippi and Ohio valleys
Paracoccidioides brasiliensis	South American blastomycosis	South America; less commonly, Central America
Coccidioides immitis	Coccidioidomycosis	USA from California to Texas; South and Central America
Histoplasma capsulatum	Histoplasmosis	Eastern and central USA; occasionally other parts of the world
Histoplasma duboisii	African histoplasmosis	Equatorial Africa
Sporothrix schenckii	Sporotrichosis	World-wide

The lesions are chronic granulomas. *Note* the similarity of this disease process to tuberculosis.

Sporotrichosis is different: it follows traumatic implantation of the fungus into the skin, and results in a chronic local pyogenic infection, with lymphatic spread and ulceration of the lymph nodes: disseminated disease is rare.

Diagnosis

Direct demonstration of the yeast-like form in suitably stained preparations of exudate (e.g. sputum, pus) or biopsy specimens.

Isolation on appropriate culture media, incubated at the correct temperature: some of the fungi grow slowly on culture.

Serology: useful in the diagnosis of histoplasmosis, coccidioido-mycosis and South American blastomycosis, but of uncertain value in the other diseases because of difficulties in interpreting the significance of antibody levels.

Treatment

Amphotericin B is the drug of choice for invasive disease. Itracon-azole is the alternative treatment, especially for long-term therapy.

Medical parasitology

48. Parasitic infections

Parasites are larger and more complex organisms than bacteria. Classified as:

- Protozoa: single-celled parasites
- Metazoa: multicelled parasites.

Infection with parasites is a major cause of morbidity and mortality in tropical and semitropical countries. In Britain infections are increasing, partly because of increasing foreign travel; also, large immigrant communities have resulted in the import of tropical parasites.

Transmission:

- *Faecal-oral*: the most common route
- *Arthropod vectors*
- *Intermediate hosts*, e.g. snails, fish, are required for the life-cycle of certain parasites.

PARASITIC INFECTIONS INDIGENOUS TO THE UK

Table 48.1 lists the main parasites that can be acquired in Britain.

TOXOCARA CANIS AND *TOXOCARA CATI* (TOXOCARIASIS)

T. canis and *T. cati* are the common roundworms of dogs and cats respectively. Humans are the *paratenic* (or incidental) hosts, in whom the parasite does not develop fully (i.e. beyond the second larval stage).

Adult worms:

Length: 5–15 cm.

Habitat: small intestine of dogs or cats (the definitive hosts).

443

Table 48.1   Parasites indigenous to the UK

Parasite	Host	Source of infection	Principal symptoms*
Nematodes (roundworms)			
Toxocara canis	Dog	Dog faeces	Often asymptomatic; sometimes visceral larva migrans
Toxocara cati	Cat	Cat faeces	Cerebral or ocular damage
Enterobius vermicularis	Human	Faecal–oral	Asymptomatic; anal pruritus
Cestodes (tapeworms)			
Echinococcus granulosus	Dogs, sheep	Animal faeces	Hydatid cysts, especially liver and lung
Trematodes (flukes)			
Fasciola hepatica	Sheep	Contaminated watercress	Hepatitis, cholangitis, cholecystitis
Protozoa			
Trichomonas vaginalis	Human	Sexual transmission	Vaginal discharge
Toxoplasma gondii	Cat	Cat faeces; raw or undercooked meat	Lymphadenopathy: congenital infection
Giardia lamblia	Human	Contaminated water	Diarrhoea
Pneumocystis carinii	Human	Unknown	Pneumonia
Cryptosporidium	? Farm animals, pets	Faecal–oral	Diarrhoea, abdominal pain, vomiting
Acanthamoeba species	Human	Corneal abrasions; contaminated contact lens solutions	Keratitis, uveitis, corneal ulceration

*Note: Symptomless infection is common with all parasites.

Pathogenesis

After ingestion, the eggs hatch in the small intestine into larvae, which then migrate, often widely, into other tissues.

Clinical features

Infection: most often symptomless.

Disease: *visceral larva migrans*, due to larval migration in the body: accompanied by eosinophilia, hepatomegaly, chronic pulmonary infection or pneumonitis – with cough and fever.

Ocular lesions (retinitis, endophthalmitis) are the commonest manifestation – usually seen in children.

Diagnosis

ELISA test, with secretory/excretory products (derived from second stage larvae maintained in vitro) as antigen.

Treatment

Albendazole; photocoagulation of ocular lesions.

Control

De-worming of pets.

ENTEROBIUS VERMICULARIS (THREADWORM)

Known as *pinworms*. Common in children: often asymptomatic, but pruritus ani is a frequent complication, and can perpetuate auto-infection because infection is via the faecal–oral route.

Adult worms:
Length: about 1 cm.
Habitat: caecum and colon.
Females: migrate to the anus and lay eggs on perianal skin.

Diagnosis

Demonstration of eggs (ova) on perianal sellotape smear, or of adult worms in faeces.

Treatment

Mebendazole, piperazine, pyrantel.

ECHINOCOCCUS GRANULOSUS (HYDATID DISEASE)

A disease of sheep-rearing communities, but rare in Britain. Dogs
– the definitive hosts – acquire infection by feeding on sheep offal
containing hydatid cysts.

Adult worms (tapeworms):

Length: about 1 cm.

Habitat: small intestine.

Pathogenesis

In the dog, adult worms mature in the small intestine producing eggs
which are excreted in the faeces.

Infection of humans is by ingestion of eggs, but humans are
accidental and intermediate hosts.

Eggs hatch in the human duodenum or small intestine into
embryos, which migrate via the portal blood supply to the liver
and, less often, the lungs.

In liver and lungs (and rarely other tissues, such as muscle, brain,
bones), larvae develop into *hydatid cysts*. The cysts may be large,
are filled with clear fluid and contain characteristic *protoscolices*
(immature forms of the head of the parasite): the protoscolices
mature into developed *scolices*, which are infective for dogs.

Clinical features

Asymptomatic infection is common, especially with hydatid disease
of the lungs; humans are surprisingly tolerant, even of large cysts
in the liver.

Symptoms include:

Hepatomegaly, with abdominal pain and discomfort; *cough*,
sometimes with haemoptysis in lung hydatid disease; *pressure*,
resulting from expanding cysts, may cause signs and symptoms in
any of the affected organs and tissues.

Rupture of cysts can cause a severe allergic reaction, such as type
I anaphylaxis.

Diagnosis

- *Scan*: ultrasound or CT
- *Serology*
- *Demonstration* of characteristic protoscolices in cysts removed
  at operation.

Treatment

For active cysts: albendazole followed by surgery. If inoperable: albendazole alone.

FASCIOLA HEPATICA (FASCIOLIASIS)

The common liver fluke of sheep and cattle.

Replicative cycle involves an intermediate host, the snail *Lymnaea trunculata*. Fasciola eggs from sheep (or cattle) develop into *miracidia*, which infect the snails: after a complex multiplication process, *cercaria* are shed from the snails onto surrounding vegetation, forming *metacercaria*. These are infectious for sheep and cattle, and also for humans.

Route of infection for humans: most often, by eating contaminated watercress.

Adult worms:

Length: 3 cm; width: 1.5 cm.

Habitat: the larger biliary passages and gall bladder.

Pathogenesis

Metacercaria, after ingestion, burrow through the wall of the duodenum and cross the peritoneal cavity to the bile ducts and liver tissue.

Clinical features

Human disease is often mild.

Symptoms may include: fever; dyspepsia; anorexia; vomiting; pain in epigastrium or right upper abdomen.

Hepatomegaly, with tenderness over liver and sometimes with disturbance of liver function; occasionally, jaundice.

Allergic reactions, such as urticaria or eosinophilia, are common.

Diagnosis

Demonstration of eggs in faeces or bile.

Treatment

Triclabendazole, bithionol.

TRICHOMONAS VAGINALIS (TRICHOMONIASIS)

A flagellated protozoon, and the major cause of vaginitis in women.
Transmission: mostly sexually transmitted from males with inapparent infection; possibly also via contaminated articles.

Clinical features

Vaginal discharge: characteristic greenish-yellow, foamy discharge, with offensive smell.

Diagnosis

Demonstration of motile parasites in wet preparations of vaginal secretion.
Culture in Fineberg's medium.

Treatment

Metronidazole, tinidazole.

TOXOPLASMA GONDII (TOXOPLASMOSIS)

A protozoon which is a parasite of all warm-blooded animals. Cats are the only definitive hosts.
In the cat: the parasite develops as sexual forms in the small intestine, and eventually oöcysts are excreted in the faeces. Trophozoites – characteristically crescent-shaped – can spread widely in cat organs and tissues, with subsequent development into cysts.
Transmission: ingestion of oöcysts shed in cat faeces, or of trophozoites or cysts in undercooked meat, e.g. pork or mutton from infected animals.

Pathogenesis

Humans – like other warm-blooded animals – are intermediate hosts. After ingestion, the protozoon, which is an obligate intracellular parasite, disseminates widely via the bloodstream. Cysts form – especially in the brain and muscles, and also in the eye.

Clinical features

Primary infection: usually symptomless, although probably always results in a generalized infection.

Symptoms: fever, myalgia, headache, fatigue and lymphadenopathy. Rarely: hepatitis, encephalitis, myocarditis, chorioretinitis.

Congenital infection

Unlike infection in later life, congenital infection is generally severe. *Typically* presents with *a triad* of disorders:

- Chorioretinitis
- Hydrocephalus or microcephaly
- Cerebral calcification.

Congenitally infected babies also have signs of generalized infection, e.g. fever, rash, jaundice and hepatosplenomegaly.

Acquired in utero, as a complication of primary infection in the mother during pregnancy. It can also cause abortion or stillbirth.

Later sequelae of congenital infection may appear months or years after infection: most often chorioretinitis, sometimes mental retardation, ocular palsy, deafness.

Immunocompromised

Reactivation of infection involves the rupture of cysts, long after primary infection, with the release of parasites. Reactivation is a serious complication of immune deficiency: a not uncommon infection in AIDS, and also reported after heart transplant.

Clinically: most often, reactivation involves the brain – *cerebral toxoplasmosis*.

Heart transplants: myocarditis has been reported after cardiac transplantation. Apparently most often due to reactivation of cysts in a donor heart in a seronegative recipient.

Diagnosis

Serology: ELISA for IgM; latex agglutination, dye and haemagglutination tests for IgG.

Demonstration of protozoan in tissues or body fluids is sometimes possible.

Treatment

Rarely necessary: most infections are self-limiting, except for toxo-plasmosis in *AIDS or choroidoretinitis*: treat with pyrimethamine, sulphadiazine and folinic acid in combination.

GIARDIA LAMBLIA (GIARDIASIS)

A flagellated protozoon, and an important cause of diarrhoea world-wide.

Route of infection: faecal–oral.

Pathogenesis

Ingestion of cysts – the resistant, infective stage – is followed by production of *trophozoites* in the upper small intestine. Trophozoites cause irritation, which leads to gastrointestinal symptoms.

Clinical features

Symptoms:

Diarrhoea: mild to severe, with characteristic light-coloured, fatty stools; abdominal pain: cramps, with flatulence and epigastric tenderness; anorexia.

Malabsorption: steatorrhoea is not uncommon, and may lead to the full-blown malabsorption syndrome.

Diagnosis

Demonstration of:

Cysts or the characteristic trophozoites, in faeces.

Trophozoites, in duodenal aspirates or biopsies.

Treatment

Metronidazole, tinidazole or mepacrine.

Epidemiology

Outbreaks due to water-borne infection have been described: cysts have been demonstrated in the water in some outbreaks.

PNEUMOCYSTIS CARINII (PNEUMOCYSTOSIS)

Taxonomy: still in dispute: some reports (based on ribosomal RNA analysis) indicate the organism is related to fungi rather than protozoa. However, it will be dealt with in this chapter as if it were a protozoon.

Life-cycle: unknown, as is the *route* of human infection – although this is most likely to be via the respiratory tract.

Pathogenesis

Pneumocystis pneumonia is the result of reactivation of latent infection.

Subclinical infection in early life is probably widespread.

Immunocompromised: symptoms are rarely (if ever) seen in immunologically competent people: pneumocystis pneumonia is a major indicator disease of AIDS.

Clinical features

Symptoms are of a severe pneumonia, with progressive dyspnoea and cyanosis leading to respiratory failure.

Diagnosis

Demonstration of the morphologically characteristic organisms in bronchial aspirates, specimens of bronchial lavage or lung biopsy, stained by methenamine–silver or by immunofluorescence with monoclonal antibody (Fig. 48.1).

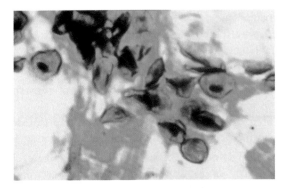

Fig. 48.1 *Pneumocystis carinii* in bronchial washing (approx. × 1000).

Treatment

Co-trimoxazole, pentamidine, atovaquone.

CRYPTOSPORIDIUM SPECIES (CRYPTOSPORIDIOSIS)

A coccidian protozoon, first recognized in 1976 as a cause of diarrhoea in the immunocompromised. Now known to be common also in normal people, and especially in children.

Animal hosts: several species of domestic animal, e.g. calves, are often infected with cryptosporidium – but not all animal cryptosporidia appear to be pathogenic for humans.

The human pathogenic species: is *Cryptosporidium parvum*.

Transmission: the infective stage is the oöcyst: small, 4–5 μm in diameter: passed in faeces.

Water-borne outbreaks are now being reported with increasing frequency.

Clinical features

Symptoms: self-limiting diarrhoea – except in the immunocompromised, in whom it can be severe and protracted, leading to an extreme degree of weight loss.

AIDS: cryptosporidiosis is one of the opportunistic infections associated with AIDS.

Diagnosis

Demonstration of oöcysts in faeces, stained with phenol auramine, modified Ziehl–Neelsen method or by immunofluorescence with monoclonal antibody.

Treatment

No highly effective treatment is available. Paromomycin may be of some benefit in AIDS-associated cryptosporidiosis.

CYCLOSPORA CAYETANENSIS (CYCLOSPORIASIS)

A newly recognized coccidian protozoon, named in 1992. The organism is indigenous to Britain, but most cases of cyclosporiasis occur in the tropics, notably in the Indian subcontinent, and in Central and South America.

Life cycle: not fully described.

Transmission: the infective stage is the oöcyst: 8–10 μm in diameter: passed in faeces. Human infection is water-borne.

Clinical features

Diarrhoea, remitting and relapsing, lasting as long as 6 weeks; malabsorption in some cases; weight loss.

Diagnosis

Demonstration of oöcysts in faeces: by microscopy of a faecal concentrate, or in a faecal smear stained by modified Ziehl–Neelsen method.

Treatment

Infection with cyclospora may be self-limiting, but where treatment is deemed necessary, co-trimoxazole is effective.

MICROSPORIDIA (MICROSPORIDIOSIS)

Obligate intracellular protozoa, characterized by resistant spores – the infective stage. Usually found as opportunistic parasites in patients with AIDS, though occasionally found in individuals with normal immunity.

Transmission: human infection is thought to be by ingestion or inhalation, or direct inoculation in the case of ocular infection.

Clinical features

The principal microsporidia infecting humans are:

- *Enterocytozoon bieneusi*: causes diarrhoea
- *Encephalitozoon (Septata) intestinalis*: causes diarrhoea
- *Nosema corneum*: causes ocular infection
- *Encephalitozoon hellem*: causes ocular infection.

Diagnosis

Histology of tissue biopsies; *microscopy* of modified trichrome-stained faecal smears.

Treatment

Albendazole is under evaluation for the treatment of gastrointestinal microsporidiosis.

Topical treatment with fumagillin or itraconazole or propamidine isethionate has been used for treatment of ocular microsporidiosis.

PARASITIC INFECTIONS NOT INDIGENOUS TO THE UK

Parasitic diseases are major causes of morbidity and mortality in tropical and undeveloped countries. Malaria is described in detail below, because of its importance if the diagnosis is missed in travellers returned from abroad. *Falciparum malaria* can be rapidly fatal if not treated promptly.

PLASMODIUM SPECIES (MALARIA)

Malaria is an important cause of death and debility throughout the tropics and subtropics.

Transmission: by the bite of anopheline mosquitoes.

The four species of plasmodia which cause malaria are shown in Table 48.2.

Life-cycle is complex, with sexual multiplication in the mosquito and asexual multiplication in human hepatocytes (exoerythrocytic schizogony) and erythrocytes (erythrocytic schizogony).

Table 48.2   The four main malaria parasites

Species	Distribution
Plasmodium vivax	The most common: found in all endemic areas and extending into subtropical and temperate zones
Plasmodium falciparum	Also common: found in most endemic areas but not in temperate zones
Plasmodium malariae	Much less common: mainly found in subtropical and temperate regions
Plasmodium ovale	Predominant in West Africa; rare in other endemic areas

Pathogenesis

Symptoms are due to:

Haemolysis, and the release of metabolites and pigment from malarial parasites:
Plugging of capillaries by parasites and infected erythrocytes.

Clinical features

Main symptoms are of intermittent recurrent fever.
Periodicity:

P. falciparum	36–48 h (malignant tertian)
P. vivax	48 h (benign tertian)
P. malariae	72 h (quartan)
P. ovale	48 h

Note: The classical regular pattern of recurrent fever can be modified by the immunological status of the patient, previous exposure to malaria, inadequate antimalarial prophylaxis and drug resistance in the infecting strain.

Incubation period:
Variable, depending on the species of *Plasmodium* and the strain within the species, and on the patient's history of previous exposure: usually 8–40 days, but can be as long as 1 year or more.

Prodrome:
Flu-like symptoms, e.g. headache, muscle pains, anorexia, photophobia, are sometimes seen at the end of the incubation period.

Malarial paroxysm:
Coincides with lysis of infected erythrocytes, and liberation of merozoites:
Rigor or shaking chill – the patient complains of feeling cold, but is in fact febrile:
Followed by feeling hot, flushed, agitated;
Severe headache and aching limbs and back are common.
Relapse: at the appropriate interval usually follows.

Complications

1. *Cerebral malaria*: a complication only of *P. falciparum* infection. Symptoms: headache and disorientation leading to coma and, if untreated, death. Cerebral infection is due to spread of the parasites to the CNS.
2. *Blackwater fever*: also most often seen in falciparum malaria. Symptoms: haemoglobinuria, due to sudden intravascular haemolysis:

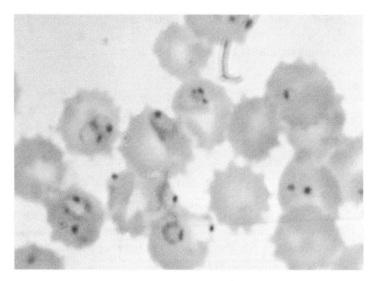

Fig. 48.2   Malarial parasites in thin blood film (approximately × 2000).

renal failure sometimes ensues, due to acute tubular necrosis as a result of renal anoxia.

3. *Proteinuria*: sometimes seen in infection with *P. malariae* when the kidneys of children are affected, producing 'quartan nephrosis', with oedema of face and limbs. This serious complication has a prolonged course.

4. *Infection of placenta* with *P. falciparum*, leading to abortion, still birth and low-weight babies; seen in tropical Africa.

5. *Tropical splenomegaly*: grossly enlarged spleen.

Diagnosis

Demonstration of parasites in thick and thin blood films, using Field's or Giemsa stain (see Fig. 48.2).

Treatment

Falciparum malaria: quinine, mefloquine or halofantrine.

Benign malaria (due to *P. vivax*, *P. ovale* and *P. malariae*): chloroquine: supplement with primaquine (if glucose-6-phosphate dehydrogenase level normal) after initial therapy, in the case of *P. vivax* and *P. ovale* infections.

Prevention

The principles of prevention are:

1. Awareness of the risk of malaria
2. Avoidance of mosquito bites
3. Chemoprophylaxis if appropriate (up-to-date guidelines are given in the British National Formulary): includes chloroquine, proguanil, mefloquine, pyrimethamine with dapsone depending on resistance in areas being visited.
4. Seeking early diagnosis
5. Treatment of febrile or flu-like illness *within 1 year* of leaving an area where malaria is endemic, even if precautions were taken.

Control

Attempts by WHO and other agencies to control malaria have been largely unsuccessful due to:

- widespread and increasing development of resistance of the plasmodia to antimalarial drugs
- increased resistance of the vector mosquitoes to insecticides
- lack of financial and political stability, preventing implementation and monitoring of control programmes.

Vaccination: various preparations, using different antigens of *P. falciparum*, are under trial.

LEISHMANIA SPECIES (LEISHMANIASIS)

Leishmaniasis is a protozoal infection found in many parts of the world, including Asia, Africa, Latin and Central America and the Middle East – but also in Europe, in Spain, France and Italy.

Several causal species have been identified, their distribution largely determined by geographical location. (See Table 48.3.)

Reservoirs: many humans, dogs, rodents and other small mammals.

Transmission: via the bite of infected sandflies.

Pathogenesis

Leishmania survive within macrophages in the human body as intracellular parasites: cell-mediated immunity determines the host response to infection, and hence the clinical manifestations of the disease.

Table 48.3   Parasites causing leishmaniasis

Species	Distribution
Old World	
Leishmania tropica	Mediterranean, Asia, Middle East
Leishmania major	Middle East, Africa, Asia
Leishmania aethiopica	Ethiopia, Kenya, South West Africa
Leishmania donovani	Asia
New World	
*Leishmania braziliensis**	Latin America
Leishmania mexicana	Mexico, Central America, Texas
Leishmania chagasi	Latin America

*Now recognized as a subgenus: *Viannia*.

Clinical features

There are three main forms of leishmaniasis:
visceral (kala-azar),
cutaneous
mucosal.

Visceral leishmaniasis (kala-azar)

Incubation period: long (3–8 months).

Symptoms: fever, weight loss with splenomegaly, hepatomegaly, anaemia, leucopenia and hypergammaglobulinaemia – protozoon-carrying macrophage infiltration is widespread throughout the reticuloendothelial system. Also seen in immunocompromised patients, e.g. with AIDS.

Causes: particularly associated with *L. donovani* (Old World) and *L. chagasi* (New World).

Cutaneous leishmaniasis

Known as 'oriental sore' in the Old World.

Symptoms: initially a papule at the site of the sandfly bite, which enlarges and ulcerates: lesions can be very large (2 cm or more in diameter) and disfiguring: a hard excrescence in the middle of the lesion is characteristic (Montpellier sign).

Diffuse cutaneous leishmaniasis is a more serious form, in which satellite lesions spread locally and to distant skin areas.

Main causes: Old World: *L. major*, *L. tropica*, *L. aethiopica*; New World: *L. braziliensis*, *L. mexicana*.

Mucosal leishmaniasis

Known as *'espundia'*.

A severe complication of cutaneous leishmaniasis, with mutilating destruction of the nose, oral cavity and pharynx where the infective process has extended to the mucous membranes of nose and mouth. *Main cause*: New World: *L. braziliensis*.

Diagnosis

Demonstration of intracellular protozoa in stained film from lesions.

Culture: of bone marrow aspirate or splenic puncture, for extracellular forms, on special media.

Skin test: intradermal inoculation of antigen from extracellular parasites (Montenegro test) to detect hypersensitivity: usually positive in established disease. Not useful in diagnosis, but helpful in epidemiological investigations.

Treatment

Sodium stibogluconate, meglumine antimonate: pentamidine as a second-line drug. Consider amphotericin B in mucosal disease.

ASCARIS LUMBRICOIDES (COMMON ROUNDWORM)

A major problem: infects around 700 million people world-wide.
Adult worms:
Length: about 20 cm.
Habitat: the small intestine.

Pathogenesis

Infection: by ingestion of eggs.

Life-cycle: larvae hatch in small intestine, from whence they migrate to liver and lungs (while growing and undergoing moults); return to small intestine as adult worms via trachea and oesophagus.

Clinical features

Symptoms accompany the infestation in two phases:

1. *Migratory phase*: about 6 weeks: often accompanied by hepatitis, pneumonitis and allergic symptoms: eosinophilia is usually present.

2. *Intestinal infection*: the presence of worms in the small intestine can cause intestinal obstruction, especially in small children.

Diagnosis

Demonstration of adult worms or – more usually – ova in faeces.

Treatment

Mebendazole, piperazine, levamisole (the latter not yet licensed in the UK).

TAENIA SAGINATA (TAENIASIS)

Humans are the only *definitive* hosts for this, the *beef* tapeworm: cattle are *intermediate* hosts.
  Adult worms:
  Length: often very long – up to 10 m.
  Structure:
* *Head* or *scolex*: with suckers, which attach to jejunal mucosa.
* *Body*, made up of segments or *proglottids*: in *T. saginata* these are characteristically elongated. Each proglottid contains both male and female organs, from which eggs are shed into the faeces.
  Habitat: small intestine.

Pathogenesis

Ingestion of *cysticerci* – an intermediate, larval form of the parasite – found in undercooked or 'measly' beef. The cysticerci mature into adult worms in the small intestine.
  Cattle develop cysticercosis of muscles after ingestion of eggs.

Clinical features

Usually symptomless: sometimes weight loss.

Diagnosis

Demonstration of proglottids or eggs in faeces.

Treatment

Praziquantel, niclosamide.

OTHER INFECTIONS NOT INDIGENOUS TO THE UK

Other important parasitic infections found in countries other than Britain are listed in Table 48.4.

Table 48.4 Other tropical parasites

Parasite	Host	Intermediate host/vector	Symptoms
Nematodes			
Hookworms:			Anaemia, gastrointestinal
Ancylostoma duodenale	Human	–	haemorrhage
Necator americanus			
Strongyloides stercoralis	Human	–	Serpiginous skin lesions, pneumonitis, enteritis
Trichuris trichiura	Human	–	Diarrhoea
Trichinella spiralis	Pigs	Human	Fever, muscle pain
Wuchereria bancrofti	Human	Mosquito	Lymphangitis,
Brugia malayi			elephantiasis
Onchocerca volvulus	Human	Blackfly	Skin nodules, ocular blindness
Loa loa	Human	Fly	Calabar swellings, subconjunctival larvae
Cestodes			
Taenia solium	Human	Pig	Cysticercosis
Trematodes			
Schistosoma mansoni	Human	Snails	Rectal bleeding, pipe-stem fibrosis of the liver,
Schistosoma japonicum			portal hypertension
Schistosoma haematobium			haematuria
Paragonimus westermani	Cats, dogs	Shellfish	Haemoptysis
Clonorchis sinensis	Cats, etc.	Fish	Cholangitis, liver abscess
Protozoa			
Entamoeba histolytica	Human	–	Amoebic dysentery with bloody diarrhoea, liver abscess
Isospora belli	Human	–	Diarrhoea
Trypanosoma rhodesiense	Cattle,	Tsetse flies	Sleeping sickness
Trypanosoma gambiense	game animals		
Trypanosoma cruzi	Various domestic/ wild animals	Bugs	Chagas' disease

Recommended reading

Benenson A S (ed) 1995 Control of communicable diseases in man, 16th edn. American Public Health Association, Washington

Department of Health 1996 Immunisation against infectious disease. HMSO, London

Greenwood D, Slack R, Peutherer J 1997 Medical microbiology, 15th edn. Churchill Livingstone, Edinburgh

Mandell G L, Bennett J E, Dolin R (eds) 1995 Mandell, Douglas and Bennett's Principles and practice of infectious diseases, 4th edn. Churchill Livingstone, New York

O'Grady F W, Lambert H P, Finch R G, Greenwood D (eds) 1997 Antibiotic and chemotherapy, 7th edn. Churchill Livingstone, Edinburgh

Index

Epidemiology (contd)
host susceptibility, 169
infection outbreaks, 168–70
measurements, 170–1
pathogenicity of organism, 169
route of spread, 169
strain differentiation, 168
surveillance, 171
Epidermophyton, 430
Epiglottitis, acute, 182
Epstein-Barr virus, 178
Erysipelas, 263, 372
Erysipeloid, 347
Erysipelothrix, 105
Erysipelothrix rhusiopathiae, 347
Erythema chronicum migrans, 145
Erythema nodosum, 372
Erythrogenic toxin, 62
Erythromycin, 387
acne vulgaris, 265
Actinomyces israelii sensitivity, 115
anthrax, 339
Bordetella pertussis sensitivity, 97, 189
Campylobacter sensitivity, 88, 202
Chlamydia psittaci pneumonia, 193
Chlamydia trachomatis genital
infection, 370
Clostridium sensitivity, 129
Corynebacterium diphtheriae
sensitivity, 104, 236
gonorrhoea, 317, 318
Haemophilus ducreyi sensitivity, 95
Haemophilus influenzae sensitivity,
94
Legionella pneumophila sensitivity,
140, 193
leptospirosis, 344
Moraxella catarrhalis sensitivity, 121
mycoplasma sensitivity, 148, 192
osteomyelitis, 311
otitis media, 180
Pasteurella multocida sensitivity, 97
streptococcal infections, 64, 174,
190
Streptococcus pneumoniae resistance,
69, 185
syphilis, 324
Vibrio cholerae sensitivity, 86
Escherichia coli, 74–5, 355
adhesive factors, 74
diarrhoeal disease, 75, 208–12
enterohaemorrhagic, 75, 211–12
enteroinvasive, 74, 75, 212
enteropathogenic, 75, 208, 209
enterotoxigenic, 75, 210
enterotoxins, 74

haemolytic uraemic syndrome,
211–12
haemorrhagic colitis, 211
identification, 74
infantile gastroenteritis, 208–10
neonatal meningitis, 256
O antigens, 74–5
pneumonia, 191
sepsis, 75
strain O157, 74, 75, 211, 212
travellers' diarrhoea (turista),
210–11
urinary tract infection, 246
vero cytotoxin (VT), 74, 211–12
Ethambutol, 109, 256, 302, 391, 392
Ethionamide, 109, 302, 392
Ethylene oxide, 49
Exogenous infection, 165
hospital-acquired infections, 349,
356, 359, 360
Exotoxins, 162
External auditory meatus flora, 154
Eye infections, 82, 327–31
Eyelid infections, 327

F (fertility) factors, 25
Fab fragments, 159
Faecal-oral transmission, 167, 199,
207, 210
Faeces
bacteria, 152–3
safe disposal, 50–1
specimen collection, 45
Fasciola hepatica, 447
Fc fragments, 159
Female genital tract flora, 154
Fever, 291
Filtration sterilization, 49
Fimbriae, 8
Fish-tank granuloma, 307
Flagella, 8, 9
Flagellin, 8
Fleming, Alexander, 5
Flucloxacillin, 58
neonatal skin sepsis, 264
osteomyelitis, 311, 312
pneumonia, 194
prosthetic joint infections, 313
toxic shock syndrome (TSS), 243
Fluconazole, 370, 427, 429
prophylaxis in immunocompromised
patients, 356
Fluorescence microscopy, 33
5-Fluorocytosine, 427, 429
Fomites, 167, 168